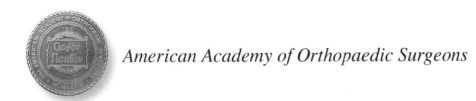
American Academy of Orthopaedic Surgeons

# OKU

## Orthopaedic Knowledge Update:

# Foot and Ankle

3

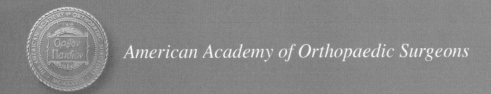

American Academy of Orthopaedic Surgeons

# OKU

## Orthopaedic Knowledge Update:

# Foot and Ankle

# 3

Edited by
E. Greer Richardson, MD

Section Editors
Bruce E. Cohen, MD
Brian G. Donley, MD
Jeffrey E. Johnson, MD
Kathleen A. McHale, MD, FACS
G. Andrew Murphy, MD
David B. Thordarson, MD

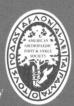

Developed by the
American Orthopaedic Foot and Ankle Society

Published 2003
by the American Academy of Orthopaedic Surgeons
6300 North River Road
Rosemont, IL 60018
1-800-626-6726

The material presented in *Orthopaedic Knowledge Update: Foot and Ankle 3* has been made available by the American Academy of Orthopaedic Surgeons for educational purposes only. This material is not intended to present the only, or necessarily best, methods or procedures for the medical situations discussed, but rather is intended to represent an approach, view, statement, or opinion of the author(s) or producer(s), which may be helpful to others who face similar situations.

Some drugs or medical devices demonstrated in Academy courses or described in Academy print or electronic publications have not been cleared by the Food and Drug Administration (FDA) or have been cleared for specific uses only. The FDA has stated that it is the responsibility of the physician to determine the FDA clearance status of each drug or device he or she wishes to use in clinical practice.

Furthermore, any statements about commercial products are solely the opinion(s) of the author(s) and do not represent an Academy endorsement or evaluation of these products. These statements may not be used in advertising or for any commercial purpose.

Third Edition
Copyright © 2004 by the
American Academy of Orthopaedic Surgeons

ISBN 0-89203-309-6

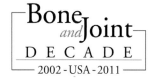

Bone *and* Joint
DECADE
2002 - USA - 2011

# Acknowledgments

## Editorial Board, OKU: Foot and Ankle 3

E. Greer Richardson, MD
Professsor
Department of Orthopaedics
University of Tennessee
The Campbell Clinic
Germantown, Tennessee

Bruce E. Cohen, MD
Foot and Ankle Center
Miller Orthopaedic Clinic
Charlotte, North Carolina

Brian G. Donley, MD
Director of Research and Education
Section of Foot and Ankle Surgery
Department of Orthopaedic Surgery
Cleveland Clinic Foundation
Cleveland, Ohio

Jeffrey E. Johnson, MD
Associate Professor
Chief, Foot and Ankle Service
Department of Orthopaedic Surgery
Barnes-Jewish Hospital
Washington University School of Medicine
St. Louis, Missouri

Kathleen A. McHale, MD, FACS
Professor of Surgery
Department of Surgery
Uniformed Services University for the Health Sciences
Bethesda, Maryland

G. Andrew Murphy, MD
Department of Orthopaedic Surgery
University of Tennessee, Memphis
The Campbell Clinic
Memphis, Tennessee

David B. Thordarson, MD
Professor of Orthopaedics
Department of Orthopaedics
University of Southern California
Los Angeles, California

## American Orthopaedic Foot and Ankle Society
### Board of Directors, 2003-2004

Glenn B. Pfeffer, MD
*President*
Mark S. Myerson, MD
*President-Elect*
James W. Brodsky, MD
*Vice President*
Robert B. Anderson, MD
*Treasurer*
Lowell H. Gill, MD
*Secretary*

Charles L. Saltzman, MD
*Secretary-Elect*
E. Greer Richardson, MD
Pierce E. Scranton Jr, MD
Michael J. Shereff, MD
*Past Presidents*
Carol C. Frey, MD
William C. McGarvey, MD
Michael S. Pinzur, MD
*Members at Large*

## American Academy of Orthopaedic Surgeons

### Board of Directors, 2003

James H. Herndon, MD
*President*
Robert W. Bucholz, MD
*First Vice President*
Stuart L. Weinstein, MD
*Second Vice President*
E. Anthony Rankin, MD
*Secretary*
Edward A. Toriello, MD
*Treasurer*
Stephen A. Albanese, MD
Leslie Altick
Frederick M. Azar, MD
Maureen Finnegan, MD
Mark C. Gebhardt, MD
Richard H. Gelberman, MD
Frank B. Kelly, MD
David G. Lewallen, MD
Peter J. Mandell, MD
Glenn B. Pfeffer, MD
Vernon T. Tolo, MD
Laura L. Tosi, MD
Gerald R. Williams, Jr, MD
Karen L. Hackett, FACHE, CAE
*(Ex Officio)*

### Staff

Mark Wieting
*Chief Education Officer*
Marilyn L. Fox, PhD
*Director, Department of Publications*
Lisa Claxton Moore
*Managing Editor*
Keith Huff
*Senior Editor*
Kathleen Anderson
*Medical Editor*
Mary Steermann
*Manager, Production and Archives*
David Stanley
*Assistant Production Manager*

Sophie Tosta
*Assistant Production Manager*
Mike Bujewski
*Database Coordinator*
Susan Morritz Baim
*Production Coordinator*
Dena Lozano
*Desktop Publishing Assistant*
Courtney Astle
*Production Assistant*
Karen Danca
*Production Assistant*

# Contributors

Jorge I. Acevedo, MD
Assistant Clinical Professor of Orthopaedics
and Rehabilitation
University of Miami
Center for Bone and Joint Surgery
West Palm Beach, Florida

Judith F. Baumhauer, MD
Associate Professor of Orthopaedics
Chief, Division of Foot and Ankle Surgery
Department of Orthopaedics
University of Rochester School of Medicine
Rochester, New York

Gregory C. Bertlet, MD, FRCSC
Clinical Assistant Professor
Department of Orthopaedics
Ohio State University
Columbus, Ohio

John T. Campbell, MD
Assistant Professor
Chief, Division of Foot and Ankle Surgery
Department of Orthopaedic Surgery
Johns Hopkins Bayview Medical Center
Baltimore, Maryland

Mark M. Casillas, MD
Clinical Assistant Professor
Department of Orthopaedics
University of Texas Health Sciences Center
at San Antonio
San Antonio, Texas

Wen Chao, MD
Orthopaedic Attending Surgeon
Department of Orthopaedic Surgery
Pennsylvania Hospital
Philadelphia, Pennsylvania

Christopher P. Chiodo, MD
Clinical Instructor of Orthopedic Surgery
Brigham Women's Hospital
Harvard Medical School
Boston, Massachusetts

Bryan D. Den Hartog, MD
Clinical Assistant Professor
University of South Dakota Medical School
Orthopaedic Surgeon
Black Hills Orthopaedic and Spine Center
Rapid City, South Dakota

Benedict F. DiGiovanni, MD
Assistant Professor
Division of Foot and Ankle Surgery
Department of Orthopaedics
University of Rochester School of Medicine
Rochester, New York

Peter C. Ferguson, MD, MSc, FRCSC
Assistant Professor
Department of Surgery
University of Toronto
Orthopaedic Surgery
Mount Sinai Hospital
Toronto, Ontario, Canada

Gregory P. Guyton, MD
Attending Physician
Departmen of Orthopaedics
Union Memorial Hospital
Baltimore, Maryland

Susan N. Ishikawa, MD
Chief, Foot and Ankle Service
Orthopaedic Surgery
Tripler Army Medical Center
Honolulu, Hawaii

Paul J. Juliano, MD
Associate Professor of Orthopedic Surgery
Department of Orthopedics
Milton S. Hershey Medical Center
Pennsylvania State College of Medicine
Hershey, Pennsylvania

John S. Kirchner, MD
Alabama Sports Medicine and Orthopaedic
Center
Birmingham, Alabama

Johnny T.C. Lau, MD, MSc, FRCSC
Assistant Professor of Orthopaedic Surgery
Department of Orthopaedics
University Health Network
Toronto Western Hospital
University of Toronto
Toronto, Ontario, Canada

William C. McGarvey, MD
Director, Foot and Ankle Surgery
Assistant Professor of Orthopaedic Surgery
Department of Orthopaedic Surgery
University of Texas Health Sciences Center
Houston, Texas

Thomas G. Padanilam, MD
Chief, Division of Foot and Ankle
Department of Orthopaedic Surgery
Medical College of Ohio
Toledo, Ohio

Steven M. Raikin, MD
Director, Foot and Ankle Service
Assistant Professor, Orthopaedic Surgery
Rothman Institute
Thomas Jefferson University Hospital
Philadelphia, Pennsylvania

Vincent James Sammarco, MD
Center for Orthopaedic Care, Inc.
Cincinnati, Ohio

James J. Sferra, MD
Head, Section of Foot and Ankle Surgery
Department of Orthopaedic Surgery
The Cleveland Clinic Foundation
Cleveland, Ohio

Naomi N. Shields, MD
Clinical Assistant Professor
Department of Orthopaedic Surgery
University of Kansas School of Medicine,
Wichita
Wichita, Kansas

C. Christopher Stroud, MD
Attending Physician
Department of Surgery
William Beaumont Hospital, Troy
Troy, Michigan

Christopher L. Tisdel, MD
Attending Staff
Department of Orthopaedic Surgery
The Cleveland Clinic Foundation
Cleveland, Ohio

Arthur K. Walling, MD
Director, Foot and Ankle Fellowship
Clinical Professor of Orthopaedics
Florida Orthopaedic Institute
Tampa, Florida

Michael R. Werner, MD
Appalachian Orthopaedics
Johnson City, Tennessee

Jay S. Wunder, MD, MSc, FRCSC
Rubinoff-Gross Chair in Orthopaedic
Oncology
University Musculoskeletal Oncology Unit
Mount Sinai Hospital
Toronto, Ontario, Canada

# Preface

This edition of *Orthopaedic Knowledge Update: Foot and Ankle* is the result of a concerted effort by its contributors to distill a large body of information into a concise, readable, and instructive volume. Over the last 20 years, clinical and laboratory research in this subspecialty of orthopaedics has grown exponentially. It is our hope that this review will pique interest in this area of orthopaedics and that patients will reap the benefits of the applied information.

I would especially like to express my gratitude to the Contributors and Section Editors for the energy and devotion they have shown in sharing their special knowledge with our readers. Thank you for many hours of hard work. I also am deeply grateful to Kay Daugherty (Campbell Foundation) and Susan Myers (Campbell Clinic) for their generous assistance in preparing this book. Also to be thanked for their conscientious efforts in editing and producing this text are the Academy publications department staff: Marilyn L. Fox, PhD, Department Director; Lisa Claxton Moore, Managing Editor; Keith Huff, Senior Editor; and Kathleen Anderson, Medical Editor, who edited the manuscripts; Sophie Tosta, who coordinated the manuscript review and permissions process; and Mary Steermann, who supervised the production efforts.

*E. Greer Richardson, MD*
*Editor*

# Table of Contents

## Section 1: Disorders of the Hallux
**Section Editor:** Brian G. Donley, MD

## Section 2: Trauma
**Section Editor:** David B. Thordarson, MD

## Section 3: Reconstruction and Acquired Disorders

**Section Editor:** Jeffrey E. Johnson, MD

## Section 4: Neurologic Disorders and Injuries

**Section Editor:** G. Andrew Murphy, MD

American Academy of Orthopaedic Surgeons

## Section 5: Arthritic Disorders
**Section Editor:** Bruce E. Cohen, MD

## Section 6: General Foot and Ankle Topics
**Section Editor:** Kathleen A. McHale, MD, FACS

*17*

# Section 1

# Disorders of the Hallux

Section Editor:
Brian G. Donley, MD

# Chapter 1

# Hallux Valgus: Adult and Juvenile

John T. Campbell, MD

## Introduction

The painful bunion is a common affliction that leads to restrictions of daily and recreational activities, difficulty in wearing fashion shoe wear, and decreased quality of life. Hallux valgus occurs in both adults and adolescents, with noteworthy distinctions in the underlying pathophysiology and necessary treatment methods. This chapter addresses both adult and juvenile hallux valgus, including etiology, clinical and radiographic evaluation, surgical decision making, and contemporary surgical techniques.

## Adult Hallux Valgus

### Pathoanatomy

The pathoanatomy of a hallux valgus deformity is apparent from the anatomic and biomechanical features of the first metatarsophalangeal (MTP) joint (Fig. 1). Metatarsus primus varus, or medial deviation of the first metatarsal, occurs in certain patients as an isolated feature in conjunction with global metatarsus adductus, or secondary to instability of the first metatarsal-cuneiform joint. This deviation leads to increased laterally directed pressure on the hallux. Many patients, however, develop metatarsus primus varus secondary to medially directed force from a laterally subluxated proximal phalanx. Valgus deformity of the first MTP joint is classified as either congruent or incongruent (Fig. 2). In a congruent deformity, inherent articular and soft-tissue balance prevents subluxation of the phalanx off the metatarsal head but not valgus angulation of the phalanx, resulting in a "balanced" congruent hallux valgus deformity. This deformity can have several components: lateral inclination of the metatarsal head chondral surface (distal metatarsal articular angle [DMAA]), lateral deviation of the proximal phalangeal shaft, lateral obliquity of the interphalangeal joint (hallux valgus interphalangeus), and rotation of the first metatarsal on its longitudinal axis (Fig. 3). An incongruent deformity consists of lateral subluxation of the joint secondary to intrinsic and extrinsic musculotendinous imbalance, usually increases in severity with time, and typically involves attenuation of the medial capsule and lateral shortening (and possible contracture) of the adductor and flexor hallucis brevis musculotendinous units, lateral capsuloligamentous contracture, and eventually pronation and lateral displacement of the phalanx. The deformity then becomes biomechanically self-perpetuating as the subluxated phalanx displaces the metatarsal medially off the sesamoids, which are statically tethered by the adductor, flexor hallucis brevis, and intermetatarsal ligament. As the deformity worsens, the entire soft-tissue sleeve displaces laterally and the abductor tendon slips plantarly, no longer exerting a stabilizing role medially. The medial eminence of the metatarsal head becomes more prominent and may cause overlying bursitis and pain.

### Etiology

Numerous etiologic factors have been proposed as contributors to the development of hallux valgus. Inappropriate shoe wear, particularly women's fashion shoe wear in which the space for the forefoot is inadequate, is believed to be an important factor in the development of hallux valgus. Previous studies have shown a higher incidence of hallux valgus deformity in populations wearing fashion shoe wear than in groups wearing sandals, wide shoes, or no shoes. Preexisting metatarsus primus varus or global metatarsus adductus caused by inappropriate shoe wear contributes to a valgus movement on the hallux. An underlying flatfoot deformity may cause repetitive valgus stress on the hallux during the toe-off phase of gait. A genetic disposition toward systemic ligamentous laxity or isolated hypermobility of the first metatarsal-cuneiform joint results in instability of the first ray, with dorsomedial subluxation of the joint and metatarsus primus varus. Inflammatory arthropathies, including rheumatoid arthritis and the seronegative spondyloarthropathies, can cause joint synovitis and attenuation of soft-tissue restraints of the MTP joint. In spastic disorders, such as cerebral palsy, the valgus deformity is secondary to muscle imbalance and lateral overpull of the hallux. Finally, traumatic disruption of the soft-tissue envelope about the hallux MTP joint is a rare cause of hallux valgus deformity.

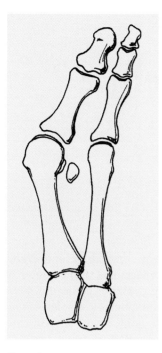

Figure 1 Hallux valgus deformity.

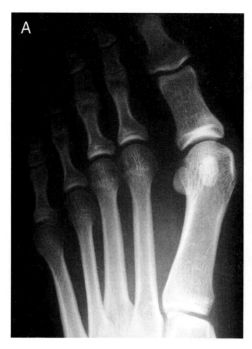

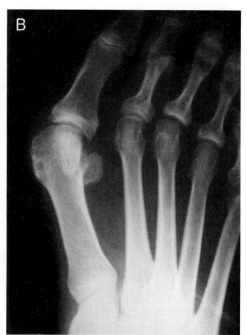

Figure 2 **A,** Congruent hallux valgus deformity. **B,** Incongruent hallux valgus deformity.

## Evaluation

### History

Onset, severity, and specific location (plantar, dorsal, or medial about the hallux MTP joint) of the patient's pain should be noted. Medial pain indicates bursal irritation, plantar pain may be indicative of sesamoid involvement, and dorsal pain implies arthritic involvement of the joint. Type of shoe wear, medical comorbidities (such as rheumatologic disorders, peripheral neuropathy, or diabetes), previous surgical procedures on the foot, family history of hallux valgus, and the patient's occupation, recreational pursuits, and sports activities all are factors that may have an impact on patient expectations, the goals of treatment, and postoperative restrictions.

### Physical Examination

Physical examination is conducted with the patient seated and again while standing. The overall alignment of the foot is visually inspected, including the arch height, hindfoot alignment (particularly valgus), and lesser toe deformities, particularly a second hammer toe deformity or a global valgus deformity of the first lesser toes at the MTP joints. Skin texture is evaluated to identify systemic disease. The presence of calluses or ulcerations indicates areas of increased pressure, pain, peripheral neuropathy, or possibly vasculitis. Pulses are palpated and cutaneous sensation is evaluated to determine the neurovascular status of the foot. Passive dorsiflexion of the ankle with the knee flexed and extended is done to identify an Achilles musculotendinous contracture. Active and passive motions of both feet are compared, focusing on the ankle, hindfoot, and metatarsal-cuneiform, MTP, and interpha-

langeal joints. Holding the hallux valgus deformity corrected while evaluating the passive dorsal and plantar motion at the first MTP joint gives an indication of the expected postoperative excursion of the joint. Passive range of motion of the first MTP joint with the joint reduced may be considerably less than with the joint subluxated. Signs of systemic hyperlaxity, such as hyperextension of the metacarpophalangeal joint of the thumb or elbow joint or hyperabduction of the thumb to the volar surface of the forearm should be documented. Hypermobility of the first metatarsal-cuneiform joint can be evaluated by stabilizing the midfoot and second and third metatarsals at their neck with one hand and translating the metatarsal in a sagittal plane with the other hand. The hallux is palpated dorsally, medially, and plantarly to localize pain resulting from arthritis, medial eminence pain or bursitis, dorsal cutaneous nerve impingement, and sesamoid involvement. Finally, the lesser toes are examined to identify hammer toe, claw toe, or crossover toe deformities. Plantar calluses under the second or third metatarsal heads may indicate hypermobility of the first metatarsal-cuneiform joint and unloading of the first ray, but they usually occur secondary to metatarsus primus varus.

### Radiographic Evaluation

Appropriate radiographic evaluation of hallux valgus requires weight-bearing views (AP, oblique, and lateral projections) to determine the true extent of the deformity. A tangential or axial sesamoid view also helps assess the degree of sesamoid subluxation or the presence of metatarsosesamoid arthrosis, particularly for congru-

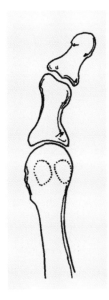
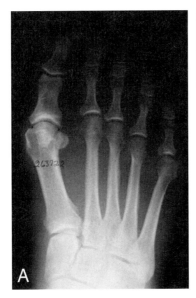
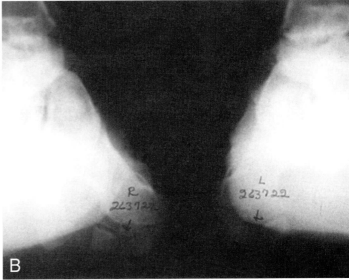

**Figure 3**  Hallux valgus interphalangeus deformity.

**Figure 4**  On AP view (**A**), sesamoids appear subluxated, but on weight-bearing view (**B**), sesamoids can be seen in their facets.

ent hallux valgus, in which the sesamoids can appear subluxated on the weight-bearing AP radiograph, yet be anatomically reduced in their facets (Fig. 4). Joint congruency and subluxation should also be noted. Next, certain angular measurements are determined to aid in defining the type and severity of the deformity (Table 1). The hallux valgus angle (HVA) is defined by the intersection of a line longitudinally bisecting the diaphysis of the first metatarsal and a line bisecting the proximal phalangeal shaft; a normal HVA measures 15° or less (Fig. 5, *A*). The first-second intermetatarsal angle ($IMA_{1-2}$) is created by axes drawn longitudinally to bisect the first and second metatarsal diaphyses; a normal $IMA_{1-2}$ measures 9° or less (Fig. 5, *B*). The DMAA identifies increased lateral obliquity of the chondral surface of the MTP joint (Fig. 5, *C*). The DMAA is measured between the longitudinal axis of the first metatarsal and a line connecting the medial and lateral edges of the chondral surface. Increased lateral obliquity with a DMAA mea-

suring greater than 15° is abnormal. A recent study showed that the HVA and $IMA_{1-2}$ measurements have good reproducibility, whereas the DMAA is a less reliable measurement among observers because of difficulty in determining the exact extent of the chondral surface edges and obtaining accurate measurements in a "congruent" joint that is now subluxated and incongruent. The proximal phalangeal articular angle (PPAA) is helpful in identifying hallux valgus interphalangeus (Fig. 5, *D*). The PPAA is subtended by a line perpendicular to the base of the proximal phalanx and a line along the longitudinal axis of the phalanx; a normal PPAA measures 10° or less.

It is clinically helpful to determine the severity of the hallux valgus deformity based on these angular measurements. Although variability and margin of error are inherent in any measurement system, Figure 6 provides a clinically useful algorithm for classifying hallux valgus deformity.

**TABLE 1 | Important Radiographic Angles in Evaluation of Hallux Valgus**

| Angle | Location | Importance | Normal |
|---|---|---|---|
| Hallux valgus angle (HVA) | Between long axes of first proximal phalanx and first metatarsal, bisecting their diaphysis | Identifies the degree of deformity at the MTP joint | ≤ 15° |
| First-second intermetatarsal angle ($IMA_{1-2}$) | Between long axes of first and second metatarsals, bisecting shafts of first and second metatarsals | Not influenced by overresection of medial eminence; not accurate for postoperative evaluation of distal osteotomies | ≤ 9° |
| Distal metatarsal articular angle (DMAA) | Angle of line bisecting metatarsal shaft with line through base of distal articular cartilage cap | Offset of angle is predisposing factor in development of hallux valgus | ≤ 15° |
| Proximal phalangeal articular angle (PPAA) | Articular angle of base of proximal phalanx in relation to longitudinal axis | Offset of angle is predisposing factor in development of hallux valgus | ≤ 10° |

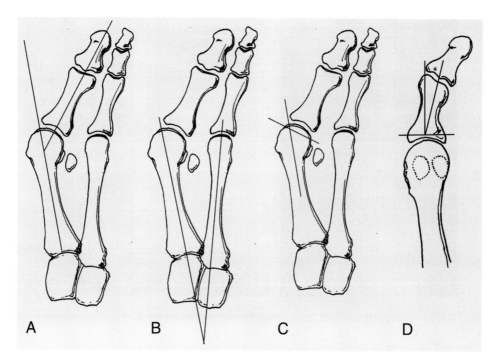

**Figure 5** Angular measurements of hallux valgus deformity. **A,** HVA. **B,** IMA$_{1-2}$. **C,** DMAA. **D,** PPAA.

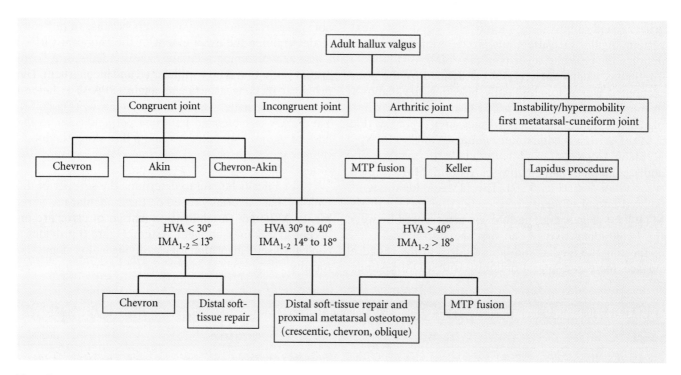

**Figure 6** Algorithm for classification and surgical treatment of adult hallux valgus.

## Nonsurgical Treatment

Nonsurgical treatment of hallux valgus often is appropriate. It is important to make the patient aware of the nature of the deformity, its relation to symptoms, and possible contributing factors. Counseling of the patient about appropriate shoe wear, including wearing low-heeled shoes with a wide toe box and soft leather uppers to re-lieve pressure over the medial bunion, is critical to successful nonsurgical treatment. Stretching the leather in the region of the bunion also may provide pain relief. Rarely, various padding devices or cushions placed over the bunion may be helpful. Strapping or splinting the hallux may partially reduce the deformity but does not provide long-term benefit. Results from a 2001 study indicate that longitudinal orthotic arch supports may assist in alleviating symptoms in patients with underlying pes planus or associated lesser metatarsalgia.

## Surgical Treatment

### Evaluation and Decision Making

Surgical treatment is chosen for hallux valgus deformity only after nonsurgical measures have failed. Occasionally, for a patient with severe deformity and pain for whom nonsurgical modalities are unlikely to provide relief, surgery may be the first method of treatment. It is vital to educate the patient regarding proper indications for and expectations after surgery. The main indication for surgery is persistent pain that limits daily activities, work duties, or recreational pursuits. Cosmesis is not considered an appropriate indication for surgical treatment.

After surgery, most patients experience pain relief and improvement in activity level. Two thirds of patients are able to resume wearing most types of shoes. Full recovery after surgery often takes 6 months or longer, with a minimum expected recovery time of 3 to 4 months. However, when the procedure is matched to the severity of the deformity, the end result usually is favorable in 80% to 85% of patients. Recent studies have shown that surgical treatment provides better pain relief, improved function, improved patient satisfaction, and better cosmesis than nonsurgical intervention.

The chosen surgical procedure must consider the fundamental components of the deformity, including removal of the prominent medial eminence, correction of the hallux valgus alignment, correction of the increased $IMA_{1-2}$, derotation of the pronated toe, reduction of the metatarsal head over the sesamoids, and correction of an excessive DMAA. Deformities should be identified radiographically as congruent or incongruent. Congruent deformities typically are treated with extra-articular procedures, such as distal metatarsal osteotomy, closing wedge proximal phalangeal (Akin) osteotomy, or a combination of the two. A congruent deformity with an increased DMAA can be corrected with a biplanar medial closing wedge chevron osteotomy, which can be augmented by an Akin phalangeal osteotomy as required.

Surgical treatment of incongruent deformities is based on the severity of the deformity. Mild deformities (HVA, < 30°; $IMA_{1-2}$, ≤ 13°) are treated with a distal chevron osteotomy or a distal soft-tissue repair. Moderate deformities (HVA, 30° to 40°; $IMA_{1-2}$, 14° to 18°) are typically treated with a distal chevron osteotomy (that can be augmented as needed with an Akin phalangeal osteotomy) or a distal soft-tissue repair in combination with a proximal metatarsal osteotomy. Severe hallux valgus deformities (HVA, > 40°; $IMA_{1-2}$, > 18°) are addressed by a distal soft-tissue repair in combination with a proximal metatarsal osteotomy or a first MTP joint arthrodesis.

Several other clinical features provide additional guidance for planning surgical treatment. First ray hypermo-

bility or instability of the first metatarsal-cuneiform joint can be corrected by a distal soft-tissue repair combined with a first metatarsal-cuneiform arthrodesis (Lapidus procedure). This metatarsal-cuneiform instability is present in approximately 5% to 10% of patients. Inflammatory arthritis of the first MTP joint is typically treated with arthrodesis, and degenerative arthritis is treated with either arthrodesis in younger, more active patients or resection (Keller) arthroplasty in more sedentary or elderly patients. Because of concerns over implant failure, synovitis, bony lysis, and shortening, implant replacement arthroplasty usually is contraindicated.

### Distal Soft-Tissue Procedure

The distal soft-tissue (modified McBride) procedure includes release of the contracted lateral structures, medial eminence resection, and medial capsulorrhaphy. Although historically performed alone, it is now typically combined with a proximal (occasionally distal) first metatarsal osteotomy. A distal soft-tissue repair is indicated for an incongruent deformity because capsulorrhaphy reduces the subluxated MTP joint. Use of this procedure in a congruent deformity can lead to iatrogenic varus subluxation of the joint, causing stiffness and arthritis. The distal soft-tissue procedure can be used alone for mild to moderate deformities (HVA, < 25°; $IMA_{1-2}$, ≤ 13°) with a flexible metatarsus primus varus. More severe metatarsus primus varus that cannot be passively corrected requires the addition of a bony procedure, such as a proximal metatarsal osteotomy or a first metatarsal-cuneiform joint fusion.

### Distal Chevron Osteotomy

The distal chevron osteotomy is appropriate for mild to moderate congruent and incongruent deformities (HVA, < 25°; $IMA_{1-2}$, ≤ 13°). When modified to become a biplanar closing wedge osteotomy, chevron osteotomy is used for congruent hallux valgus with an increased DMAA (> 15°) (Fig. 7).

Osteonecrosis of the capital fragment after chevron osteotomy occurs in fewer than 10% of patients. Progressive sclerosis and cyst formation of the head fragment should alert the surgeon to possible osteonecrosis. However, apparent early osteonecrosis (mottling and cystic changes in the first metatarsal head) usually resolves in 4 to 6 months. Hallux valgus may recur after chevron osteotomy if the procedure is done to correct a more severe deformity than is indicated.

### Proximal Metatarsal Osteotomy

Proximal metatarsal osteotomy and a distal soft-tissue procedure are indicated for moderate to severe incongruent hallux valgus deformities (HVA, ≥ 25°; $IMA_{1-2}$, ≥ 14°). The proximal osteotomy provides more correction of metatarsus primus varus than a distal osteotomy (eg, a chevron osteotomy). Proximal metatarsal osteoto-

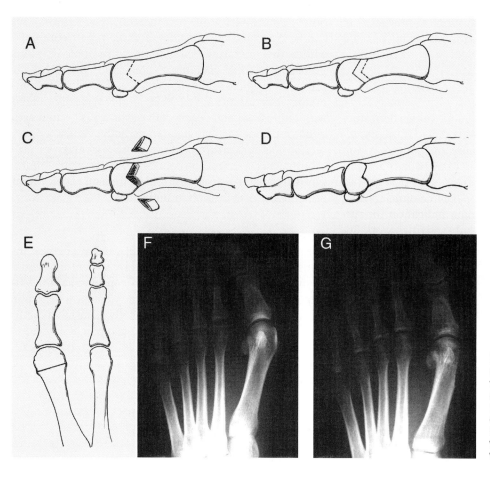

Figure 7 Biplanar closing wedge chevron osteotomy. **A,** Lateral view of osteotomy site, with first cut templated (dotted line). **B,** Lateral view of second cut (dotted line). **C,** Removal of medially based wedges from chevron osteotomy site. **D,** Lateral view after reduction. **E,** AP view of correction. **F,** Preoperative weight-bearing radiograph. **G,** Postoperative weight-bearing radiograph.

mies vary, but each produces good pain relief and deformity correction, including the proximal chevron and crescentic osteotomies, as well as the oblique (Ludloff) osteotomy (Figs. 8 and 9). Each is performed in combination with a distal soft-tissue repair as detailed previously.

Overcorrection of deformity with creation of iatrogenic hallux varus is possible if the intermetatarsal angle is overreduced. Dorsiflexion malunion can lead to disabling transfer metatarsalgia of the lesser toes.

### Metatarsal-Cuneiform Arthrodesis
Arthrodesis of the first metatarsal-cuneiform joint is indicated for instability or hypermobility of the first ray in conjunction with metatarsus primus varus. This arthrodesis is done in combination with a distal soft-tissue repair as described previously (Fig. 10).

Complications after first metatarsal-cuneiform joint arthrodesis include nonunion, malunion, and transfer metatarsalgia. Nonunion rates of 10% to 15% have been reported, but not all nonunions are symptomatic. Revision arthrodesis in situ or with tricortical bone block graft may be necessary when the nonunion is painful or unstable or deformity recurs. Elevation of the first ray should be avoided during arthrodesis positioning and screw fixation. Transfer metatarsalgia, which results from shortening or elevation of the first ray, typically is managed with

a custom-made orthotic device with a Morton's extension to engage the hallux and improve first ray weight transmission; plantar flexion osteotomy may be needed for severe deformity.

### Akin Proximal Phalangeal Osteotomy
The medial closing wedge (Akin) osteotomy of the proximal phalanx achieves an extra-articular correction of valgus deformity but does not address metatarsus primus varus or decrease the $IMA_{1-2}$. Akin osteotomy can be used alone to treat hallux valgus interphalangeus and as an adjunct to other techniques for correcting congruent deformities, including the distal chevron osteotomy, proximal metatarsal osteotomies, and the Lapidus procedure (Fig. 11). However, Akin osteotomy should not be used as the sole method of correcting a hallux valgus deformity.

Insufficient correction or recurrent deformity may indicate improper patient selection for Akin osteotomy. Nonunion of the osteotomy is uncommon; when it does occur, it usually is asymptomatic despite its radiographic appearance.

### Keller Resection Arthroplasty
Resection arthroplasty of the hallux MTP joint is indicated for hallux valgus with arthritic involvement. This

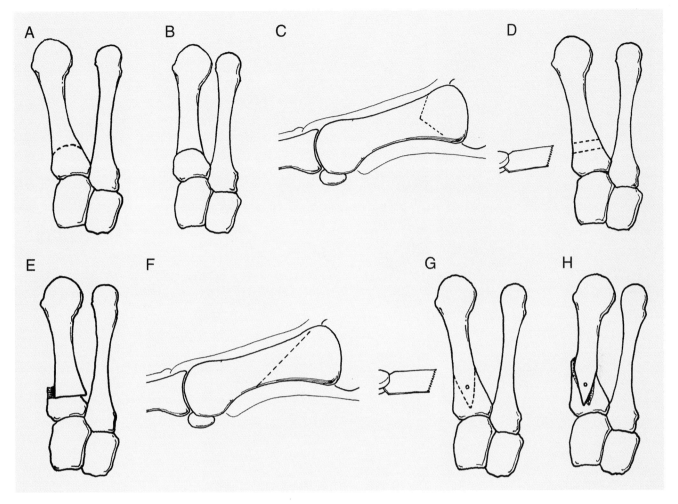

**Figure 8** Proximal metatarsal osteotomies. Preoperative **(A)** and postoperative **(B)** views of a crescentic osteotomy. **C,** Lateral view of a proximal chevron osteotomy. AP views before **(D)** and after **(E)** a proximal chevron osteotomy. **F,** Lateral view of an oblique (Ludloff) osteotomy. AP views before **(G)** and after **(H)** an oblique (Ludloff) osteotomy.

procedure is appropriate treatment for elderly, sedentary, or low-demand patients but is contraindicated for younger, more active patients, who are better treated with MTP joint arthrodesis.

### MTP Joint Arthrodesis
Arthrodesis of the first MTP joint is indicated for patients with severe deformities (HVA > 40°) and for those with arthritic involvement of the first MTP joint (Fig. 12). Arthrodesis provides excellent deformity correction along with durable pain relief, making it an excellent option for patients with rheumatoid arthritis and inflammatory arthropathies and for patients with neurologic disorders or spastic conditions such as cerebral palsy. MTP joint arthrodesis may be appropriate as a salvage option after failure of other bunion surgeries.

Malunion after MTP joint arthrodesis occurs in approximately 10% of patients and can result from initial malpositioning at the time of surgery or dorsal elevation of the toe postoperatively secondary to inadequate fixation, delayed union, or poor bone stock. Such malposi-

tioning leads to increased stress on the interphalangeal joint, which can ultimately become arthritic. Methods to alleviate this situation include a custom-made orthotic device with a Morton's extension (to improve capture and weight bearing of the hallux) and lamb's wool or gel spacers (to relieve impingement of the second toe). If these are insufficient, revision surgery may be necessary to reposition the toe.

## Juvenile Hallux Valgus
### Pathophysiology
Hallux valgus deformity in juveniles or adolescents is a pathophysiologic entity distinct from that in adults. Juvenile or adolescent hallux valgus usually is a congruent deformity that is less likely to progress than an incongruent deformity (Fig. 13). Hallux valgus in juveniles also has less severe angular deformity (HVA, $IMA_{1-2}$), less pronation, and less sesamoid malposition than that in adults. Although the symptoms of juvenile hallux valgus may be exacerbated by tight shoe wear, this is considered less

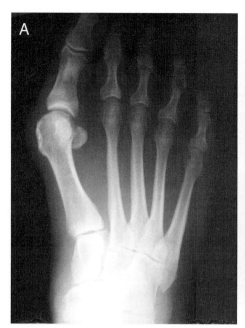
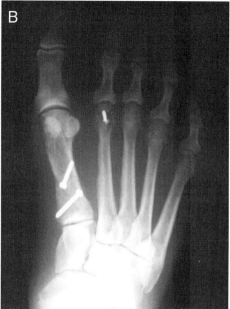

**Figure 9** Weight-bearing radiographs before **(A)** and after **(B)** an oblique (Ludloff) osteotomy and distal soft-tissue repair.

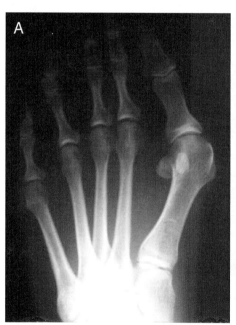
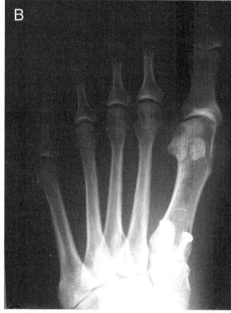

**Figure 10** Weight-bearing radiographs before **(A)** and after **(B)** a first metatarsal-cuneiform arthrodesis and distal soft-tissue repair (Lapidus procedure).

of a causative factor in young patients than in older patients. In addition, adolescent patients with hallux valgus rarely have an overly large medial eminence or arthritic involvement of the first MTP joint. They often have open physes (Fig. 14) and other contributing intrinsic foot deformities (such as metatarsus adductus). Furthermore, adolescents may have unrealistic expectations, especially about the cosmetic result, which may make treatment more difficult.

### Etiology

Contributing factors for juvenile hallux valgus include pes planus, contracture of the Achilles tendon (secondary to laterally directed force on the hallux with gait), generalized ligamentous laxity or hypermobility (resulting in instability of the first metatarsal-cuneiform joint and elevation of the first ray), residual metatarsus adductus or metatarsus primus varus, a first metatarsal with increased intrinsic obliquity of the chondral surface and large DMAA, and hallux valgus interphalangeus. Juvenile hallux valgus occurs more commonly in girls than in boys.

### Nonsurgical Treatment

As in the adult patient, treatment begins with nonsurgical measures. Education and counseling of the patient and parents are critical, especially because the young patient may

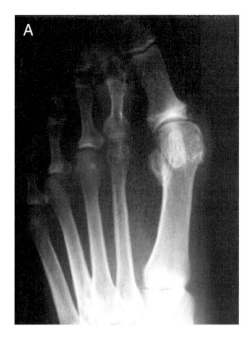
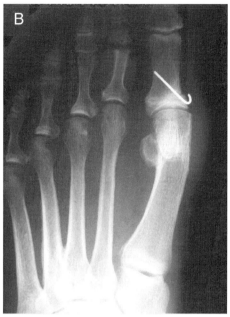

**Figure 11** Weight-bearing radiographs before **(A)** and after **(B)** combined distal chevron and closing wedge proximal phalangeal (Akin) osteotomies.

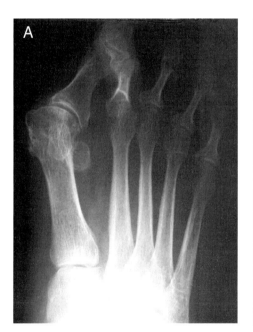
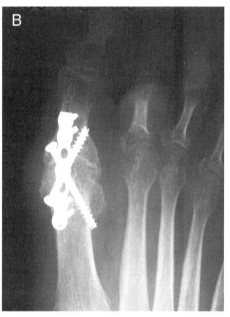

**Figure 12** Weight-bearing radiographs before **(A)** and after **(B)** MTP arthrodesis. The preoperative radiograph shows the arthritic involvement of the MTP joint.

not adequately comprehend or accept such issues. Discussion of contributing factors focuses on the underlying foot anatomy and generalized ligamentous laxity. It is also necessary to explain appropriate expectations regarding pain relief, cosmesis, risk of progression, and appropriate surgical indications. It is important to explain the contribution of tight shoe wear in exacerbating symptoms. Shoes with a wide toe box and low heel and the use of foam or gel padding devices may relieve bunion pain caused by shoe compression.

Specific interventions include stretching of the leather upper of the shoe (to decompress direct pressure over the bunion), a custom-made medial longitudinal arch support, and routine heel cord stretching for young patients with pes planus and hallux valgus. Nonsteroidal anti-inflammatory medications may diminish pain, particularly when the patient has bursitis over the medial MTP joint region.

## Surgical Treatment
### Evaluation and Decision Making
Several specific considerations related to juvenile or adolescent hallux valgus affect surgical decision making, timing, and technique. The presence of open physes at the phalangeal or first metatarsal base not only indicates that the foot has not reached skeletal maturity and maximal growth, but it may preclude osteotomies or arthrodeses in those areas to avoid growth disturbances. Recurrence

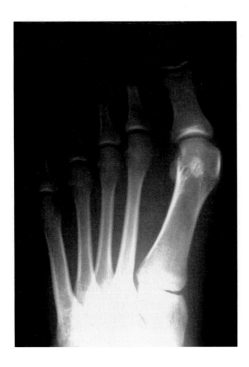

Figure 13 Juvenile hallux valgus deformity.

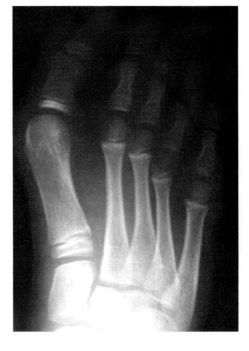

Figure 14 Juvenile hallux valgus with open physes.

of deformity is frequent after bunion surgery in adolescents, which may be indicative of generalized soft-tissue laxity in young patients or improper selection of the surgical procedure. Finally, the surgeon must cautiously assess the patient's ability to comply with the necessary postoperative restrictions and appropriate shoe wear; young patients may be prone to noncompliance because of peer pressure, improper expectations, and emotional immaturity. Such factors should prompt careful evaluation of the patient's symptoms and expectations, ensure an adequate trial of nonsurgical treatment, and possibly delay surgical treatment until the foot has reached skeletal maturity.

The exact location and severity of pain must be determined, as well as the extent to which it limits daily activities and recreational and athletic pursuits. Shoe wear and cosmetic expectations also are explicitly discussed with the patient and family. The patient is examined while seated and again while standing to assess the degree of deformity and the presence of pes planus and associated lesser toe abnormalities. Palpation of the first ray localizes the pain about the MTP joint, and manipulation of the hallux determines the degree of flexibility of the valgus alignment. Signs of systemic hypermobility, such as hyperextension of the metacarpophalangeal joints or abduction of the thumb to the volar forearm, are sought, and the first MTP joint is vertically stressed to identify instability. As for adult hallux valgus, weight-bearing radiographs are obtained, MTP joint congruency is evaluated, and angular measurements (including the HVA, $IMA_{1-2}$, DMAA, and PPAA) are made. The presence of underlying metatarsus adductus and open physes is also documented.

Surgical treatment of juvenile or adolescent bunions must correct the valgus alignment and any incongruency

of the joint, decrease the metatarsus primus varus, and remove the medial eminence. Evidence of first ray instability or hypermobility requires stabilization of the metatarsal-cuneiform joint. As in adult patients, juvenile hallux valgus can be differentiated into congruent deformities and incongruent deformities (Fig. 15). Deformities can then be categorized into different levels of severity based on the radiographic angular measurements.

In juveniles, congruent deformities are more common than incongruent. For mild (HVA, $< 30°$; $IMA_{1-2}$, $\leq 13°$) congruent hallux valgus, a distal metatarsal osteotomy is appropriate. For moderate (HVA, $30°$ to $40°$; $IMA_{1-2}$, $14°$ to $18°$) congruent deformities, a combined chevron-Akin procedure can achieve extra-articular correction. Severe (HVA, $> 40°$; $IMA_{1-2}$, $> 18°$) congruent deformities, unusual in adolescents or juveniles, require combined procedures, such as Akin-proximal metatarsal osteotomy or Akin-medial cuneiform wedge osteotomy. Congruent hallux valgus with an HVA $> 35°$ and an $IMA_{1-2} > 16°$ is rare.

Incongruent deformity occurs infrequently in juvenile patients. Mild (HVA, $< 30°$; $IMA_{1-2}$, $\leq 13°$) incongruent deformities are approached with a distal chevron osteotomy, or a distal soft-tissue repair. Moderate to severe (HVA, $> 30°$; $IMA_{1-2}$, $\geq 14°$) incongruent deformities are typically treated with a distal soft-tissue repair combined with a proximal metatarsal or medial cuneiform osteotomy. A closing wedge (Akin) phalangeal osteotomy is appropriate as an isolated procedure only for hallux valgus interphalangeus; it also can enhance correction of the overall deformity when combined with a proximal metatarsal osteotomy or metatarsal-cuneiform joint arthrodesis.

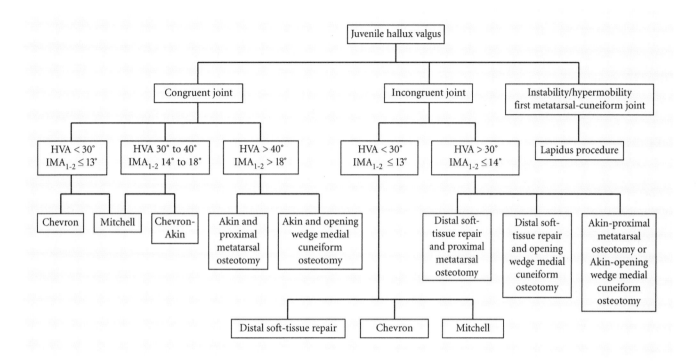

Figure 15  Algorithm for classification and surgical treatment of juvenile hallux valgus.

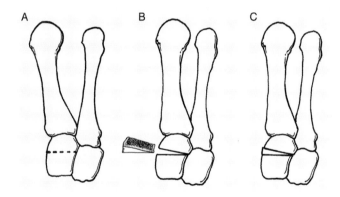

Figure 16  Opening wedge medial cuneiform osteotomy. **A,** Osteotomy site. **B,** Insertion of bone graft wedge. **C,** After correction.

### Proximal Metatarsal Osteotomy/Medial Cuneiform Osteotomy

Proximal osteotomy of the first metatarsal or the medial cuneiform is combined with a distal soft-tissue repair for moderate to severe incongruent deformities. However, if used for a congruent deformity, these procedures may result in overcorrection of the joint and iatrogenic varus alignment. Congruent deformities are better corrected by multiple osteotomies, which allow extra-articular correction without causing subluxation of the MTP joint. The proximal metatarsal osteotomies can be done similar to those in adults, but if the proximal physis of the first metatarsal remains open, proximal osteotomy may cause growth arrest, shortening, and lesser toe metatarsalgia. In such instances, an

opening wedge osteotomy of the medial cuneiform provides similar correction of the metatarsus primus varus and avoids injury to the first metatarsal physis (Fig. 16). Cuneiform osteotomy also is indicated in patients with increased obliquity of the first metatarsal-cuneiform joint.

### Metatarsal-Cuneiform Joint Arthrodesis

Arthrodesis of the first metatarsal-cuneiform joint is indicated in juvenile and adolescent patients with instability or laxity of this articulation, often caused by generalized ligamentous hypermobility. If the proximal physis of the first metatarsal is still open, arthrodesis of the first metatarsal-cuneiform joint may cause physeal injury, growth arrest, and shortening of the first ray, delaying the arthrodesis until physeal closure is recommended. When pain or functional limitation is severe, medial cuneiform osteotomy can be combined with distal soft-tissue repair, but metatarsal-cuneiform joint instability may persist.

### Multiple Osteotomies

Multiple osteotomies are indicated for moderate to severe congruent deformities that require extra-articular procedures for correction. A distal chevron osteotomy, a proximal metatarsal osteotomy, or an opening wedge medial cuneiform osteotomy, combined with a proximal phalangeal closing wedge (Akin) osteotomy can provide more improvement of great toe alignment than can be obtained with a single osteotomy. In general, the proximal osteotomy is done first, and then the second osteotomy, which fine tunes the degree of correction, is completed. Triple osteotomies (proximal and distal first metatarsal and phalangeal) rarely may be indicated in adolescent hallux valgus. If the physis is open, an opening wedge osteotomy of the medial cuneiform combined with a distal metatarsal ostetomy to correct an increased DMAA (not uncommon in adolescent hallux valgus) and a phalangeal closing wedge osteotomy may be needed for complete correction of a severe deformity.

## Summary

The evolving understanding of the contributing factors and the subtleties of hallux valgus deformity have led to refinements in surgical planning and techniques. The next generation of study on hallux valgus will likely focus on outcomes research to validate current approaches. With careful clinical and radiographic evaluation, use of appropriate indications and surgical decision making, and meticulous technique, the orthopaedic surgeon can achieve satisfactory results with minimal complications in most patients.

## Annotated Bibliography

### Adult Hallux Valgus

Coughlin MJ, Freund E: The reliability of angular measurements in hallux valgus deformities. *Foot Ankle Int* 2001;22:369-379.

Twenty-four surgeons independently measured standard angular parameters on a uniform set of radiographs of hallux valgus. The HVA and $IMA_{1-2}$ measurements showed good interobserver reproducibility, whereas the presence of congruency and the DMAA were found to be less reproducible because of difficulty in accurately measuring the exact limits of the chondral surface of the metatarsal head. The authors warn that comparing studies regarding various surgical methods should be interpreted cautiously because of this lack of reproducibility.

Glasoe WM, Allen MK, Saltzman CL: First ray dorsal mobility in relation to hallux valgus deformity and first intermetatarsal angle. *Foot Ankle Int* 2001;22:98-101.

This case-controlled study compared the $IMA_{1-2}$ to dorsal mobility of the first metatarsal under standardized loading in patients with hallux valgus and control subjects. Although a marginal correlation was noted between $IMA_{1-2}$ and dorsal mobility, the patients with hallux valgus had significantly greater dorsal mobility than the controls, supporting the premise that first ray instability may contribute to hallux valgus.

Sammarco GJ, Idusuyi OB: Complications after surgery of the hallux. *Clin Orthop* 2001;391:59-71.

This article presents a systematic review of decision making and contemporary surgical techniques for the management of recurrent hallux valgus and other common complications after bunion surgery.

Thordarson DB, Rudicel SA, Ebramzadeh E, et al: Outcome study of hallux valgus surgery: An AOFAS multicenter study. *Foot Ankle Int* 2001;22:956-959.

This multicenter prospective study used clinical outcome scoring instruments to assess the results of hallux valgus surgery on 195 patients. The authors found significant improvements in patients' pain, function, and satisfaction after surgical correction.

Torkki M, Malmivaara A, Seitsalo S, et al: Surgery vs orthosis vs watchful waiting for hallux valgus: A randomized controlled trial. *JAMA* 2001;285:2474-2480.

This randomized, controlled multicenter study compared observation, orthotic management, and surgical treatment for symptomatic hallux valgus in 209 patients. At the 6-month follow-up, patients treated with orthotic devices and with surgery had improved pain levels compared with the control patients. At the 12-month follow-up, the surgery group showed continued improvement in regard to pain, shoe wear limitations, and function, whereas the beneficial effects of orthotic devices appeared to have diminished.

Trnka HJ, Zembsch A, Easley ME, Salzer M, Ritschl P, Myerson MS: The chevron osteotomy for correction of hallux valgus: Comparison of findings after two and five years of follow-up. *J Bone Joint Surg Am* 2000;82:1373-1378.

The authors studied the results of chevron osteotomy for the treatment of mild to moderate hallux valgus in 43 patients followed for 5 years. There was no difference in patients' clinical outcome scoring or radiographic parameters between 2 and 5 years after surgery, indicating the durability of this procedure. There was also no difference in outcomes between patients younger than 50 years and older patients.

Veri JP, Pirani SP, Claridge R: Crescentic proximal metatarsal osteotomy for moderate to severe hallux valgus: A mean 12.2 year follow-up study. *Foot Ankle Int* 2001;22:817-822.

Twenty-five patients treated with proximal crescentic metatarsal osteotomy and distal soft-tissue repair were evaluated at 1- and 12.2-year follow-up. Ninety-four percent of the patients reported that they would undergo the surgery again. There was no loss of correction of the HVA or intermetatarsal angle on radiographic evaluation over that period, and the overall recurrence rate was 11%.

### Juvenile Hallux Valgus

Aronson J, Nguyen LL, Aronson EA: Early results of the modified Peterson bunion procedure for adolescent hallux valgus. *J Pediatr Orthop* 2001;21:65-69.

Double osteotomies of the first metatarsal were fixed with a medial plate and screws, and an osteoperiosteal distally based flap was used to correct MTP joint subluxation in 16 adolescent patients (18 feet). All osteotomies healed, but deformity recurred in three feet in which the original deformity was inadequately corrected. The HVA was corrected from an average 34° to 16°, and the $IMA_{1-2}$ was improved from 14° to 6°. At minimum 1-year follow-up, no patient had requested plate removal.

Coughlin MJ, Carlson RE: Treatment of hallux valgus with an increased distal metatarsal articular angle: Evaluation of double and triple first ray osteotomies. *Foot Ankle Int* 1999;20:762-770.

Eighteen patients (21 feet) with high DMAAs were treated by combinations of distal closing wedge metatarsal osteotomy, proximal metatarsal or opening wedge cuneiform osteotomy, and closing wedge phalangeal osteotomy. This approach showed good correction of deformity with an 81% patient satisfaction rate.

Nery C, Barroco R, Ressio C: Biplanar chevron osteotomy. *Foot Ankle Int* 2002;23:792-798.

Of 32 patients (54 feet) ranging in age from 11 to 66 years, 90% were satisfied with their results after biplanar chevron osteotomy. HVA was improved from an average of 25° to 14°, IMA$_{1-2}$ from 12° to 8°, and DMAA from 15° to 5°.

Talab YA: Hallux valgus in children: A 5-14 year follow-up study of 30 feet treated with a modified Mitchell osteotomy. *Acta Orthop Scand* 2002;73:195-198.

Surgical modifications included diverging trapezoidal cuts, plantar displacement of the head, release of the lateral collateral ligament and adductor insertion, and Kirschner wire fixation of the osteotomy. At average follow-up of 8 years, there were no nonunions, osteonecrosis, or deformity recurrences; all patients were satisfied with their cosmetic results, could wear regular shoes, and had no physical restrictions. Only two patients reported occasional pain, which was believed to be caused by transfer metatarsalgia.

## Classic Bibliography

Coughlin MJ: Hallux valgus. *J Bone Joint Surg Am* 1996;78:932-966.

Frey C, Jahss M, Kummer FJ: The Akin procedure: An analysis of results. *Foot Ankle* 1991;12:1-6.

Geissele AE, Stanton RP: Surgical treatment of adolescent hallux valgus. *J Pediatr Orthop* 1990;10:642-648.

Hattrup SJ, Johnson KA: Chevron osteotomy: Analysis of factors in patients' dissatisfaction. *Foot Ankle* 1985;5: 327-332.

Mann RA, Rudicel S, Graves SC: Repair of hallux valgus with a distal soft-tissue procedure and proximal metatarsal osteotomy: A long-term follow-up. *J Bone Joint Surg Am* 1992;74:124-129.

Peterson HA, Newman SR: Adolescent bunion deformity treated with double osteotomy and longitudinal pin fixation of the first ray. *J Pediatr Orthop* 1993;13:80-84.

Piggott H: The natural history of hallux valgus in adolescence and early adult life. *J Bone Joint Surg Br* 1960;42: 749-760.

Richardson EG: Keller resection arthroplasty. *Orthopedics* 1990;13:1049-1053.

Sangeorzan BJ, Hansen ST Jr: Modified Lapidus procedure for hallux valgus. *Foot Ankle* 1989;9:262-266.

Sim-Fook L, Hodgson AR: A comparison of foot forms among the non-shoe and shoe-wearing Chinese population. *J Bone Joint Surg Am* 1958;40:1058-1062.

# Chapter 2

# Disorders of the First Ray

Thomas G. Padanilam, MD

## Introduction

Disorders of the first ray are a frequent cause of foot and ankle problems. Pathology of the first ray can lead to alterations in gait and cause significant pain and disability, especially in younger patients and athletes. This chapter focuses on the evaluation and treatment of hallux rigidus, turf toe injuries, and sesamoid disorders. Initial treatment of these conditions usually is nonsurgical, but surgery may be necessary to relieve persistent symptoms.

## Hallux Rigidus

The term hallux rigidus is used to describe a degenerative arthritic process that causes a functional limitation of motion of the first metatarsophalangeal (MTP) joint. Although a generalized decrease in motion is noted, dorsiflexion is especially limited by a mechanical block caused by periarticular osteophytes. Terms such as hallux limitus, dorsal bunion, hallux dolorosus, and metatarsus primus elevatus have been used to describe various components of this disorder.

Hallux rigidus affects approximately 2.5% of the adult population, second only to hallux valgus in frequency of conditions affecting the first MTP joint. In adolescents, hallux rigidus often is associated with a swollen joint that is limited at the extremes of motion. Localized chondral or osteochondral lesions in the articular cartilage of the metatarsal head have been implicated in having an etiologic role. Hallux rigidus is more common in adults than in adolescents and has more generalized degenerative changes that tend to progress with increasing age.

### Etiology, Anatomy, and Pathophysiology

The primary etiology of hallux rigidus has not been determined. The typical presentation of an isolated arthritis suggests that local pathologic alteration in the first MTP joint causes the degenerative changes. The most common cause is trauma that may occur as a result of a single injury such as an intra-articular fracture or a crush injury. Either type of injury can cause an acute compression injury to the MTP joint as a result of either forced hyperextension or forced plantar flexion with resultant chondral or osteochondral injury. What initially is believed to be

an acute sprain or turf toe injury can lead to chronic pain and progressive loss of motion. More commonly, hallux rigidus is caused by repetitive microtrauma that injures the articular cartilage. Over time, a generalized bony proliferation occurs about the joint, especially at the dorsolateral aspect of the metatarsal head. The medial aspect of the joint usually is spared until later in the process. MTP joint motion is limited by a dorsal osteophyte that blocks dorsiflexion. Pain associated with hallux rigidus is secondary to joint synovitis, movement at the degenerated joint, impingement from the dorsal osteophytes with dorsiflexion, and stretching of synovium, capsule, and digital nerves over the dorsal osteophytes during forced plantar flexion.

Anatomic variations of the foot believed to contribute to the development of hallux rigidus include a pronated foot, a long first metatarsal, elevation of the first metatarsal (metatarsus primus elevatus), a long, slender foot, and a flat metatarsal head. However, reproducible data confirming these anatomic variants as causative in the etiology of hallux rigidus are not available. Systemic conditions such as gout and rheumatoid arthritis can lead to limitation of motion and loss of articular cartilage of the first MTP joint, simulating clinically and even radiographically the common idiopathic form of hallux rigidus.

### Clinical Presentation

Patients usually experience an insidious onset of activity-related pain at the first MTP joint and report swelling and stiffness of the joint. Limitation of dorsiflexion leads to greater difficulty with such activities as running, squatting, and walking up an incline. Wearing high-heeled shoes is difficult because the MTP joint is forced into dorsiflexion. The increased bulk associated with the dorsal osteophytes can lead to irritation from shoe wear. Paresthesia along the medial aspect of the joint or into the first web space may be caused by compression of the dorsal cutaneous nerves between the osteophyte and the shoe. Patients with osteochondral lesions may note a sensation of persistent clicking or catching with range-of-motion assessment. Lateral forefoot pain can be caused by a supinated gait that is adopted to avoid push-off on the great toe.

The findings on physical examination vary with disease severity. The most common finding is limitation of dorsiflexion associated with pain. In the early stages of the disease, a generalized thickening around the first MTP joint may cause little limitation of motion, but over time, osteophytes on the dorsal aspect become more prominent and dorsiflexion more limited, with pain resulting from proximal phalangeal abutment on the eburnated metatarsal head. Two or more prominent ridges of bone along the dorsal aspect of the metatarsal head and frequently along the dorsolateral base of the proximal phalanx are easily palpable. Tenderness to palpation often is noted along the MTP joint, particularly at its dorsolateral aspect. Occasionally, dorsal osteophyte proliferation may prevent the hallux from assuming a neutral position (hallux flexus) and secondarily cause elevation of the first metatarsal.

Axial loading of the joint usually is not painful unless joint degeneration is severe or osteochondral lesions are present. Passive plantar flexion of the joint may be painful because of stretching of the extensor hallucis longus and brevis, the MTP joint capsule, and inflamed synovium over the dorsal osteophytes. Stresses on the interphalangeal joint are increased as MTP joint motion decreases, which can lead to a secondary hyperextension deformity of the interphalangeal joint and possibly an associated plantar callus under this joint. Alterations in gait occur relatively late in the disease process and are caused by supination of the forefoot, which the patient adopts to avoid weight bearing on the painful hallux. This alteration in gait can cause tenderness along the lesser metatarsal heads with transfer callosities. Sesamoid symptomatology usually is absent.

### Radiographic Findings

Radiographic evaluation should consist of weight-bearing AP, lateral, and oblique views of the foot. The AP view often shows nonuniform narrowing of the joint space with widening and flattening of the first metatarsal head. On the AP view, marginal osteophytes are commonly seen on adjacent bony surfaces at the lateral aspect of the joint. The degree of degenerative changes may be overestimated from the AP view because osteophytes may overlie the joint space, leading to a false impression of articular wear. Osteochondral injuries occur along the central and dorsolateral portions of the metatarsal head. The lateral radiograph shows the degree of dorsal osteophyte formation as well as the presence of loose bodies. The oblique view allows evaluation of the more plantar aspect of the metatarsal head. This view can be useful in assessing the degree of joint involvement because the plantar aspect of the joint often is spared until more advanced stages of the disease process. The diagnosis of hallux rigidus is made by physical examination and plain radiographs. Occasionally, a bone scan or CT is useful in de-

tecting osteochondral injuries and early degenerative changes. MRI can also be useful in identifying chondral injuries to the articular cartilage; however, MRI is so sensitive to chondral injury that an overestimation of articular injury is possible.

### Classification

Hallux rigidus has been classified into three grades based on radiographic findings. There is some controversy as to the usefulness of the classification system because the degree of degenerative changes seen on radiographs does not necessarily correlate with symptoms. In grade 1 (mild) hallux rigidus, the joint space is maintained and there is minimal osteophyte formation. The grade 2 (moderate) stage shows some joint space narrowing with osteophyte formation on the metatarsal head. Spurring also may be seen at the dorsal and lateral aspects of the base of the proximal phalanx and dorsal aspect of the metatarsal head. The oblique radiograph usually reveals sparing of the plantar aspect of the joint. Associated subchondral sclerosis or cysts may accompany the joint space narrowing. In grade 3 (severe) hallux rigidus, significant joint space narrowing and extensive osteophyte formation around the periphery of the joint are seen. Large dorsal osteophytes and intra-articular loose bodies may be present. Involvement of the metatarsal-sesamoid joint is rare.

### Nonsurgical Treatment

The decision to use nonsurgical treatment depends on the patient's symptoms and the extent of degenerative changes. Patients with mild synovitis and generalized soft-tissue thickening can be treated with nonsteroidal medications and rest. The hallux can be taped to limit dorsiflexion, provide a compressive dressing, and facilitate resting of the joint. Several commercially available orthotic devices can be used to increase rigidity of the medial forefoot area of the shoe, thus limiting MTP motion, minimizing dorsiflexion impingement pain, and decreasing the stress across the joint. An intra-articular steroid injection may provide some pain relief, but repeated injections can accelerate the degenerative process.

Significant dorsal osteophytes, present in more advanced stages of hallux rigidus, can limit the space available for orthoses. An extra-depth shoe with a deep toe box will accommodate large dorsal osteophytes. In addition, a shoe with a stiff-soled rocker bottom or a metatarsal bar is often helpful. These footwear modifications, although effective, are somewhat cumbersome, are not curative, and patient acceptance varies considerably.

### Surgical Treatment

Surgical treatment may be indicated for patients with persistent pain despite nonsurgical treatment. It is important to educate patients regarding surgical outcomes to maximize patient satisfaction. Although hallux rigidus is a pro-

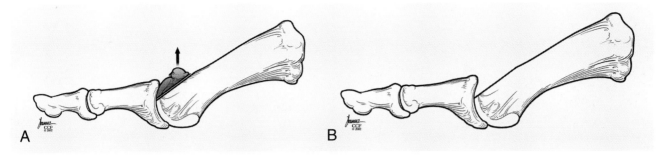

**Figure 1** **A,** Lateral view of the first metatarsal with suggested resection of both the dorsal osteophyte and a portion of the metatarsal head (gray-shaded area). **B,** Lateral view of the first metatarsal after resection. *(Reproduced with permission from the Cleveland Clinic Foundation, Cleveland, OH.)*

gressive disease process and the joint can be expected to deteriorate over time, the patient's symptoms may not progress. A study evaluating the natural history of hallux rigidus involved 27 patients for whom surgical treatment had been recommended but who declined treatment at the time. At an average follow-up of 14 years, 77% of patients who had refused surgical treatment were satisfied with their decision. Radiographic deterioration was noted in all patients who were examined during follow-up; however, 21 of 27 patients judged their symptoms to be the same.

No procedure will restore normal anatomy and range of motion of the joint; surgical goals should be relief of dorsal impingement and lessening of associated synovitis. The surgical procedure chosen depends on the patient's age, activity level, expectations, and degree of joint involvement. Surgical options include synovectomy with débridement of osteochondral or chondral lesions, cheilectomy with or without dorsiflexion osteotomy of the proximal phalanx, resection arthroplasty, arthrodesis, and interpositional arthroplasty.

### Joint Débridement and Synovectomy
Joint débridement and synovectomy may be indicated in patients with an acute chondral or osteochondral injury of the metatarsal head. These patients do not have any secondary changes such as dorsal osteophytes that would require removal. Typically, a cartilage flap is found along the dorsal margin of the joint. The flap is débrided to stable cartilage. For small defects, drilling of exposed bone may stimulate fibrocartilage ingrowth. Larger areas of exposed bone along the dorsal aspect of the joint may benefit from a limited cheilectomy. Some surgeons recommend arthroscopic evaluation and débridement of the joint, which presumably minimizes the soft-tissue injury associated with open treatment. No studies are available comparing arthroscopic with open treatment of these injuries.

### Cheilectomy
For patients whose symptoms are primarily the result of mechanical impingement of the proximal phalanx on the dorsal osteophytes of the metatarsal head, cheilectomy is the procedure of choice. Resection of the dorsal aspect of the metatarsal head along with the osteophyte is effective in relieving the pain associated with impingement and improving dorsiflexion. The technique involves either a dorsal or medial approach to the MTP joint to expose the dorsal osteophytes. Because osteophyte formation is more common on the lateral aspect of the joint, it is important that the lateral side is adequately débrided. In addition to osteophyte removal, most authors recommend removing 25% to 33% of the metatarsal head to achieve 70° to 90° of joint dorsiflexion, measured intraoperatively (Fig. 1). Postoperative range of motion usually is less than that seen at the time of surgery. Inadequate resection has been associated with poor results.

The degree of degenerative changes that preclude a good result with cheilectomy is controversial. Most surgeons believe that patients with grade 1 hallux rigidus are good candidates for the procedure, but conflicting data exist regarding patients with grades 2 and 3 disease. One study attempted to classify results of cheilectomy on the basis of radiographic grade with significant improvement noted in all grades. However, the average improvement in patients with grade 3 hallux rigidus was less than that in patients with grade 1 or 2 of the disease. Another recent study suggested that patients older than 60 years with predominantly extra-articular symptoms may be good candidates for cheilectomy regardless of radiographic grade. Advantages of cheilectomy include preservation of joint motion (albeit limited) and a shorter recovery time compared with fusion. This procedure also does not preclude a later arthrodesis or resection arthroplasty if cheilectomy fails to adequately relieve symptoms.

### Dorsiflexion Osteotomy of the Proximal Phalanx
A dorsal closing wedge proximal phalangeal osteotomy can be useful in the treatment of hallux rigidus (Fig. 2). Typically, MTP joint plantar flexion is not affected because the dorsal half of the joint is more commonly involved than the plantar aspect. A phalangeal osteotomy changes the arc of motion such that plantar motion is de-

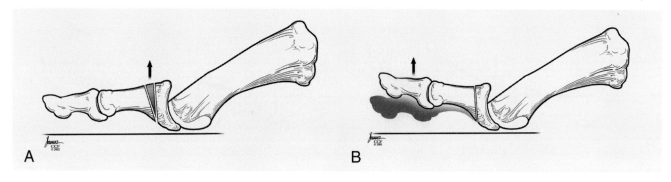

**Figure 2 A,** Lateral view of the proximal phalanx showing location of the dorsal closing wedge proximal phalangeal osteotomy. A cheilectomy was also performed. **B,** Dorsiflexion increases as a result of the dorsal closing wedge osteotomy. (*Reproduced with permission from the Cleveland Clinic Foundation, Cleveland, OH.*)

creased and dorsiflexion is increased. This procedure creates a more functional range of motion for the hallux. Recently, there has been interest in combining phalangeal osteotomy with cheilectomy. Cheilectomy will relieve the pain associated with dorsal impingement, while osteotomy will place the joint in a position that allows more functional range of motion. One study reviewed the results of this combination of procedures in 20 patients at an average follow-up of 5 years and found a 96% patient satisfaction rate and a 100% union rate of the proximal phalanx. The authors concluded that a phalangeal osteotomy combined with a cheilectomy significantly improved patient outcomes in the treatment of hallux rigidus. The necessity of a dorsal closing wedge osteotomy of the proximal phalanx can be determined intraoperatively and added to the procedure if cheilectomy does not allow adequate dorsiflexion (30° to 40°).

### Resection Arthroplasty
Resection arthroplasty of the first MTP joint consists of removal of the base of the proximal phalanx and is intended to provide decompression and improve motion of an arthritic joint. Resection of the base of the proximal phalanx destabilizes the joint by removing the attachment of the plantar plate and the flexor hallucis brevis, which can lead to a cock-up deformity of the first toe, instability of the first ray, weakness during push-off, excessive shortening of the hallux, and transfer metatarsalgia. Because of these potential complications, resection arthroplasty usually is reserved for elderly and more sedentary patients.

To decrease the risk of some of the complications associated with resection arthroplasty, a modification of the technique that involves capsular interposition has been suggested. In this modified technique, less than 25% of the proximal phalanx is resected, the short flexors are reattached to the base of the proximal phalanx, and the extensor hallucis brevis and dorsal capsule are interposed between the metatarsal head and base of the proximal phalanx. A study of this procedure in 30 patients showed that 28 were satisfied with the outcome. Range of motion improved an average of 40°, and no complications with

transfer metatarsalgia, weakness during push-off, malalignment, or shortening of the hallux were found. This procedure appears to be a suitable alternative treatment for advanced cases of hallux rigidus even in an active patient population.

### Arthrodesis
Arthrodesis of the MTP joint is the most commonly used procedure for severe hallux rigidus and remains the definitive procedure for pain relief; however, stabilization of the joint requires the sacrifice of joint motion. It is generally agreed that the toe should be fused in approximately 10° to 15° of valgus and should not touch the second toe. Optimally, 20° to 30° of dorsiflexion relative to the first metatarsal or 10° to 15° of dorsiflexion relative to the plantar aspect of the foot should be obtained in the sagittal plane.

Many methods for fixation and bone preparation have been advocated; the use of flat cuts and a cone and cup technique both have had high success rates. Fixation methods included compression screws, pins, sutures, staples, and a dorsal minifragment plate. Fusion rates have ranged from 70% to 100%. Complications associated with arthrodesis include malalignment, nonunion, and arthritis of the interphalangeal joint. Degeneration of the interphalangeal joint has been reported after MTP joint fusion in up to 15% of patients, although this condition is of limited clinical significance because most patients are not symptomatic. Excessive dorsiflexion may lead to pain at the tip of the toe, over the interphalangeal joint, and beneath the first metatarsal head. Excessive plantar flexion can cause increased pressure at the tip of the toe. However, excessive dorsiflexion is better tolerated than excessive plantar flexion.

### Interpositional Arthroplasty
The role of prosthetic replacement of the MTP joint remains unclear. Its lack of superiority to resection arthroplasty or arthrodesis and its significant complication rate have limited its role in the treatment of patients with hallux rigidus.

## Turf Toe Injuries

Turf toe is a term used to describe injuries to the first MTP joint that vary in both severity and the structures injured. Injuries to the periarticular structures of the hallux can lead to significant functional disability. Initial symptoms include pain with push-off and running. Long-term complications include a lack of push-off strength, hallux rigidus, hallux valgus, and a hallux cock-up deformity. The true incidence of injury is difficult to measure, but occurrences in college athletic programs have ranged from four to six injuries per year.

### Mechanism of Injury

The mechanisms of injury include hyperextension, hyperflexion, and valgus stress. The most commonly reported mechanism of injury to the MTP joint of the great toe is hyperextension. This typically involves an axial load on a foot fixed in equinus. A force applied to the heel causes forefoot dorsiflexion resulting in hyperextension at the hallux MTP joint. This hyperextension can lead to a spectrum of injuries from partial tearing of the plantar plate to dislocation. With dorsal dislocation of the hallux, the insertion of the flexor hallucis brevis can avulse, producing an intrinsic minus or clawed hallux. In addition, as the plantar structures are torn from the plantar surface of the base of the proximal phalanx, the dorsal edge of the proximal phalanx may compress into the dorsal articular surface of the metatarsal head, producing an osteochondral shear or compression articular injury. Hyperflexion is the second most common mechanism of injury to the MTP joint of the great toe and has been reported in dancers and football, beach volleyball, and basketball players. Hyperflexion of the MTP joint causes tearing of the dorsal capsule and possibly compression or shear injury to the plantar aspect of the metatarsal head or the proximal phalanx. Because of its frequency in beach volleyball players, this injury has been termed sand toe. The third most common mechanism of injury to the MTP joint of the hallux is valgus force applied to the MTP joint when the forefoot is firmly planted and is internally rotated during push-off to decelerate and change directions suddenly. This results in injury to the plantar medial structures and occasionally the medial sesamoid that can lead to the development of traumatic hallux valgus and bunion formation.

### Etiology

The most commonly postulated etiologic factors in turf toe injuries are the type of playing surface and the flexibility of the patient's shoe. One study reported that 83% of professional football players sustained their initial turf toe injuries on artificial turf. Some investigators have speculated that the hardness of aging artificial turf contributes to these injuries. However, clinical findings do not show a difference between new and old artificial turf as causative factors in turf toe injuries. The shoe-surface interface has been suggested as a factor in these injuries. The increased friction between the shoe and the turf may cause the forefoot to become fixed, while external forces cause a hyperextension of the MTP joint. The type of shoe wear also is thought to play a role in turf toe injuries. Traditional shoe wear used on grass surfaces had a steel plate in the sole of the shoe for attachment of the cleats; this plate limited forefoot motion. The shoes worn on artificial turf are lighter and more flexible, which is thought to provide less protection against these injuries. Another factor implicated in turf toe injury is that players with increased ankle dorsiflexion may be more at risk for this injury because they tend to place the MTP joint in a position where hyperextension is likely.

Other causative factors for injury include decreased MTP joint range of motion; the team position played by an athlete; the age, weight, and number of years of sports participation of an athlete; and the existence of pes planus and a flat metatarsal head. The role of these factors in the development of an MTP joint injury is undetermined.

### Physical Examination

The spectrum of injury to anatomic restraints about the MTP joint and the severity of injury to these structures require detailed examination. The best time to evaluate these patients is immediately after injury, when swelling and discomfort are at a minimum. It is important to determine as precisely as possible the mechanism of injury. The amount and location of swelling and ecchymosis, the overall alignment of the hallux, and whether the MTP joint is reduced clinically and radiographically should be noted. Palpation of the dorsal capsule, medial and lateral collateral ligaments, and the plantar aspect of the MTP joint including the sesamoids will localize the most severely injured structures. The hallux MTP joint should be evaluated for range of motion and compared with the contralateral side. Hypermobility or gross instability of the joint or mechanical block to motion from chondral, osteochondral, or soft-tissue interposition should be evaluated. Varus and valgus stress testing will delineate the integrity of the collateral ligaments, and a dorsoplantar drawer test of the MTP joint will aid in determining the status of the plantar and dorsal structures. Evaluation of MTP joint motion against resistance aids in determining the status of the intrinsic and extrinsic tendons that cross the joint. The patient's ability to bear weight on the injured toe either comfortably or with only mild discomfort is very helpful in determining the severity of the injury. With an acute injury, pain may limit evaluation of strength and stress testing of the joint. Any suggestion of an intrinsic minus position of the hallux with the MTP joint extended and the interphalangeal joint flexed (compared with the contralateral hallux) is an ominous sign. In this situation, it is important to identify plantar plate avulsion from the base of the proximal phalanx or rupture of one or both tendon insertions of the flexor hallu-

**TABLE 1 | Classification of Turf Toe Injuries**

| Grade | Pathology | Findings | Activity Level |
|-------|-----------|----------|----------------|
| 1 | Incomplete tear of capsule | Localized plantar or medial tenderness<br>Minimal swelling and ecchymosis | Continued sports participation usually is possible |
| 2 | Partial tear of capsule | More diffuse tenderness<br>Moderate swelling and ecchymosis<br>Some decrease in range of motion<br>Moderate pain with ambulation | Unable to play for 3 to 14 days |
| 3 | Complete tear of capsuloligamentous complex | Severe diffuse tenderness<br>Marked swelling<br>Moderate to severe ecchymosis<br>Limited range of joint motion<br>Inability to bear weight normally | May require 4 to 6 weeks before return to activity |

cis brevis onto the sesamoids.

Radiographic evaluation should include weight-bearing AP and lateral views and a non–weight-bearing oblique view, as well as a sesamoid axial view. Radiographs should be evaluated for sesamoid fractures, impaction fractures, capsular avulsions, and diastasis of bipartite sesamoids. Because complete plantar plate rupture can allow proximal migration of the sesamoids, the distance from the distal aspect of the sesamoid to the MTP joint on the injured side should be measured and compared with the contralateral side. The difference between sides should be less than 3 mm for the medial sesamoid and 2.7 mm for the lateral sesamoid. One method for evaluating joint subluxation, sesamoid migration, and separation of a bipartite sesamoid is a forced dorsiflexion lateral view obtained after a local anesthetic block. Varus or valgus stress views can be useful to determine collateral ligament injury. Additional studies such as bone scanning can be used to detect stress fractures of the sesamoids. MRI recently has been shown to be beneficial in defining the extent of chondral and soft-tissue injury associated with turf toe. The classification of turf toe injuries is based on the severity of injury (Table 1).

### Nonsurgical Treatment

The treatment of MTP joint injuries varies depending on the nature and severity of the injury. Initial treatment usually consists of rest, ice, compression, and elevation (the RICE protocol). Analgesics and anti-inflammatory medication can be useful for grade 1 and 2 injuries; grade 3 injuries require a walker boot or a short leg cast with a toe extension. Early joint motion can begin within 3 to 5 days of injury if symptoms permit. Athletes with grade 1 injuries usually can return to their sport with little or no loss of playing time. These athletes may benefit from taping of the toe to prevent hyperextension, the use of a spring carbon fiber steel plate in the forefoot region of the shoe, or a custom shoe insert with a Morton's extension. Grade 2 injuries usually result in 3 to 14 days of lost

playing time. Treatment is similar to that for grade 1 injuries. Grade 3 injuries can result in 4 to 6 weeks of lost playing time. The MTP joint is immobilized until it is stable and then joint mobilization is begun. Return to athletic activities is based on the patient's comfort level and the type of activity. Generally, an athlete should have 50° to 60° of painless dorsiflexion before returning to competitive sport.

### Surgical Treatment

Surgical treatment of turf toe injuries seldom is necessary. Surgical intervention should be considered for loose bodies in the MTP joint, large cartilage flaps, sesamoid fractures or bipartite sesamoids with diastasis, retraction of the sesamoids and traumatic bunion, or progressive hallux valgus. The acute repair or reconstruction of these injuries can be done through a medial, medial and plantar, or J-incision technique. Care must be taken to protect the proper branch of the medial plantar nerve and the medial side of the pulp of the hallux, which lies adjacent to the medial edge of the medial sesamoid. The sesamoids are advanced and repaired to either soft tissue at the base of the proximal phalanx or through drill holes in the base of the proximal phalanx. Diastasis of a bipartite sesamoid often can be treated with excision of the distal pole and reattachment of the soft tissue to the proximal pole. If one of the sesamoids is fragmented, excision may be necessary. Careful dissection around the sesamoid margins often can preserve some tendinous continuity from the flexor hallucis brevis to the proximal phalanx. If no continuity of the tendon or the plantar plate can be preserved, an abductor hallucis transfer to restore flexion power and to act as a plantar restraint to dorsiflexion may be needed. Late reconstructions are quite difficult, and abductor hallucis transfer is often needed.

## Sesamoid Disorders

There has been an increasing recognition of the role of sesamoids in clinical problems related to the hallux. The surge in enthusiasm for athletic activities has caused an increase in sesamoid-related problems. Despite their small size, these bones can be a source of disabling pain. The sesamoids function to absorb and transmit weight-bearing pressure, reduce friction, protect the flexor hallucis longus (FHL) tendon, and serve as a fulcrum to increase the mechanical force of the flexor hallucis brevis tendon. Because more than 50% of the body weight can be transmitted through the first MTP joint, the sesamoids are vulnerable to injury from traumatic and repetitive stresses.

### Anatomy

The two sesamoids of the MTP joint are within the tendons of the flexor hallucis brevis. Each sesamoid articulates with the metatarsal head through matched congruent sulci, which are separated by an osteocartilaginous ridge (the crista). The two hallucal sesamoids are held together by the intersesamoid ligament and by the plantar plate, which attaches to the base of the proximal phalanx. The FHL tendon glides between and immediately plantar to the two sesamoids. Because the medial (tibial) sesamoid usually is larger than the lateral (fibular) sesamoid and is more impacted by weight bearing, it is the more frequently injured. The medial sesamoid is the attachment site for the abductor hallucis, and the lateral sesamoid is the attachment site for the oblique head of the adductor hallucis and the deep transverse metatarsal ligament. The medial sesamoid is bipartite in approximately 10% of the population; the lateral sesamoid rarely is bipartite. In 25% of patients with a bipartite medial sesamoid, the condition is bilateral.

### Clinical Presentation

Patients may report generalized pain around the hallux, but often the pain is more localized to the plantar aspect. Usually there is an insidious onset of symptoms over weeks, with a gradual progression of pain, swelling, and discomfort with motion, especially dorsiflexion. A patient with a sesamoid fracture may recall a single traumatic event. Patients often report difficulty walking and shift their weight to the outer border of the foot to avoid bearing weight on the painful sesamoids. Stair climbing and athletic activities may provoke symptoms. In addition, patients may report neuritic symptoms and numbness if the digital nerve is compressed.

### Physical Examination

Tenderness is present along the plantar aspect of the first MTP joint. Using palpation, it is difficult to isolate one sesamoid from the other or from the FHL tendon because of the close proximity of these structures. Moderate joint effusion may be present, which further restricts motion of the MTP joint while increasing pain and decreasing function. In patients with localized tenosynovitis of the FHL tendon, tenderness is exacerbated by resisted

plantar flexion of the hallucal interphalangeal joint. A Tinel sign may be elicited when nerve compression is present. The foot should be inspected for a cavus deformity, which often is associated with a plantar flexed first ray that places more axial load on the sesamoids, particularly the medial one. The presence of any callus should be noted.

### Radiographic Examination

Radiographs for sesamoid evaluation usually include AP, lateral, medial and lateral oblique, and axial sesamoid views. The AP and lateral views can be useful for the detection of sesamoid fractures, bipartite sesamoids, and proximal retraction of the sesamoids that occur with turf toe injuries. The lateral oblique view allows evaluation of the lateral sesamoid and osteochondral injury to the dorsal surface of the metatarsal head. The medial sesamoid is best seen on the medial oblique view. The axial sesamoid view is useful for evaluating osteochondritis of the sesamoid and the degree of degenerative changes between the sesamoid and the metatarsal head. If the radiographs are normal and there is persistent pain, a bone scan is indicated. Appropriate scintigraphic views are important to distinguish between sesamoid and MTP joint pathology. Consultation between the orthopaedic surgeon and the nuclear medicine physician clarifies the particular view needed. A sesamoid abnormality may be obscured on an AP bone scan if there are degenerative or posttraumatic changes in the MTP joint. The PA, lateral, or oblique views with collimation will help distinguish the source of the pathology. Interpreting data from a bone scan should be done with caution; increased activity has been reported in 26% to 29% of asymptomatic persons (particularly elite athletes). A significant difference in the radioisotope uptake between one foot and the other is an indication that injury has occurred. MRI also can be useful to evaluate the presence of osteomyelitis, fractures, FHL tendinitis, and osteochondritis.

### Differential Diagnosis

Sesamoiditis is a generic term that refers to multiple etiologies, such as sesamoid fractures, osteochondritis, infection, arthritis, intractable plantar keratoses, osteonecrosis, digital nerve compression, and tendinitis. The medial sesamoid is involved more often than the lateral because of its larger size and the more force it absorbs.

### Nonsurgical Treatment

Nonsurgical treatment is indicated for most closed sesamoid injuries. Nonsurgical treatments focus on reducing the weight borne under the first metatarsal head and include limitation of activities, avoiding the wear of high-heeled shoes, and the use of a weight-relieving pad, rocker sole, or metatarsal bar. Taping to limit dorsiflexion can sometimes be effective in reducing the symptoms during athletic activities, and periodic shaving of keratotic lesions can keep them from becoming painful. Steroid injections may be helpful. Treatment of acute sesamoid fractures is controversial, with some authors recommending the use of a short leg cast (extending beyond the toes) for 4 to 6 weeks, while others prefer a stiff-soled shoe or boot with padding around the sesamoid.

### Surgical Treatment

Surgical treatment should be considered for patients whose symptoms have not improved after 3 to 12 months of nonsurgical treatment. Sesamoid sparing procedures have been recommended to avoid complications associated with sesamoid excision. Good healing and preservation of function have been reported after bone grafting of sesamoid nonunions in a small number of patients. For patients with a plantar flexed first ray, dorsiflexion osteotomy of the first metatarsal should be considered. Excision of the sesamoid often is the best option for treatment of sesamoid symptoms that are not relieved by exhaustive nonsurgical treatment. As a general rule, only one sesamoid should be excised to avoid claw toe deformity. The medial sesamoid is approached through a medial incision, whereas the lateral sesamoid can be reached by a dorsal or plantar approach. The plantar approach to the lateral sesamoid is technically easier. It is important to protect the digital nerves, which are in close proximity to the sesamoids, and to maintain the capsular and ligamentous sleeve in order to minimize the risk of an associated deformity, such as hallux valgus, hallux varus, or clawed hallux. Sesamoid excision can provide significant improvement for the patient; however, pain relief is complete in only 50% to 80% of patients. Other possible complications of sesamoid excision are loss of motion, plantar flexion weakness, an intractable plantar keratosis over the remaining sesamoid, and neuroma formation.

## Summary

Hallux rigidus, turf toe, and sesamoid injuries all can cause debilitating pain and functional limitations. Appropriate treatment depends on accurate identification of the etiology and pathology of each of these conditions. Although initial treatment usually is nonsurgical, surgery may be required for persistent symptoms. Surgical treatment of hallux rigidus may require joint débridement and synovectomy, cheilectomy, dorsiflexion osteotomy of the proximal phalanx, or MTP joint arthroplasty or arthrodesis for severe joint degeneration. Turf toe injuries seldom require surgical treatment, except for grade 3 complete tears of the capsuloligamentous complex. Sesamoid symptoms unrelieved by prolonged nonsurgical treatment may be alleviated by sesamoid excision, but complete pain relief is obtained in only 50% to 80% of patients.

## Annotated Bibliography

### Hallux Rigidus

Easley ME, Davis WH, Anderson RB: Intermediate to long-term follow-up of medial-approach dorsal cheilectomy for hallux rigidus. *Foot Ankle Int* 1999;20:147-152.

The authors evaluated results of cheilectomy through a medial approach in 52 patients at an average follow-up of 5 years and concluded that this procedure can effectively provide relief of pain and improve function, despite progression of generalized first MTP joint arthritic degeneration.

Feltham GT, Hanks SE, Marcus RE: Age-based outcomes of cheilectomy for the treatment of hallux rigidus. *Foot Ankle Int* 2001;22:192-197.

In a retrospective study of patients treated with cheilectomy, good outcomes were reported in patients older than 60 years. Extra-articular symptoms were predominant regardless of radiographic grade.

Hamilton WG, O'Malley MJ, Thompson FM, Kovatis PE: Capsular interposition arthroplasty for severe hallux rigidus. *Foot Ankle Int* 1997;18:68-70.

Outcomes of a modified resection arthroplasty that involved interposition of the dorsal capsule and extensor hallucis brevis were reported; this was determined to be a reliable method for the treatment of severe hallux rigidus.

Horton GA, Park YW, Myerson MS: Role of metatarsus primus elevatus in the pathogenesis of hallux rigidus. *Foot Ankle Int* 1999;20:777-780.

In a comparison of 100 feet with hallux rigidus to controls, no difference in metatarsal elevation was found.

Lau JT, Daniels TR: Outcomes following cheilectomy and interpositional arthroplasty in hallux rigidus. *Foot Ankle Int* 2001;22:462-470.

This is a retrospective study of patients who underwent cheilectomy with proximal phalangeal osteotomy and interpositional arthroplasty. The authors concluded that cheilectomy/phalangeal osteotomy was reliable, whereas interpositional arthroplasty was a salvage procedure with less predictable results.

Smith RW, Katchis SD, Ayson LC: Outcomes in hallux rigidus patients treated nonoperatively: A long-term follow-up study. *Foot Ankle Int* 2000;21:906-913.

The authors attempted to define the natural history of hallux rigidus. Significant radiographic progression over time was found, but clinically most patients did not notice a significant increase in symptoms.

Thomas PJ, Smith RW: Proximal phalanx osteotomy for the surgical treatment of hallux rigidus. *Foot Ankle Int* 1999;20:3-12.

The authors reported a 96% satisfaction rate and 100% union rate of the proximal phalanx. They concluded the combination of cheilectomy and phalangeal osteotomy significantly improved results in the treatment of hallux rigidus.

### Turf Toe Injuries

Watson TS, Anderson RB, Davis WH: Periarticular injuries to the hallux metatarsophalangeal joint in athletes. *Foot Ankle Clin* 2000;5:687-713.

The authors present a review of the anatomy, mechanisms of injury, and treatment options for periarticular injuries to the hallux MTP joint.

### Sesamoid Disorders

Anderson RB, McBryde AM Jr: Autogenous bone grafting of hallux sesamoid nonunions. *Foot Ankle Int* 1997; 18:293-296.

The results of this study showed good outcomes in 19 of 21 patients who underwent bone grafting of the medial sesamoid. The authors concluded that sesamoid preservation should be attempted.

Richardson EG: Hallucal sesamoid pain: Causes and surgical treatment. *J Am Acad Orthop Surg* 1999;7:270-278.

A review of the evaluation and treatment options for various disorders of the sesamoid is presented.

## Classic Bibliography

Aper RL, Saltzman CL, Brown TD: The effect of hallux sesamoid resection on the effective moment of the flexor hallucis brevis. *Foot Ankle Int* 1994;15:462-470.

Chisin R, Peyser A, Milgram C: Bone scintigraphy in the assessment of hallucal sesamoids. *Foot Ankle Int* 1995;16: 291-294.

Clanton TO, Butler JE, Eggert A: Injuries to the metatarsophalangeal joints in athletes. *Foot Ankle* 1986;7: 162-176.

Clanton TO, Ford JJ: Turf toe injury. *Clin Sports Med* 1994;13:731-741.

Clayton ML, Ries MD: Functional hallux rigidus in the rheumatoid foot. *Clin Orthop* 1991;271:233-238.

Coughlin MJ: Sesamoid pain: Causes and surgical treatment. *Instr Course Lect* 1990;39:23-35.

Dietzen CJ: Great toe sesamoid injuries in the athlete. *Orthop Rev* 1990;19:966-972.

Hattrup SJ, Johnson KA: Subjective results of hallux rigidus following treatment with cheilectomy. *Clin Orthop* 1988;226:182-191.

Jahss MH: Traumatic dislocations of the first metatarsophalangeal joint. *Foot Ankle* 1980;1:15-21.

Leventen EO: Sesamoid disorders and treatment: An update. *Clin Orthop* 1991;269:236-240.

Mann RA: Hallux rigidus. *Instr Course Lect* 1990;39: 15-21.

Mann RA, Clanton TO: Hallux rigidus: Treatment by cheilectomy. *J Bone Joint Surg Am* 1988;70:400-406.

Rodeo SA, O'Brien S, Warren RF, Barnes R, Wickiewicz TL, Dillingham MF: Turf-toe: An analysis of metatarsophalangeal joint sprains in professional football players. *Am J Sports Med* 1990;18:280-285.

Sammarco GJ: Turf toe. *Instr Course Lect* 1993;42: 207-212.

# Chapter 3

# Hallux Varus: Acquired

Mark M. Casillas, MD

## Introduction

Varus angulation of the hallux metatarsophalangeal (MTP) joint produces a spectrum of deformity and associated impairment of the first ray. Hallux varus may be acquired or congenital. This chapter focuses on acquired hallux varus, with specific attention to pathogenesis, prevention, evaluation, and management of the deformity.

## Anatomy

The first MTP joint is composed of the first metatarsal head, the hallucal proximal phalangeal base, and the sesamoids. The MTP joint is stabilized by bony, ligamentous, and musculotendinous structures. The bony stability is provided by the size and topography of the metatarsal head. A flat or pointed head imparts inherent resistance to angular deflection of the proximal phalangeal base, whereas a round head provides minimal stability. The sagittal groove is a prominent bony trough delineating the medial extent of the articular surface of the metatarsal head from the medial eminence (Fig. 1). The metatarsal head medial to the groove buttresses and resists medial angulation of the proximal phalanx.

Soft-tissue stability is provided by the MTP joint capsule and its associated ligamentous and tendinous structures. The tissues provide both static and dynamic stability to the joint. The plantar plate represents a confluence of capsule, ligaments, sesamoids, and tendons. Four intrinsic foot tendons (flexor hallucis brevis medial and lateral heads, extensor hallucis brevis, abductor hallucis, and adductor hallucis) provide dynamic stabilization to the MTP joint.

Hallux varus is defined as varus angulation of the first MTP joint or a hallux-first metatarsal angle of 0° or less. Sagittal plane deformity also may occur and includes varying degrees of extension of the first MTP joint and flexion of the first interphalangeal (IP) joint. Axial deformity is typically marked by supination of the hallux. The malaligned hallux is not capable of full weight transfer. This functional deficit may overload the lesser MTP joints and produce a transfer callosity, particularly under the second and/or third metatarsal heads.

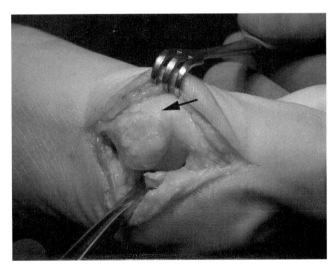

**Figure 1** Medial exposure of the hallux metatarsal head with identification of the sagittal groove (arrow).

## Incidence

Acquired hallux varus can be idiopathic or related to a specific traumatic injury to the dynamic or static joint stabilizers or related to a specific inflammatory (eg, rheumatoid arthritis and osteoarthritis) or neurologic (eg, Charcot-Marie-Tooth disease and polio) disease process. Iatrogenic hallux varus, however, is the most common form of the deformity. The incidence of iatrogenic hallux varus varies by the type of hallux valgus repair and by report. A review of the literature suggests that the incidence of hallux varus after simple bunionectomy is between 2% and 13%. The McBride procedure with a lateral sesamoid excision is the repair most commonly associated with hallux varus.

## Pathogenesis

Hallux varus usually is produced by a lack of static support, with or without associated imbalance of the dynamic forces that act across the MTP joint. These forces are both linear and rotational, and both the intrinsic and extrinsic musculotendinous structures crossing the MTP joint are capable of accentuating the established deformity.

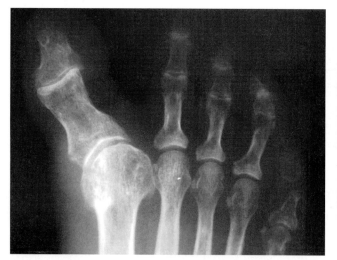

**Figure 2** Iatrogenic hallux varus subsequent to lateral sesamoid excision.

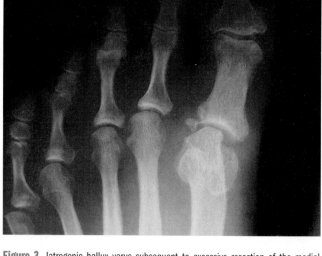

**Figure 3** Iatrogenic hallux varus subsequent to excessive resection of the medial eminence.

The pathogenesis of iatrogenic hallux varus typically is multifactorial, but some more common causes can be identified and avoided. Excessive tightening of the medial joint capsule, excessive resection of the medial eminence, and overcorrection of the intermetatarsal angle contribute to the tendency to produce hallux varus deformity. Even subtle errors, in combination, are capable of producing hallux varus.

### Excessive Release of Lateral Structures

The lateral side of the MTP joint is stabilized by the lateral capsule and ligaments, the adductor hallucis tendon, the lateral head of the flexor hallucis brevis, and the lateral sesamoid. Removal of the lateral sesamoid is of particular concern because it commonly requires weakening of all of the entire lateral joint stabilizers (lateral capsule, flexor hallucis brevis, and adductor tendon) (Fig. 2). It also produces a sizable defect in the plantar plate through which the metatarsal head may pass.

When deemed necessary, the lateral release is done sequentially—the adductor release is done first and followed by capsular release, which itself can be done gradually. If valgus deformity persists, lateral sesamoid excision may be indicated, even though it is known to contribute to the development of hallux varus deformity.

### Excessive Tightening of the Medial Joint Capsule

Medial capsular repair involves the repair of two separate structures—the tibial sesamoidal ligament (plantarmedial) and the medial collateral ligament (approximately midline). Overcorrection of either or both may contribute to hallux varus. Excessive tightening of the tibial sesamoidal ligament produces a medial subluxation of the sesamoid apparatus, which allows the flexor hallucis brevis to produce a varus vector across the MTP joint. Excessive tightening of the medial collateral ligament

produces overt varus angulation or medial subluxation of the MTP joint or both. Once present, these deformities may progress, particularly if the medial eminence resection was aggressive. This complication can be prevented by careful resection and repair of these two structures. If too much medial capsule is resected, surgical repair becomes exponentially more difficult. The use of intraoperative radiographs or fluoroscopy is particularly useful in the assessment of joint congruity, angulation, and sesamoid apparatus position. Clinical examination and direct inspection of the sesamoid position are recommended.

### Excessive Resection of the Medial Eminence

The stability of the hallucal proximal phalanx is influenced by the presence of sufficient buttressing by the metatarsal head. Of particular importance is the preservation of the sagittal groove. The loss of the sagittal groove causes significant loss of bony resistance to varus deformity (Fig. 3).

The most predictable way to avoid this complication is to identify the sagittal groove before medial eminence resection and to make sure that resection preserves the groove and approximately 1 to 2 mm of metatarsal head medial to it. This ensures the maintenance of adequate medial support for the proximal phalangeal base.

### Overcorrection of the Intermetatarsal Angle

A proximal osteotomy combined with a distal soft-tissue procedure is a reproducible and effective method for bunion correction. It allows reduction of the intermetatarsal angle through an osteotomy of the metatarsal base. Overreduction of the intermetatarsal angle increases the tendency of the sesamoid apparatus to subluxate medially, which results in a varus-producing vector through the intrinsic musculature. In a large series of patients treated with proximal osteotomy and distal soft-tissue procedures, hallux varus occurred most often in those with greater intermetatarsal angle correction and in some patients with overcorrection of the intermetatarsal angle. This complication is avoided by careful alignment of the metatarsal before placement of fixation and careful clinical and radiographic evaluation after fixation. To correct the first-second intermetatarsal angle to 5° or less is inviting hallux varus.

## Evaluation

The evaluation begins with a pertinent history that includes surgical history, cosmetic concerns, location of foot pain, functional concerns, occupation, and athletic activities. Most patients with hallux varus are asymptomatic, and concerns about the appearance of the foot and the inability to wear shoes comfortably are more common than concerns about pain related to the hallux varus deformity. Difficulty wearing shoes usually is related to the great toe varus, although it can be related to the dorsal abutment caused by the prominent IP joint. The IP joint often becomes dorsally prominent because of the extension that occurs at the MTP joint and the resultant flexion at the IP joint. This deformity also limits shoe wear, especially when the deformity is fixed. Often, the extensor hallucis longus tendon is medially bowstrung and taut. The longer the patient has had the deformity, the more likely it is that the range of motion of the MTP and IP joints is restricted. Decreased function of the first ray may result in painful keratotic lesions (particularly at the plantar aspect of the second metatarsal head) or development of a synovitis of the second MTP joint caused by overload at this joint. With plantar palpation of the MTP joint, a medially displaced tibial sesamoid sometimes can be identified.

All components of the deformity must be examined and the location of any tenderness noted. It is important to document the range of motion of the MTP and IP joints because this will be a major factor in choosing the appropriate surgical procedure. Before any surgical procedure, vascular and neurologic status must be thoroughly documented.

The radiographic evaluation of hallux varus includes weight-bearing AP and lateral views, a non–weight-bearing oblique view, and a sesamoid axial view to determine the degree of varus deformity, arthrosis, extension of the MTP joint, flexion of the IP joint, and MTP joint and sesamoid subluxation. The presence or absence of the lateral sesamoid is also documented. A weight-bearing AP radiograph with the hallux taped or wrapped with the lesser toes may provide additional information regarding the passive correctability of the MTP joint.

## Classification

Hallux varus is classified by the type of muscle imbalance present or by the type and location of the deformity. Ac-

quired hallux varus can be described as static or dynamic. Static deformity is not associated with an inherent muscle imbalance and usually is not progressive. Dynamic deformity is associated with disruption of the adductor hallucis and flexor hallucis brevis (lateral head) musculotendinous units and usually is progressive.

Classification based on the deformities associated with hallux varus is helpful for surgical planning because it identifies the soft-tissue and bony abnormalities that require correction. It is important to identify both sagittal plane deformity (extension at the MTP joint or flexion at the IP joint) and axial plane deformity (varus at the MTP joint). Deformities at the MTP and IP joints also are classified as fixed or flexible (passively correctable).

## Nonsurgical Treatment

Ideally, prevention of acquired hallux varus begins early after hallux valgus correction. Splints and taping are used to reduce any varus deformity and maintain a slight valgus position. If dressings fail to maintain an acceptable correction, early surgical revision is favored over delayed surgical reconstruction. However, initial treatment of chronic acquired hallux varus is directed to pain relief. A shoe with a wide, flexible, extra-deep toe box may be sufficient. Local padding and taping also may provide relief related to specific areas of contact between the hallux and the shoe. If arthritic complaints predominate, a carbon fiber insert can be used to decrease motion at the MTP joint.

## Surgical Treatment

Surgical treatment of hallux varus is directed toward restoration of the alignment and function of the first ray. Soft-tissue release always is required and may be combined with osseous reconstruction. To choose the appropriate treatment for hallux varus, the IP and MTP joints must be evaluated in both the axial and sagittal planes, and the joints must be evaluated to determine whether the deformities are flexible or fixed. The foot also must be evaluated clinically and radiographically for degenerative arthritis because, with the exception of arthroplasty and arthrodesis, this condition precludes all surgical treatment.

### Soft-Tissue Release

The release of tight medial capsuloligamentous-tendinous soft tissues is required for every hallux varus correction. The medial exposure is achieved using a V to Y or inverted U capsulotomy. The joint is then débrided and articular adhesions are resected. An extensor hallucis longus (EHL) tenolysis is done if the tendon is tethered medial to the midline. When adequate correction is obtained, the medial capsule is repaired in a lengthened position, the abductor hallucis is lengthened with the capsu-

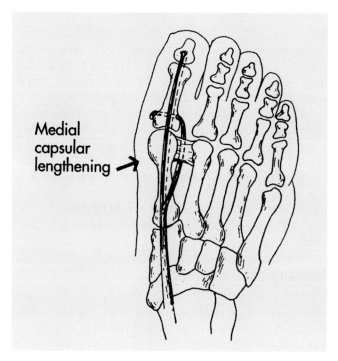

Figure 4  Split EHL tendon transfer for correction of flexible hallux varus deformity. The lateral two thirds of the EHL tendon is detached distally and transferred deep to the intermetatarsal ligament and into the proximal phalanx. *(Reproduced with permission from Mann RA, Coughlin MJ: Adult hallux valgus, in Coughlin MJ, Mann RA (eds): Surgery of the Foot and Ankle, ed 7. St. Louis, MO, Mosby, 1999, pp 150-269.)*

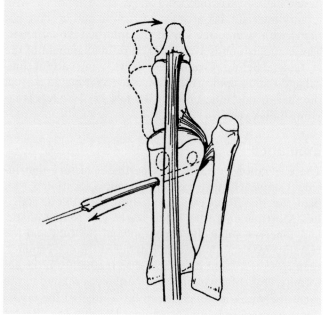

Figure 5  Extensor hallucis brevis tenodesis for correction of flexible hallux varus. The extensor hallucis brevis is transected near the muscle tendon junction, then routed deep to the intermetatarsal ligament and into the metatarsal head. *(Reproduced with permission from Juliano PJ, Myerson MS, Cunningham BW: Biomechanical assessment of a new tenodesis for correction of hallux varus. Foot Ankle Int 1996;17:17-20.)*

lar release, and the EHL tendon and both sesamoids (with the flexor hallucis longus between them) are returned to their anatomic positions. It is essential to reproduce normal balance of the extrinsic and intrinsic muscles as they course across the MTP joint. The sesamoids must rest in their facets. If the tibial sesamoid cannot be relocated in its facet, it must be excised if the lateral sesamoid is still present. An arthrodesis of the MTP joint must be done if the lateral sesamoid is absent and the tibial sesamoid cannot be reduced into its facet.

### Tendon Transfer

Transfer of the EHL tendon is a reliable means of correcting a flexible, nonarthritic hallux varus deformity. The method was first described as a complete EHL transfer to the base of the hallucal proximal phalanx, with an IP joint arthrodesis to correct IP joint flexion deformity. The transfer is routed deep to the intermetatarsal ligament, which serves as a pulley for the transfer.

Several technique modifications have been described. The most useful is the split-EHL tendon transfer, which preserves the medial third of the EHL tendon and transfers the lateral two thirds as described previously. The remnant of EHL tendon may be shortened to reduce IP joint flexion. Arthrodesis of the IP joint is useful when arthritic or fixed IP joint flexion contractures are present. However, arthrodesis of the IP joint should be avoided, if possible, because MTP joint arthrodesis is likely to be required if hallux varus

correction fails. The combination of MTP and IP joint arthrodeses is not desirable because of the excessive stiffness produced in the first ray. Even well-positioned arthrodeses of both joints are tolerable only in low-demand patients.

### Tenodesis

Extensor hallucis brevis tenodesis is one of several methods of lateral collateral ligament reinforcement. The tenodesis is accomplished by detaching the extensor hallucis brevis proximally and routing the free end deep to the intermetatarsal ligament and into the first metatarsal head (Figs. 4 and 5). Biomechanical evaluation suggests that extensor hallucis brevis tenodesis restores the joint's ability to resist varus force.

### Metatarsal Osteotomy

If the etiology of the hallux varus includes an overcorrected first-second intermetatarsal angle after a proximal osteotomy, the malpositioned osteotomy must be corrected. The potential for further shortening of the first ray should be considered. Correction of the intermetatarsal angle is best accomplished through a proximal crescentic osteotomy with medial angulation of the metatarsal. A distal soft-tissue release and repair, as previously described, also must be done to rebalance the MTP joint in 10° to 15° valgus.

### Reverse Akin Osteotomy

Mild residual varus deformity can be corrected with a proximal phalangeal base osteotomy. Because the correction is the opposite of that produced by a classic Akin osteotomy, the procedure is termed a reverse Akin osteotomy. A lateral closing wedge osteotomy is placed just distal to the concave articular surface of the proximal phalanx. Fixation is accomplished with nonabsorbable or stainless steel sutures. Only mild, completely correctable deformities that have shown no propensity to worsen over many months should be treated with this type of osteotomy.

### Keller Resection Arthroplasty
Marked hallux varus deformity can be treated with Keller resection arthroplasty. The procedure includes resection of the proximal phalangeal base that significantly, if not totally, destroys the intrinsic insertions onto the hallux. The result is an intrinsic minus deformity-extension of the MTP joint and flexion of the IP joint. Also, the ability of the hallux to transfer weight is significantly diminished, and the potential for a transfer lesion at the lesser rays is increased. Therefore, the Keller procedure is restricted to low-demand patients with significant deformity and loss of joint function.

### MTP Joint Arthrodesis
Arthrodesis is perhaps the most common surgical solution for symptomatic hallux varus. It allows reproducible positioning of the hallux MTP joint and thus reestablishes the first ray as a stable weight-bearing unit. Arthrodesis is indicated for an arthritic MTP joint or rigid deformity without arthritis. The procedure is accomplished through a dorsal or medial approach. Internal fixation usually is with interfragmentary screws, a dorsal plate, or both. The position is set to 15° valgus and 15° extension relative to the plantar surface of the foot and neutral axial rotation. The procedure may be complicated by delayed union or nonunion of the arthrodesis, poor positioning of the arthrodesis, and shoe wear limitations related to the fixed dorsiflexion of the hallux.

## Summary
Hallux varus is most commonly a complication of hallux valgus repairs and probably is not completely avoidable. Contributing factors include overresection of the medial eminence, overplication of the medial capsule, overcorrection of the intermetatarsal angle, overrelease of the lateral structures, and excision of the lateral sesamoid. Hallux varus may be associated with sagittal and axial plane deformities. Initial treatment focuses on accommodative shoe wear. Surgical treatment of chronic deformity is reserved for symptomatic deformities, and the choice of procedure depends on the flexibility of the MTP and IP joints and the uniplanar or multiplanar components of the deformity. A variety of joint-sparing procedures are effective. If indicated, resection arthroplasty or MTP joint arthrodesis is a reasonable surgical option.

## Annotated Bibliography
### Anatomy, Incidence, Pathogenesis, Evaluation, Classification
Donley BG: Acquired hallux varus. *Foot Ankle Int* 1997; 18:586-592.

This excellent review of the literature related to acquired hallux varus discusses incidence, anatomy, pathogenesis, and treatment options.

Mann RA, Coughlin MJ: Adult hallux valgus, in Coughlin MJ, Mann RA (eds): *Surgery of the Foot and Ankle,* ed 7. St. Louis, MO, Mosby-Year Book, 1999, pp 150-269.

This chapter provides a comprehensive and logical approach to hallux valgus surgery in which complications, including hallux varus, are discussed in detail. The split EHL transfer is described and illustrated along with other treatment options.

Richardson EG: Complications after hallux valgus surgery. *Instr Course Lect* 1999;48:331-342.

This comprehensive review describes common complications after surgery on the hallux, including hallux varus, and discusses etiology, evaluation, and treatment options.

Sammarco GJ, Idusuyi OB: Complications after surgery of the hallux. *Clin Orthop* 2001;391:59-71.

This comprehensive review also describes common complications after surgery on the hallux, including hallux varus, and discusses etiology, evaluation, and treatment options.

Trnka HJ, Zettl R, Hungerford M, Muhlbauer M, Ritschl P: Acquired hallux varus and clinical tolerability. *Foot Ankle Int* 1997;18:593-597.

In a retrospective study of 16 patients (19 feet) with iatrogenic hallux varus, the mean deformity was 10.1° of varus at a mean follow-up of 18.3 years. Only patients with extreme varus deformity (16° to 24°) were dissatisfied.

### Treatment
Lau JTC, Myerson MS: Technique tip: Modified split extensor hallucis tendon transfer for correction of hallux varus. *Foot Ankle Int* 2002;23:1138-1140.

In this modified technique of EHL tendon transfer, the latter half of the tendon is released proximally, which allows it to function as a static tenodesis. Tensioning of the tenodesis does not affect the remaining function of the EHL tendon and may provide a more reliable correction of static hallux varus deformity.

Rochwerger A, Curvale G, Groulier P: Application of bone graft to the medial side of the first metatarsal head in the treatment of hallux varus. *J Bone Joint Surg Am* 1999;81:1730-1735.

At average follow-up of 8.6 years, results were satisfactory in six of seven feet treated with a bone graft screwed onto the medial aspect of the metatarsal head. The authors recommend this technique for flexible hallux varus caused by excessive bone removal during bunionectomy.

## Classic Bibliography

Hawkins FB: Acquired hallux varus: Cause, prevention and correction. *Clin Orthop* 1971;76:169-176.

Johnson KA, Spiegl PV: Extensor hallucis longus transfer for hallux varus deformity. *J Bone Joint Surg Am* 1984;66: 681-686.

Juliano PJ, Myerson MS, Cunningham BW: Biomechanical assessment of a new tenodesis for correction of hallux varus. *Foot Ankle Int* 1996;17:17-20.

Miller JW: Acquired hallux varus: A preventable and correctable disorder. *J Bone Joint Surg Am* 1975;57:183-188.

Myerson MS, Komenda GA: Results of hallux varus correction using an extensor hallucis brevis tenodesis. *Foot Ankle Int* 1996;17:21-27.

Skalley TC, Myerson MS: The operative treatment of acquired hallux varus. *Clin Orthop* 1994;306:183-191.

# Section 2

# Trauma

Section Editor:
David B. Thordarson, MD

# Chapter 4

# Fractures and Dislocations of the Talus and Subtalar Joint

Benedict F. DiGiovanni, MD

Judith F. Baumhauer, MD

## Introduction

Trauma to the talus and subtalar joint often results in severe injuries that can be devastating, require extended recovery times, and cause serious functional impairment. The complexity of talar anatomy and the precarious blood supply in this area of the foot contribute to the challenges encountered during treatment. Although talar injuries are relatively uncommon (approximately 1% of all fractures), talar fractures are the second most common tarsal bone injury after calcaneal fractures.

## Anatomy and Blood Supply

The talus is divided into three main anatomic regions: the head, neck, and body. The unique shape of the talus predisposes it to complex injury patterns. The transverse diameter of the body is wider anteriorly than posteriorly, which allows for increased joint stability with ankle dorsiflexion. The talar neck angles medially, with a variable angle of declination that averages 24°. The talar head articulates with the navicular distally and with the anterior facet of the calcaneus inferiorly. Hindfoot motion is complex and is essential for optimal function. The talonavicular joint is central to this function and contributes most of hindfoot motion.

About 70% of the talus is covered by articular cartilage. With the exception of the extensor digitorum brevis, the talus lacks muscular origins or insertions. This lack of soft-tissue attachments limits indirect perfusion of the talar body and causes it to be vulnerable to osteonecrosis. The intraosseous and extraosseous blood supply of the talus has been studied extensively (Fig. 1), and complete intraosseous arterial continuity among all regions of the talus has been found to occur only 60% of the time. When present, this extensive intraosseous arterial confluence allows survival of the talus after marked displacement or soft-tissue damage. The extraosseous blood supply is derived from the three main arteries of the distal leg. These arteries, in order of importance, are the posterior tibial, the anterior tibial, and the peroneal. The artery of the tarsal canal, a branch of the posterior tibial artery, provides most of the blood supply to the talar body. The artery of the tarsal sinus, formed from contributions of the anterior tibial and peroneal arteries, is the main contributor to the talar head and neck. The artery of the tarsal canal and the artery of the tarsal sinus form a vascular ring around the talar neck and sinus tarsi. The deltoid artery, which is located within the deep portion of the deltoid ligament, is an important source of extraosseous circulation to the talar body.

## Talar Neck Fractures

### Incidence

Fractures of the talar neck account for about 50% of all talar fractures. Most are the result of motor vehicle accidents or falls from a height. Associated injuries are common, with 19% to 28% of patients having associated foot or ankle fractures and approximately 67% having other bone or soft-tissue injuries. Open fractures occur more commonly in association with significantly displaced fractures or fractures with extruded, devitalized bodies.

### Mechanism

Excessive dorsiflexion of the foot against a stationary tibia is the predominant mechanism of injury. The narrow, less dense neck of the talus impacts against the broad, strong, anterior margin of the tibia, resulting in a fracture of the talar neck between the middle and posterior facets of the talus. As forces progress, excessive ankle dorsiflexion leads to rupture of the posterior capsule and ligaments of the ankle and subtalar joints, resulting in either subluxation or dislocation of the talar body from the subtalar and tibiotalar articulations. With inversion added to dorsiflexion, a common mechanism of injury, the neck may strike the medial malleolus, resulting in medial neck comminution and subsequently medial foot and talar head subluxation or dislocation through the subtalar joint. When the talar body dislocates, it usually is still attached to the deltoid ligament, resulting in posteromedial displacement adjacent to the Achilles tendon and often compressing the neurovascular bundle and stretching the overlying skin. With the less common dorsiflexion and eversion force, the foot and talar head will subluxate or dislocate laterally.

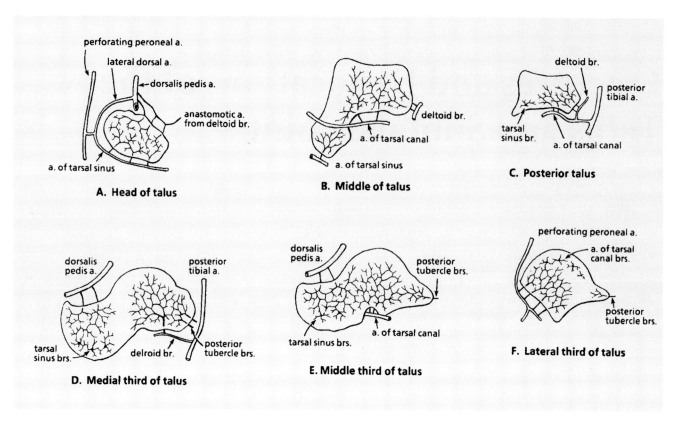

A. Head of talus

B. Middle of talus

C. Posterior talus

D. Medial third of talus

E. Middle third of talus

F. Lateral third of talus

**Figure 1** Regional vascular anatomy of the talus. a.= artery; br.= branch; brs.= branches. *(Reproduced from Adelaar RS: Fractures of the talus, in Greene WB (ed): Instructional Course Lectures XXXIX. Park Ridge, IL, American Academy of Orthopaedic Surgeons, 1990, pp 147-156.)*

In the laboratory, it has been difficult to re-create talar neck fractures by excessive dorsiflexion alone. One study found that vertical compression through the calcaneus also was necessary. Clinically, the association of medial and lateral malleolar fractures with talar neck fractures supports the concept of the importance of rotational forces. In another study, it was noted that 26% of patients with talar neck fractures had associated medial malleolar fractures. A fracture of the medial or lateral malleolus associated with a displaced talar neck fracture further compromises the prognosis.

### Fracture Classification

In 1970, Hawkins published a classic study in which a classification system was presented that was prognostic and correlated with blood supply disruption. Talar neck fractures were classified as type I, type II, or type III. Canale and Kelly described a fourth fracture type. These classification systems were derived from findings on plain radiographs obtained at initial injury presentation.

A type I fracture is a nondisplaced fracture of the talar neck. The talus remains anatomically positioned in the subtalar joint and ankle joint, and minimal potential for blood supply disruption at the talar neck exists. If there is doubt that the fracture is nondisplaced, a CT scan is indicated. If displacement is noted on CT scan, then the fracture should be reclassified as type II.

A type II fracture is a displaced talar neck fracture with subtalar joint subluxation or dislocation. The foot and calcaneus most often are displaced medially, and the ankle joint is not affected. Two of the main sources of blood supply to the talus may be injured: the vessels entering at the talar neck (sinus tarsi vessels) and the tarsal canal vessels entering the talar neck and body.

A type III fracture is characterized by a displaced fracture of the talar neck with associated displacement of the talar body from both the subtalar and tibiotalar joints. These typically are the result of high-energy injuries, with dislocation of the talar body from the mortise. More than half are open fractures, and all three sources of blood supply usually are damaged. The deltoid branch of the tarsal canal artery may be the only remaining blood supply to the talar body.

A type IV fracture includes subluxation or dislocation of the body from the subtalar and tibiotalar joints as well as subluxation or dislocation of the talar head at the talonavicular joint. Type IV fractures are rare; when they do occur, the outcome is frequently poor.

### Clinical and Radiographic Evaluation

Significant dorsal swelling of the midfoot and hindfoot usually is present in patients with talar neck fractures. With displaced fractures, normal contours of the ankle are distorted, and small, open wounds can go unnoticed

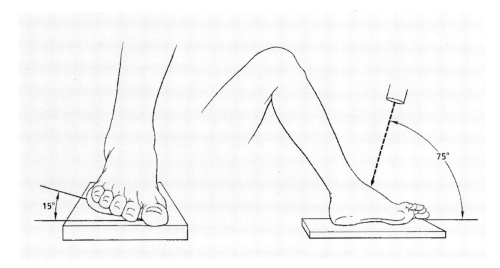

**Figure 2** Canale and Kelly modified AP view of the talar neck. *(Adapted with permission from Canale ST, Kelly FB Jr: Fractures of the neck of the talus: Long-term evaluation of seventy-one cases. J Bone Joint Surg Am 1978;60:143-156.)*

without careful inspection. Occult injuries, such as those to the thoracolumbar spine, have been associated with talar fractures and should be ruled out.

Standard radiographs include AP, oblique, and lateral foot views. Orthogonal ankle radiographs are obtained to evaluate associated ankle injuries. A modified AP view of the foot allows for optimal evaluation of talar neck angulation and shortening (Fig. 2), and it is particularly helpful when evaluating displacement and classifying fractures as either type I or type II.

CT can be helpful for further defining the extent of injury to the talus. Axial and semicoronal images can add useful information about fracture patterns and the extent of comminution. Sagittal and coronal images aid surgical planning and may be most helpful to surgeons who do not frequently treat these complex injuries.

### Treatment

A stable anatomic reduction is the main goal of treatment. One report defines an acceptable reduction as displacement of less than 5 mm and malalignment of less than 5°. More recent studies indicate that any displacement or malalignment can have a significant negative impact on foot function. In a cadaveric model of varus malunion, 17° of varus malrotation resulted in a 30% loss of subtalar motion. In another study, displacement as small as 2 mm significantly changed the subtalar joint contact characteristics. Dorsal and varus displacement created the greatest changes in contact stress, particularly at the posterior facet. These findings emphasize the importance of anatomic reduction for optimal function.

### Type I Fractures

Nondisplaced fractures can be treated in a non–weight-bearing short leg cast for 6 to 8 weeks. Close monitoring with follow-up radiographs is necessary during the first few weeks to assess whether displacement occurs. If the fracture displaces when the ankle is placed in neutral po-

sition, then it is a type II fracture, which requires surgical treatment. If the fracture does not displace after 6 to 8 weeks in a non–weight-bearing short leg cast, progressive weight bearing is then begun, with advancement based on the radiographic presence of bridging trabecular bone.

### Type II Fractures

Type II fractures are unstable and require surgical treatment to achieve a stable anatomic reduction (Fig. 3). Controversy exists as to whether a type II fracture represents a surgical emergency. Most authors agree that the minimal level of treatment should include immediate closed reduction to relieve tension on the soft tissues. A near anatomic or anatomic closed reduction is the goal to preserve the remaining blood supply, which includes avoiding venous congestion. The technique of closed reduction includes foot plantar flexion (particularly at the midfoot/forefoot), followed by manipulation of the heel into varus or valgus to correct initial displacement. The ankle needs to be immobilized in plantar flexion to maintain the reduction. If a near anatomic closed reduction cannot be achieved acutely, then surgical intervention is indicated.

The goal of surgical treatment is a stable, anatomic reduction. Closed reduction with percutaneous screw fixation is an option; however, it is difficult to accurately evaluate rotational alignment and proper neck length with intraoperative plain radiographs or fluoroscopy. Most authors recommend open reduction and rigid internal fixation, which allows better visualization of the fracture to accomplish an anatomic reduction.

Anteromedial, anterolateral, and posterolateral approaches have been described for reduction of talar neck fractures. The goal of any approach is optimal exposure of the fracture without further damage to the blood supply. The anteromedial incision is used alone or more often combined with the anterolateral approach. The posterolateral approach is used most often for fluoroscopic

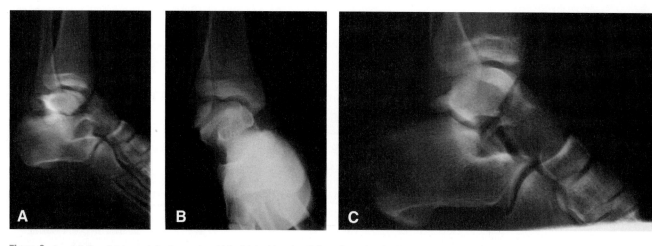

Figure 3   **A** and **B**, Type II talar neck fracture; note subtalar joint subluxation. **C**, Immediate closed reduction to protect soft tissues and vessels (followed later by early surgical stabilization).

screw placement from the talar body into the talar neck or head fragment.

The anteromedial approach can be made through the interval between the tendons of the extensor hallucis and tibialis anterior or between the tendons of the tibialis anterior and tibialis posterior. The main advantage of the first option is direct exposure of the medial and superior aspects of the talar neck after reduction. The main disadvantage is the potential for further vascular injury by disruption of medial vessels. If the fracture extends proximally into the talar body, either approach can be extended proximally and a medial malleolar osteotomy can be done to increase exposure. The addition of the anterolateral approach to the anteromedial approach allows for more complete exposure of the fracture as well as access to the subtalar joint to carefully inspect its anatomic reduction. There often is less comminution on the lateral side of the talar neck, which facilitates the reduction. In addition, the anterolateral aspect of the talar neck is frequently preserved and is an ideal area for screw placement.

A posterolateral approach is made between the Achilles tendon and the fibula. It does not expose the fracture but allows for posterior screw insertion through the deep interval between the flexor hallucis longus and peroneus brevis tendons. The posterolateral tubercle of the talus is located, and screws are inserted there from posterolateral to anteromedial. Two screws most commonly are used. In a biomechanical study, superior mechanical strength was reported with posterior to anterior screw insertion when compared with anterior to posterior screw placement. The main drawback of the posterolateral exposure is the lack of direct view of the talar neck to confirm anatomic reduction. It is common for the posterolateral exposure to be used in combination with an anterior approach. Patients are placed in a semilateral position to access both incisions.

Screw fixation is superior to Kirschner wire (K-wire) fixation alone to achieve stable anatomic reduction. Solid-

core screw fixation is preceded by provisional K-wire fixation. Cannulated screws are used most commonly. In comminuted fractures, the screws should not be placed in compression (for example, lagged) to prevent medial impaction with resultant varus malunion. Titanium screws should be strongly considered because they are compatible with MRI. The use of headless screws obviates the potential problem of prominent screw heads leading to posterior ankle impingement or interference with talonavicular joint function when inserted front to back. Bioabsorbable implants are available, but little information exists regarding their use to treat talar neck fractures.

Ideally, internal fixation achieves a stable reduction with minimal comminution. Range-of-motion exercises are begun when the soft tissues are well healed. Patients should wear a fracture boot and not bear weight until fracture healing is evident on radiographs, usually about 8 to 12 weeks. Weight bearing in the fracture boot is continued until complete healing is achieved.

### Type III Fractures

Immediate surgical treatment is required for type III talar neck fractures. Closed reduction rarely is successful. Urgent open reduction is required to relieve tension on the soft tissues, which include the skin and neurovascular structures. The reduction process often is challenging, and complete muscle relaxation can greatly assist the reduction process. To assist with traction and manipulation, a transverse calcaneal pin is placed in the tuberosity. Most commonly, the talar body is displaced posteromedially and tethered by the deltoid ligament. Associated medial malleolar fractures occur frequently and facilitate reduction of the body fragment into the ankle mortise. If intact, a medial malleolar osteotomy may be necessary. Initial ankle dorsiflexion and then plantar flexion with eversion of the calcaneus opens the medial joint of the ankle. Pressure is applied to the body fragment to move it laterally and anteriorly to achieve reduction into the ankle joint. Levering the talar body into place with a

**TABLE 1 | Talar Neck Fractures: Reported Complication Rates**

| Fracture Pattern | Osteonecrosis (%) | Posttraumatic Arthritis (%) | Malunion (%) |
|---|---|---|---|
| Type I | 0-13 | 0-30 | 0-10 |
| Type II | 20-50 | 40-90 | 0-25 |
| Type III IV | 80-100 | 70-100 | 18-27 |

*(Reproduced from Fortin PT, Balazsy JE: Talus fractures: Evaluation and treatment. J Am Acad Orthop Surg 2001;9:114-127.)*

strong periosteal elevator also may help reduce the ankle joint. The medial subtalar joint dislocation is reduced with laterally directed pressure on the calcaneus.

Extensive comminution is common at the medial aspect of the talar neck; attention is directed to an anatomic reduction, while taking care to avoid a varus malunion. The accessory lateral incision can be helpful by allowing direct observation of the lateral neck, which is usually less comminuted, aiding in accurate reduction as well as better exposure of the subtalar joint reduction. After reduction, a gap often exists at the site of medial comminution that can be filled with bone graft. A postoperative regimen similar to that for type II talar neck fractures is used.

### Type IV Fractures

The treatment protocol for type IV fractures is the same as for type III fractures, but with the addition of reduction of the talonavicular joint. K-wires often are used to maintain anatomic reduction of the talonavicular joint and are removed at 6 weeks postoperatively. Postoperative treatment is similar to that used after type III injuries.

### Wound Complications

Skin necrosis, a serious complication, frequently is associated with types III and IV injuries. The goals of treatment of open fractures are soft-tissue healing, bony union, and avoidance of infection. Authors of a study of severe, open talar fractures reported that the final result correlated with the occurrence of infection. An extruded talar body with no soft-tissue attachments that was replaced into the ankle mortise also correlated with a high rate of infection and poor results.

### Osteonecrosis

The incidence of osteonecrosis of the talar body also has been shown to increase with severity of the injury (Table 1). The Hawkins sign, which can be an early indicator of sufficient blood supply to the body of the talus, appears as a subchondral linear radiolucency of the talar dome on AP radiographs of the ankle. Its presence suggests bone resorption, which is an active process requir-

ing vascularity. The Hawkins sign typically appears at 6 to 8 weeks after injury and may be seen only on the medial side because of an intact deep deltoid branch, indicating blood flow medially and partial osteonecrosis. If this sign is present, the blood supply is intact and extensive osteonecrosis should not develop. The absence of a Hawkins sign does not necessarily indicate the development of osteonecrosis.

Radiographic evidence of osteonecrosis can indicate a relative increase in talar bone density 3 to 6 months after injury. Loss of blood supply and the presence of osteonecrosis are not absolutely predictive of a poor outcome. MRI is more helpful than CT in the diagnosis and quantification of osteonecrosis. Marrow elements in trabecular bone are predominately fat cells and are responsible for the high signal on T1-weighted images. Marrow necrosis is an early sign of osteonecrosis, and T1-weighted images are sensitive (decreased signal) to these early changes. The role of MRI in detecting osteonecrosis after open reduction and internal fixation of talar neck fractures has been recently reported. In patients with more than 50% body involvement detected on MRI, plain radiographic findings correlated well with MRI findings. However, inconsistent correlation was noted in those with less than 50% body involvement detected on MRI. This suggests that at a minimum of 3 weeks after injury MRI can play a significant role in identifying patients who are at risk of collapse secondary to osteonecrosis, which may in turn help guide treatment recommendations.

Treatment of osteonecrosis is aimed at preventing segmental talar body collapse. Revascularization may take 2 years or longer to occur. To our knowledge, outcome studies on osteonecrosis to help direct treatment have not been done. Invasive procedures, such as revascularization, core decompression, and subtalar arthrodesis, currently are not recommended. No consensus exists as to the optimal method of protected weight bearing while maintaining function. Recommendations may be based on the extent of osteonecrosis, and serial MRIs may help direct the type and duration of treatment. Extended periods of no weight bearing during the revascularization period is one option, but patients often have difficulty complying with such a protracted treatment regimen (up to 2 years). Protected weight bearing with a patellar tendon-bearing brace to alleviate weight to the ankle-hindfoot joints or wearing a sport ankle brace that prevents varus or valgus stress are other options. At a minimum, activities such as running or cutting maneuvers should be restricted.

Fortunately, many patients with isolated osteonecrosis do not experience late segmental collapse. Segmental collapse occurs more commonly in patients with more extensive involvement and may be treated with a salvage procedure. One such procedure is the Blair fusion (or the modified Blair fusion as described by Lionberger and associates). The talar head, which is still vascularized even with extensive talar body osteonecrosis, is preserved and used during this procedure. After excision of the avascular body, a slot graft from the tibia is fitted into the talar head and a small portion of the talar neck. The Lionberger modification of the Blair fusion uses posterior tibial to anterior talar head cancellous screws. Other salvage options include a tibiotalocalcaneal fusion with a posterior bone graft between the tibia and dorsal calcaneus and a tibiocalcaneal fusion in conjunction with a partial talectomy. The tibiotalocalcaneal or tibiocalcaneal fusion has been more commonly used recently and allows arthrodesis of the head and neck of the talus to the anterior tibia.

### Malunion and Posttraumatic Arthritis

The incidence of malunion and posttraumatic arthritis increases as the Hawkins stage increases (Table 1). A varus malunion is the most common type of malunion, occurring after as many as 50% of displaced talar neck fractures. As the energy of the injury increases, more medial neck comminution occurs, and achievement of a truly anatomic reduction with rigid fixation becomes more challenging, particularly through a single incision anteromedially. Varus malunion leads to a significant decrease in hindfoot motion; an awkward, high-energy–demanding gait; and lateral column foot pain with subsequent functional limitations. Corrective osteotomy has been suggested as a treatment option for symptomatic varus malunion, but its efficacy is still under investigation.

The development of posttraumatic arthritis depends on the extent of articular cartilage damage at the time of the injury and the quality of the reduction. Early advanced posttraumatic degenerative joint disease typically occurs within the first 18 to 24 months after injury. Reconstructive procedures are based on the location and extent of the degenerative joint disease and often are guided by preoperative CT evaluations. Selective joint injection with a local anesthetic is another helpful diagnostic tool. Salvage options include isolated subtalar arthrodesis, isolated ankle arthrodesis, and combined fusions.

## Talar Body Fractures

### Dome Fractures

Dome fractures are complex talar body fractures and usually are subclassified by fracture pattern as transverse, sagittal, or coronal. Plain radiographs often are diagnostic, but accurate definition of a dome fracture usually is blocked by the medial and lateral malleoli. CT can help diagnose a suspected talar fracture when plain radiographs show no evidence of injury or help further define the fracture pattern. Even without dislocation of the talus, clinically significant osteonecrosis of the talus occurs in about 25% of dome fractures.

Surgical treatment usually is required to achieve anatomic reduction. Anteromedial or anterolateral surgical approaches often are suboptimal, and medial and occa-

sionally lateral malleolar osteotomies may be necessary. A medial malleolar osteotomy technique that was recently described that can aid exposure of displaced talar body fractures. Anatomic reduction is followed by rigid fixation, based on the same principles used for talar neck fractures.

### Posterior Process Fractures

The posterior process of the talus is composed of the posteromedial and posterolateral tubercles. The posterior third of the deltoid ligament and the posterior talotibial ligament insert on the posteromedial process. Although fractures of the posteromedial process are rare, the diagnosis is often missed. Delayed diagnosis leads to functional limitations that may require excision of the process. There currently is no consensus regarding the optimal treatment for small, acutely diagnosed fractures, but they are often treated with immobilization and surgery later if persistent symptoms develop. Large, displaced fractures, however, are treated with open reduction and internal fixation. Posteromedial process (corner) fractures of the talus are particularly difficult to see with plain films. If the magnitude of injury and clinical findings do not correlate with plain radiographic findings, a CT scan should be ordered.

The posterolateral tubercle (Stieda's process) is larger than the posteromedial tubercle and projects farther posteriorly. It is more frequently injured than the posteromedial tubercle because of its size. The posterior talofibular ligament inserts on the posterolateral tubercle, and the posterolateral tubercle also functions as the lateral border of the fibro-osseous canal for the flexor hallucis longus tendon.

Several mechanisms of injury for fractures of the posterolateral tubercle have been described. Inversion of the ankle can injure the posterior talofibular ligament and in turn can cause an avulsion fracture at the talar insertion. Forced dorsiflexion of the tibiotalar joint with torsion of the posterior talofibular ligament also has been suggested as a mechanism of injury. A third mechanism proposed is direct impingement of the posterolateral tubercle against the posterior tibia secondary to forced plantar flexion at the tibiotalar joint.

It often is difficult to detect an acute fracture of the posterolateral process of the talus. Initially, plain radiographs often are unremarkable because it is difficult to see the posterolateral talus. However, lateral radiographs of the foot and/or ankle may demonstrate an acute fracture. If a posterolateral process fracture is suspected, a CT scan with sagittal reconstructions can be helpful.

A more typical presentation is a patient with chronic ankle pain after an initial diagnosis and treatment for a lateral ankle sprain. Forced passive plantar flexion of the ankle often re-creates the type of pain the patient experiences with stair climbing or prolonged walking. A nonunited fracture of the posterior lateral tubercle of the ta-

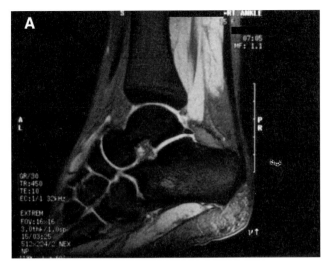 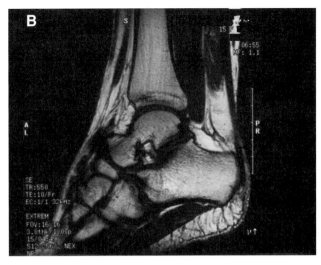

**Figure 4** T2- (**A**) and T1- (**B**) weighted MRI scans show signal changes at the talus posterolateral process in a patient with chronic posterior ankle pain.

lus may be difficult to distinguish from a symptomatic os trigonum. A CT scan is less helpful with an old fracture. Technetium 99m ($^{99m}$Tc) bone scanning may aid in distinguishing these two conditions. However, a recent study found that it is not uncommon for $^{99m}$Tc bone scans to demonstrate increased uptake in the posterior ankle of active individuals without posterior ankle pain. MRI may be more useful for diagnosing a symptomatic nonunited fracture of a posterolateral process of the talus (Fig. 4). A diagnostic injection of 1 mL of 1% lidocaine into this area may aid the confirmation of a clinical suspicion before surgical intervention.

Acute injuries usually are immobilized in short leg casts with protection from full weight bearing for 4 to 6 weeks. If a displaced large fragment is noted, open reduction with internal fixation may be indicated. Nonunited fractures may require surgical excision of the nonunited fragment. Results after excision of the nonunited fragment are typically good.

### Lateral Process Fractures

Fractures of the lateral process of the talus are fairly common, occurring about 25% as often as talar body fractures. The most common mechanism of injury is axial compression with dorsiflexion and external rotation. A high association with snowboarding has been reported (snowboarder's fracture). A prospective review of foot and ankle snowboarding injuries noted no correlation between boot type (soft, hybrid, or hard) and the overall foot and ankle injury rate. A high number of lateral process talar fractures was noted (15% of ankle injuries and 34% of all ankle fractures). Many of these fractures are not seen on routine plain radiographs; in retrospect, however, they can be seen as comminution on ankle AP views. Anterolateral ankle pain in snowboarders should raise suspicion for possible occult lateral process fracture, and a CT scan should be obtained if there is doubt.

Acute, nondisplaced fractures are treated with a non–weight-bearing short leg cast with the foot in slight equinus for 6 to 8 weeks. Displaced acute fractures with large fragments should be treated by open reduction and internal fixation. Small fragments from comminuted, acute fractures may be excised. More commonly, these fractures are immobilized for a few weeks and the fragments are excised at a later date if the patient is still symptomatic. With delayed diagnosis, results are less predictable. Despite late fragment excision, persistent pain and symptomatic subtalar arthritis can occur because these are articular fractures.

### Osteochondral Fractures of the Talus

Osteochondritis dissecans, transchondral talar dome fracture, and talar osteochondral defect refer to osteochondral fractures of the talus. The etiology of these fractures frequently is associated with trauma. However, idiopathic talar osteochondral defects can occur. Talar osteochondral defects are associated with acute ankle sprains in 0.9% to 6.5% of patients. A higher incidence has been noted in patients with chronic lateral ankle instability. The average age group affected is 20 to 30 years, with bilateral lesions noted in 10%.

Medial and lateral talar osteochondral defects are the most common osteochondral lesions of the talus, although medial osteochondral defects occur more frequently than lateral lesions. These medial fractures typically are cup shaped, frequently deep, located posteriorly, and may be associated with trauma. They also are more often nondisplaced than lateral. Trauma is more commonly associated with lateral lesions, particularly ankle inversion injuries. Lateral osteochondral defects usually are located in the middle or anterior talus and are shallow and wafer shaped. Lateral lesions are more commonly displaced and are more symptomatic than medial lesions. Lateral lesions also have a poor healing potential.

**TABLE 2 | Talar Osteochondral Defects: MRI Classification**

| | |
|---|---|
| Stage I: | Subchondral trabecular compression, marrow edema on MRI with plain radiographs normal |
| Stage II: | Incomplete separation of fragment |
| Stage IIA: | Formation of subchondral cyst |
| Stage III: | Unattached, nondisplaced fragment with presence of synovial fluid around the fragment |
| Stage IV: | Displaced fragment |

*(Reproduced with permission from Anderson IF, Crichton KJ, Grattan-Smith T, Cooper RA, Brazier D: Osteochondral fractures of the dome of the talus. J Bone Joint Surg Am 1989;71: 1143-1152.)*

**TABLE 3 | Talar Osteochondral Defects: CT Classification**

| | |
|---|---|
| Stage I: | Cystic lesion dome of talus, with intact roof |
| Stage IIA: | Cystic lesion extending to surface talar dome |
| Stage IIB: | Open articular surface with overlying nondisplaced fragment |
| Stage III: | Nondisplaced lesion with lucency |
| Stage IV: | Open lesion with displaced fragment |

*(Reproduced with permission from Heinen GT, Ferkel RD: Arthroscopy of the ankle and subtalar joints. Foot Ankle Clin 1999;4:4:833-864.)*

Clinical presentation typically includes localized ankle pain with swelling and clicking. Often a sensation of instability is reported, with a history of recent or remote ankle sprain. Radiographs demonstrate displaced fragments, but other lesions often are not appreciated. In addition, plain radiographs often underestimate the extent of an osteochondral injury. In medial lesions with no history of trauma, radiographs of the contralateral asymptomatic ankle are justified to rule out a congenital talar dome abnormality. CT reveals most lesions and is particularly helpful to further define known lesions. MRI provides better information about the condition of the cartilage as well as associated soft-tissue abnormalities, both intra-articular and extra-articular.

One classification system for transchondral fractures of the talus, developed in 1959 by Berndt and Harty, comprises four stages based on plain radiographs: stage 1 includes compression of the subchondral bone without a break of the cartilage (7%), stage 2 includes incomplete lesions with partial fragment detachment (25%), stage 3 includes complete lesions but no fragment displacement (40%), and stage 4 includes complete lesions with a displaced fragment or loose body (28%). Although this classification system aids in initial evaluation, it has a poor correlation with arthroscopic findings.

Another classification system uses MRI findings to identify talar dome lesions (Table 2). CT findings also have been used to classify these lesions. The stages of this classification system correspond to those described by Berndt and Harty, but they also account for the degree of osteonecrosis, subchondral cysts, and fragment separation.

The decision whether to use CT or MRI to identify these fractures often is based on surgeon preference. CT allows better bone definition than MRI, and it is preferred by some authors when the presence of an osteochondral defect lesion has been suggested by plain radiographic findings (Table 3). MRI is preferred by others because it provides more specific information about the status of cartilage as well as potential associated soft-tissue pathology.

Arthroscopic surgery allows direct examination of the cartilage. The surgical grading system outlined in Table 4 is based on articular cartilage findings at the time of arthroscopic surgery. Because the arthroscopic appearance of the lesion often does not correlate with the results of preoperative staging studies, the surgical findings should guide final treatment plans.

Treatment recommendations are based on the age of the lesion and the status of the cartilage fragment. Nondisplaced, acute lesions can be treated with a non–weight-bearing cast for 6 weeks. Displaced, acute lesions should be treated with early arthroscopic surgery. Long-term prognoses for nonsurgical treatment of loose or detached lesions suggest that few will heal and arthritic changes will occur. Ankle arthroscopy obviates the need for malleolar osteotomy in most lesions. Acute, large fragments can be reduced and fixed, possibly with bioabsorbable pins, but more commonly, fixation of acute and chronic lesions is not possible, and the surgical procedure must include fragment excision, curettage of necrotic bone at the crater, and drilling or microfracture technique to promote the formation of fibrocartilage (Fig. 5). In addition, hypertrophic synovium and scar are débrided to treat associated soft-tissue impingement lesions. Small- or medium-sized flap tears typically are débrided and stabilized. Large flap tears can be treated with fixation with bioabsorbable pins and drilling of the bed of the lesion. Retrograde drilling of the lesion through the medial or lateral tubercle of the talus under fluoroscopic and arthroscopic observation has been reported. This technique reduces the chance of articular cartilage damage, while still bone grafting of lesions with intact cartilage.

Postoperative treatment includes short-term immobilization (7 to 10 days) followed by non–weight-bearing

**TABLE 4 | Surgical Grading of Articular Cartilage Defects**

| | |
|---|---|
| Grade A | Articular cartilage is smooth and intact, but soft |
| Grade B | Articular cartilage has a rough surface |
| Grade C | Fibrillations/fissures are present |
| Grade D | A flap is present or bone is exposed |
| Grade E | A loose, nondisplaced fragment is present |
| Grade F | A displaced fragment is present |

*(Reproduced with permission from Heinen GT, Ferkel RD: Arthroscopy of the ankle and subtalar oints. Foot Ankle Clin 1999;4:4:833-864.)*

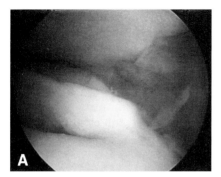 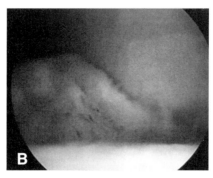 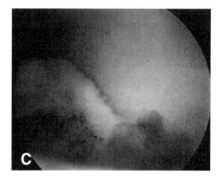

**Figure 5**  **A**, Arthroscopic visualization of a posttraumatic lateral talar osteochondral defect. **B**, Fragment excision with curettage of necrotic bone at crater. **C**, K-wire drilling or microfracture technique. Bleeding is noted at the base of crater after drilling, and the tourniquet is then released.

range-of-motion exercises for 6 weeks. The mechanical symptoms often are greatly improved, and short- and intermediate-term results are encouraging. Arthroscopic treatment using mosaicplasty and chrondrocyte transplantation techniques are examples of newer surgical methods that are currently undergoing clinical trials. These methods may hold particular promise for patients in whom initial débridement with microfracture or drilling results in unsatisfactory outcome and additional surgery is needed.

New techniques also are being developed for the treatment of symptomatic, earlier-stage lesions. Soft cartilage lesions and flap tears also can be treated with various arthroscopic techniques. Flap tears often are accompanied by corresponding hypertrophic synovitis and scar, which can be treated with arthroscopic débridement. In addition, drilling often is recommended to promote vascularization and healing. For medial lesions, this involves drilling through intact distal tibia cartilage, which may contribute to future degenerative changes.

## Subtalar Dislocations

Dislocations of the subtalar joint are rare. The frequency of these injuries has increased over the last decade, particularly in association with motor vehicle accidents. A subtalar dislocation is a simultaneous dislocation of both the talocalcaneal and talonavicular joints. It is believed that this pattern of injury occurs because the strong calcaneonavicular ligaments remain intact, while the weaker talocalcaneal and talonavicular ligaments and capsule rupture. The classification of this particular injury depends on the direction of the foot in relation to the talus. The most common types are medial and lateral subtalar joint dislocations. Anterior and posterior subtalar dislocations have been described but are extremely rare.

Eighty percent of subtalar dislocations are medial. The mechanism of injury is forceful inversion of the foot with the sustentaculum tali acting as a fulcrum. Although most subtalar dislocations are the result of high-energy injuries, they also have been associated with playing basketball. Lateral subtalar dislocation, seen only in high-energy

injuries, occurs in about 15% of patients and is the result of the forceful eversion of the foot.

Because this particular type of injury is so rare, diagnosis of an acute injury may be delayed. Clinical deformity is noted, but it may be mistakenly diagnosed as an ankle dislocation or fracture-dislocation. Prompt recognition and reduction of these injuries are important to avoid soft-tissue or neurovascular compromise. Plain radiographs of the ankle and foot should be obtained. Although AP ankle radiographs usually reveal the dislocation pattern (Fig. 6), the full set of radiographs should be carefully reviewed for the presence of associated fractures.

Closed reduction usually can be accomplished with the use of intravenous sedation. The reduction maneuver includes knee flexion to relieve the gastrocnemius-deforming force and countertraction to the thigh while the surgeon grasps the heel and forefoot. The deformity is accentuated and then reversed. The foot is subsequently placed in plantar flexion, and digital pressure is applied at the talar head to reduce the talonavicular component. A palpable reduction typically is appreciated as the hindfoot joints return to their normal positions. Range of motion and stability are then tested. In most patients, a stable reduction is achieved with a full range of motion.

An irreducible reduction is usually the result of interposed anterior soft tissues. With medial subtalar dislocations, the most common block to a successful closed reduction occurs when the talar head buttonholes through the anterior soft tissues (for example, through the extensor digitorum brevis muscle, the inferior extensor retinaculum, or the talonavicular ligament and joint capsule). The posterior tibial tendon most commonly blocks reduction of a lateral subtalar dislocation. Failure to achieve reduction by closed manipulation is more common in lateral than medial subtalar dislocations.

Associated fractures are present in at least 50% of these injuries, and they often are undetected during initial examination. CT is helpful in detecting associated injuries. In one study, previously undetected associated injuries were identified with CT in 44% of patients, and these findings altered

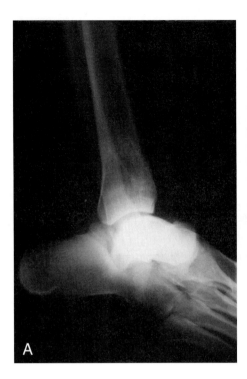
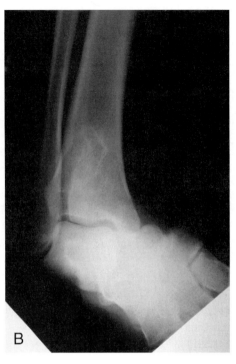

**Figure 6** **A**, Medial subtalar dislocation on lateral radiograph. **B**, Injury pattern more readily apparent on AP ankle radiograph.

the course of treatment for these patients. CT is a useful tool and should be considered in the evaluation of all subtalar dislocations after successful closed or open reduction.

Treatment after reduction usually includes immobilization for 3 to 4 weeks in a weight-bearing short leg cast, after which range-of-motion exercises are begun. Loss of subtalar joint motion is the most common complication of this injury, even though most patients have excellent passive motion immediately after reduction. The only group in which a trend toward increased risk of instability has been identified is young women with generalized ligamentous laxity. This group of patients should be immobilized for 6 weeks after reduction.

Functional results after the surgical repair of subtalar dislocations depend on a number of factors. Low-energy medial subtalar dislocations have a good prognosis, but the prognosis becomes less favorable as the energy associated with the injury increases. High-energy injuries have increased rates of associated fractures, posttraumatic arthritis, and soft-tissues injuries. In a long-term study of 15 open subtalar dislocations, significant soft-tissue injuries were also noted, including 10 injuries to the tibial nerve (of which 7 resulted in causalgia) and 5 lacerations of the posterior tibial artery. Five of 15 resulted in osteonecrosis of the talar body, all of which required arthrodesis. Ten dislocations were lateral and five medial. Because significant functional limitations were noted in most of these patients, the authors of this study cautioned physicians about the distinct severity of open subtalar dislocations.

## Summary

The complex anatomy and precarious blood supply of the talar and subtalar joints make fractures and dislocation in these areas difficult to treat and prone to complications. Anatomic reduction and stable function are required because even small amounts of malalignment can result in functional impairment.

## Annotated Bibliography

### Talar Neck Fractures

Elgafy H, Ebraheim NA, Tile M, Stephen D, Kase J: Fractures of the talus: Experience of two level 1 trauma centers. *Foot Ankle Int* 2000;21:1023-1029.

Of 60 talar fractures, 48 had surgical treatment and 12 had nonsurgical management. The average follow-up period was 30 months (range, 24 to 60 months). Subtalar arthritis developed in 32 fractures (53.3%), and ankle arthritis developed in 15 fractures (25%). Fractures of the body of the talus were associated with the highest incidence of degenerative joint disease of both the subtalar and ankle joints. Osteonecrosis developed in 10 fractures (16.6%), most often after Hawkins type II and III fractures of the talar neck. Assessment with three rating systems showed that talar process fractures had the best results followed by talar neck fractures and then talar body fractures.

Fortin PT, Balazsy JE: Talus fractures: Evaluation and treatment. *J Am Acad Orthop Surg* 2001;9:114-127.

In this article, the authors review the etiology, treatment, and outcome of talar fractures.

Kitaoka HB, Patzer GL: Arthrodesis for the treatment of arthrosis of the ankle and osteonecrosis of the talus. *J Bone Joint Surg Am* 1998;80:370-379.

Arthrodesis was done at the level of the ankle only in 3 patients and in both the ankle and the subtalar joint in 16. External fixation was used in 13 patients, internal fixation was used in 4, and no fixation was used in 2. Supplemental bone graft from the iliac crest was used in 14 patients, and local bone graft was used in 5. Clinical results were excellent in 7 patients, good in 6, fair in 3, and poor in 3. The use of rigid fixation and bone grafting had a rate of success approximating that reported for primary arthrodesis in patients who do not have osteonecrosis.

Monroe MT, Manoli A II: Osteotomy for malunion of a talar neck fracture: A case report. *Foot Ankle Int* 1999;20: 192-195.

The authors describe a surgical technique for osteotomy of the talar neck with insertion of a tricortical iliac crest bone graft to correct malunion deformity.

## Talar Body Fractures
Abramowitz Y, Wollenstein R, Barzilay Y, et al: Outcome of resection of a symptomatic os trigonum. *J Bone Joint Surg Am* 2003;85:1051-1057.

Forty-one patients with os trigonum syndrome whose symptoms were not relieved after nonsurgical treatment underwent excision of symptomatic os trigonum. The authors report that an os trigonum can be excised using a posterolateral approach with satisfactory results. Sural nerve injury was the main complication of this procedure.

Boon AJ, Smith J, Zobitz ME, Amrami KM: Snowboarder's talus fracture: Mechanism of injury. *Am J Sports Med* 2001;29:333-338.

Fracture of the lateral process of the talus in snowboarders has been thought to result from pure dorsiflexion and inversion combined with axial loading. The authors hypothesized, however, that external rotation is a key component of the mechanism of injury. Ten cadaver ankles were mounted on a materials testing machine in a position of fixed dorsiflexion and inversion. All ankles were loaded to failure axially, with or without combined external rotation. No fractures occurred after axial loading in dorsiflexion and inversion, but fractures of the lateral process of the talus occurred in six of eight specimens when similarly loaded with external rotation added.

DiGiovanni BF, Fraga CJ, Cohen BE, Shereff MJ: Associated injuries found in chronic lateral ankle instability. *Foot Ankle Int* 2000;21:809-815.

In 61 patients who underwent primary ankle lateral ligament reconstruction for chronic instability, no patient was found to have an isolated lateral ligament injury. Fifteen different associated injuries were noted. The injuries found most often by direct inspection included peroneal tenosynovitis, 47 of 61 patients (77%); anterolateral impingement lesion, 41 of 61 patients (67%); attenuated peroneal retinaculum, 33 of 61 patients (54%); and ankle synovitis, 30 of 61 patients (49%). Other less common but significant associated injuries included intra-articular loose body, 16 of 61 patients (26%); peroneus brevis tear, 15 of 61 patients (25%); talus osteochondral lesion, 14 of 61 patients (23%), and medial ankle tendon tenosynovitis, 3 of 61 patients (5%).

Hamilton WG, Chao W: Posterior ankle pain in athletes and dancers. *Foot Ankle Clin* 1999;4:811-832.

The authors review the etiologies and treatment of posterior ankle pain in athletes and dancers.

Heinen GT, Ferkel RD: Arthroscopy of the ankle and subtalar joints. *Foot Ankle Clin* 1999;4:4:833-864.

The authors review the indications, instrumentation, techniques, and outcomes of arthroscopy of the ankle and subtalar joints.

Kirkpatrick DP, Hunter RE, Janes PC, Mastrangelo J, Nicholas RA: The snowboarder's foot and ankle. *Am J Sports Med* 1998;26:271-277.

Data from 3,213 snowboarding injuries were collected from 12 Colorado ski resorts; 491 (15.3%) were ankle injuries and 58 (1.8%) were foot injuries. Ankle injuries included 216 fractures (44%) and 255 sprains (52%). Thirty-three (57%) of the foot injuries were fractures and 16 (28%) were sprains. The remaining injuries were soft-tissue injuries, contusions, or abrasions. An unexpectedly high number of fractures of the lateral process of the talus was noted.

Sopov V, Liberson A, Groshar D: Bone scintigraphic findings of os trigonum: A prospective study of 100 soldiers on active duty. *Foot Ankle Int* 2000;21:822-824.

Radionuclide whole-body skeletal imaging and physical examination of the foot were carried out in 100 consecutive soldiers on active duty referred for evaluation of suspected stress injury of the lower limbs, back pain, and other skeletal trauma. Among 200 feet, 27 (13.5%) showed an increased uptake of $^{99m}$Tc methylene diphosphonate ($^{99m}$Tc MDP) in the os trigonum region. Only 10 of these 27 feet (37%) had a symptomatic os trigonum. These results suggest that increased uptake of $^{99m}$Tc MDP in the os trigonum region is a frequent finding among active soldiers and is of limited value in detecting symptomatic os trigonum.

Taranow WS, Bisignani GA, Towers JD, Conti SF: Retrograde drilling of osteochondral lesions of the medial talar dome. *Foot Ankle Int* 1999;20:474-480.

Sixteen patients (16 ankles) with symptomatic osteochondral lesions of the medial talar dome were treated arthroscopically with percutaneous retrograde drilling through the sinus tarsi. The surgical technique allows preservation of intact articular cartilage, in contrast to traditional methods. Mean improvement in American Orthopaedic Foot and Ankle Society scores was 25 points. There were no surgical complications. Short-term results were comparable to results reported with other available techniques.

Ziran BH, Abidi NA, Scheel MJ: Medial malleolar osteotomy for exposure of complex talar body fractures. *J Orthop Trauma* 2001;15:513-518.

The authors describe a technique of medial malleolar osteotomy used in a small series of patients to gain access to the talar body in situations in which the traditional approaches did not provide adequate exposure.

### Subtalar Dislocations

Bibbo C, Lin SS, Abidi N, et al: Missed and associated injuries after subtalar dislocation: The role of CT. *Foot Ankle Int* 2001;22:324-308.

A review of subtalar joint dislocations revealed that most of these injuries occurred in men (78%) with a mean age of 29 years. The right lower extremity was most frequently injured (87.5%). The subtalar joint dislocation was initially diagnosed in all patients using plain radiography. In 100% of patients, CT identified additional injuries missed in initial plain radiographs. In 44% of patients, new information gathered by CT dictated a change in treatment.

## Classic Bibliography

Alexander AH, Lichtman DM: Surgical treatment of transchrondral talar dome fractures (osteochondritis dissecans): Long-term follow-up. *J Bone Joint Surg Am* 1980; 62:646-652.

Berndt AL, Harty M: Transchondral fractures (osteochondritis dissecans) of the talus. *J Bone Joint Surg Am* 1959;41:988-1020.

Blair HC: Comminuted fractures and fracture-dislocation of the body of the astragalus. *Am J Surg* 1943;59:37-43.

Canale ST: Fractures of the neck of the talus. *Orthopedics* 1990;13:1105-1115.

Canale ST, Kelly FB Jr: Fractures of the neck of the talus: Long-term evaluation of seventy-one cases. *J Bone Joint Surg Am* 1978;60:143-156.

Comfort TH, Behrens F, Gaither DW, et al: Long-term results of displaced talar neck fractures. *Clin Orthop* 1985; 199:81-87.

Daniels TR, Smith JW, Ross TI: Varus malalignment of the talar neck: Its effect on the position of the foot and on subtalar motion. *J Bone Joint Surg Am* 1996;78:1559-1567.

Dennis MD, Tullos HS: Blair tibiotalar arthrodesis injuries to the talus. *J Bone Joint Surg Am* 1980;62:103-107.

Hawkins LG: Fracture of the lateral process of the talus: A review of thirteen cases. *J Bone Joint Surg Am* 1965;47: 1170-1175.

Hawkins LG: Fractures of the neck of the talus. *J Bone Joint Surg Am* 1970;52:991-1002.

Heppenstall RB, Farahvar H, Balderston R, et al: Evaluation and management of subtalar dislocations. *J Trauma* 1980;20:494-497.

Johnson RP, Collier D, Carerra GF: The os trigonum syndrome: Use of bone scan in the diagnosis. *J Trauma* 1984; 24:761-764.

Lionberger DR, Bishop JO, Tullos HS: The modified Blair fusion. *Foot Ankle* 1982;3:60-62.

Marsh JL, Saltzman CL, Iverson M, Shapiro DS: Major open injuries of the talus. *J Orthop Trauma* 1995;9: 371-376.

McDougall A: The os trigonum. *J Bone Joint Surg Br* 1955;37:257-265.

Peterson L, Romanus B, Dahlberg E: Fracture of the collum tali: An experimental study. *J Biomech* 1976;9: 277-279.

Sarrafian SK: *Anatomy of the Foot and Ankle: Descriptive, Topographic, Functional.* Philadelphia, PA, Lippincott, 1983, pp 18, 52-53, 94.

Thordarson DB, Triffon MJ, Terk MR: Magnetic resonance imaging to detect avascular necrosis after open reduction and internal fixation of talar neck fractures. *Foot Ankle Int* 1996;17:742-747.

Turner W: A secondary astragalus in the human foot. *J Anat Physiol* 1882;17:82-83.

Veazey BL, Heckman JD, Galindo MJ, McGanity PL: Excision of ununited fractures of the posterior process of the talus: A treatment for chronic posterior ankle pain. *Foot Ankle* 1992;13:453-457.

Zimmer TJ, Johnson KA: Subtalar dislocations. *Clin Orthop* 1989;238:190-194.

# Chapter 5

# Calcaneal Fractures

Michael R. Werner, MD

## Introduction

Intra-articular calcaneal fractures are serious injuries that frequently result in functional disability. The calcaneus is the most frequently fractured tarsal bone, with 60% of tarsal fractures and 1% to 2% of all fractures involving the calcaneus. Calcaneal fractures are one of the few intra-articular fractures for which surgical treatment remains controversial. Seventy-five percent of calcaneal fractures are intra-articular and up to 10% are bilateral. Most calcaneal fractures occur in men age 25 to 45 years. Some studies report that up to 70% of these injuries occur at the workplace.

Both nonsurgical and surgical treatment of calcaneal fractures have been advocated. Initially, all calcaneal fractures were treated nonsurgically. Even though it was recognized early that a calcaneal fracture was a serious injury, most authors recommended nonsurgical management. Surgical treatment included primary subtalar fusion or closed reduction with pins and plaster. Although good results with surgical treatment have been reported as early as the 1940s and 1950s, optimal treatment is still a matter of controversy, with many patients reporting problems with morning stiffness and long-term running despite the treatment used.

## Mechanism of Injury

Seventy-five percent of calcaneal fractures are intra-articular (involving the subtalar joint), and 25% are extra-articular. The two main mechanisms of injury are axial load and avulsion forces. Axial load is the more common mechanism of injury and typically results from a fall from a height or a motor vehicle accident.

Essex-Lopresti described two types of intra-articular calcaneal fractures: joint depression-type and tongue-type. Both are caused by axial compression and start with the oblique primary fracture line running from anterolateral superiorly to posteromedial inferiorly and involving some amount of the posterior facet. With both types of fracture, the lateral process of the talus acts as a wedge at the crucial angle of Gissane. The fracture is caused by a shearing force because the tuberosity of the calcaneus is

lateral to the mechanical axis of the leg and divides the calcaneus into a sustentaculum piece and a tuberosity piece. From the primary fracture line, the secondary fracture line determines if a joint depression-type or tongue-type calcaneal fracture exists. In a joint depression-type fracture, the secondary fracture line runs superior from the primary line and exits behind the posterior facet. In addition, portions of the posterior facet are impacted and typically rotated up to 90° or more into the body of the calcaneus. If the secondary fracture line runs posteriorly from the primary fracture line and out the back of the tuberosity of the calcaneus, then a tongue-type fracture exists. A portion of the lateral aspect of the posterior facet remains attached to the tongue fragment.

In a 1993 cadaver study, calcaneal fractures were experimentally reproduced by dropping weights down a rod through the top of the tibia and thereby causing axial compression injuries. Because two primary fracture lines were observed, these results confirmed earlier theories about the mechanism of injury and the fracture patterns produced. One fracture line divided the calcaneus into medial and lateral portions, and the other ran from medial to lateral starting at the angle of Gissane and divided the calcaneus into anterior and posterior portions. A superior medial fragment (also know as the "constant fragment"), a superior lateral fragment with portions of the posterior facet, an anterolateral fragment (also known as the "blowout fragment"), an anterior main fragment with the calcaneocuboid joint, and the posterior tuberosity were identified. Open fractures of the calcaneus are relatively uncommon and are surgical emergencies requiring irrigation and débridement.

## Physical Examination

On physical examination, typical findings include significant swelling, acute deformity with rapid onset of fracture blisters, and ecchymosis of the heel and arch. The heel appears shorter and wider than normal and the blowout fragment may impinge on the peroneal tendons. The heel also is in a varus position, and the tuberosity is frequently elevated. Sural nerve injury is also common.

Twenty-six percent to 70% of patients with calcaneal fractures have associated injuries, and any fall from over 2 feet should raise suspicion of a calcaneal fracture. Lumbar spine fractures occur in 3% to 12% of patients with calcaneal fractures and ipsilateral lower extremity fractures occur in 10%.

A calcaneal fracture is always accompanied by surrounding soft-tissue trauma, with soft-tissue disruption proportional to the amount of force absorbed. Frequently, lateral skin creases are absent, and surgery should be delayed until these creases return. Skin creases should occur over the lateral heel when the ankle is dorsiflexed and everted (wrinkle test), indicating that edema has resolved. Compartment syndrome occurs in approximately 10% of patients and can lead to clawing of the lesser toes. Severe pain and swelling should raise suspicion of a compartment syndrome; definitive diagnosis is by direct measurement of compartment pressures, and fasciotomies should be done immediately when indicated.

## Imaging/Radiographic Evaluation

### Plain Radiographs

Plain radiographs for evaluation of calcaneal injuries include a lateral view of the foot and ankle, Harris axial view, and AP view of the foot. The lateral image is used to classify the fracture as joint depression or tongue-type and to measure the Böhler angle. This angle is formed by the intersection of a line drawn from the highest point on the posterior tuberosity to the highest point on the posterior facet and a line drawn from the highest point on the posterior facet and the highest point on the anterior process of the calcaneus and usually is between 20° to 40°. A double density frequently appears on the lateral view, indicating the piece of displaced and rotated posterior facet. The lateral view often gives a better indication of the amount of displacement of the posterior facet fragment than a CT scan and shows lateral extension of the fracture into the calcaneocuboid joint. The AP view of the foot also can be used to evaluate the calcaneocuboid joint. The Harris view allows measurement of the amount of heel varus, medial wall displacement, and shortening. Intraoperatively, Broden views can be used to evaluate the reduction of the posterior facet. Rotating the leg internally 45° and angling the x-ray beam from vertical toward horizontal in 10° increments from 10° to 40° is the recommended technique for Broden views.

### Computed Tomography

CT is recommended for preoperative evaluation, fracture classification, and surgical planning, particularly for displaced articular fractures of the calcaneus. Both coronal and transverse CT scans are useful. Ideally, these should be obtained with the patient's knee flexed 90° and the foot flat on the table. This position will help minimize nonorthogonal images. CT allows for better visualization of the articular surfaces and allows classification that ad-

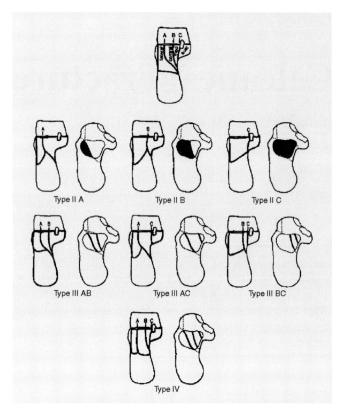

**Figure 1** CT classification of intra-articular calcaneal fractures. It is important that the coronal section analyzed includes the widest point of the articular surface (the sustentaculum tali). *(Reproduced with permission from Sanders R: Intra-articular fractures of the calcaneus: Present state of the art. J Orthop Trauma 1992;6:252-265.)*

dresses prognosis and outcomes as used in the classification system described by Sanders and associates. Coronal CT scans show the number and location of posterior facet fragments, but do not allow as accurate a determination of this displacement as do lateral scans. Calcaneal widening, shortening, and displacement of the lateral wall and impingement of the peroneal tendons also can be determined and the tuberosity fragment can be evaluated for varus deformity on both coronal and transverse CT scans. Finally, sustentacular fracture(s) and adduction or varus of the tuberosity can be appreciated on transverse CT scans of the calcaneocuboid joint.

In 1990, a classification based on CT scans that identified calcaneal fractures as either type I nondisplaced, type II displaced, or type III comminuted was developed. In 1993, Sanders and associates described a classification system based on CT scans that is widely used today (Fig. 1). On coronal and axial CT scans of the widest section of the posterior facet, the talus is divided into three equal columns by two lines, and then a third line is drawn medial to the most medial line continuous with the medial border of the posterior tuberosity, separating the sustentaculum tali from the posterior facet. The fractures are classified with a number indicating the number of posterior facet pieces and then with a letter indicating the line(s) creating those pieces.

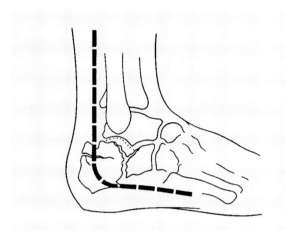

Figure 2 The extensile right angle lateral approach to the calcaneus. The longitudinal limb of incision is made just anterior to the Achilles tendon to avoid damage to the sural nerve. The inferior limb of the incision is made at the junction of the plantar and dorsal skin and ends just proximal to the base of the fifth metatarsal. This incision also avoids the angiosome that supplies the arterial blood flow to the lateral hindfoot skin. *(Reproduced with permission from Sanders R, Hansen ST, McReynolds IC: Trauma to the calcaneus and its tendon, in Jahss M (ed):* Disorders of the Foot and Ankle: Medical and Surgical Management, *ed 2. Philadelphia, PA, WB Saunders, 1991, pp 2326-2360.)*

## Treatment

Nondisplaced calcaneal fractures usually are treated non-surgically. The treatment of displaced calcaneal fractures remains controversial, but CT has improved fracture evaluation and has allowed outcome studies with valid post-operative comparisons. Since the advent of CT, a number of studies have reported good results after both closed and open treatment of all types of calcaneal fractures. The best outcomes have been reported in patients with anatomically reduced Sanders type II fractures and those with tongue-type fractures. Poorer outcomes have been weakly associated with older patients (older than 50 years), men, overweight patients with strenuous jobs (particularly workers' compensation patients), and those with bilateral fractures or fractures resulting from polytrauma. Some studies have shown a faster return to work and less long-term foot pain after surgical intervention, but there have been relatively few studies comparing surgical and nonsurgical treatment of intra-articular calcaneal fractures.

### Open Reduction and Internal Fixation

Numerous techniques have been described to surgically repair calcaneal fractures, including percutaneous reduction and open reduction through medial, lateral, combined medial and lateral, extensile lateral, and sinus tarsi approaches. The currently preferred method is open reduction and internal fixation (ORIF) through an extensile lateral approach for Sanders types II and III intra-articular calcaneal fractures if no medical contraindication to surgery exists. Recently, interest has been revived in the sinus tarsi approach (the so-called minimally inva-

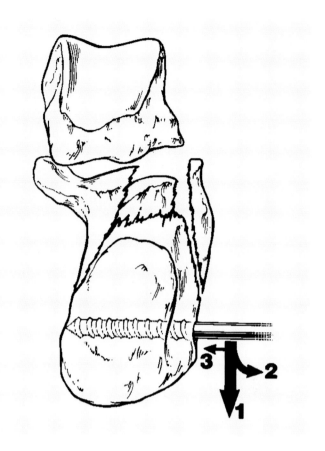

Figure 3 Indirect reduction of the tuberosity of the calcaneus. A Schanz pin is placed in the tuberosity fragment, and three arrows indicate its relative motion. The three components of the reduction are also illustrated as the tuberosity fragment is moved plantarly, medially, and in a slight valgus position to reestablish its normal alignment. *(Reproduced with permission from Sangeorzan BJ, Benirschke SK, Carr JB: Surgical management of fracture of the os calcis.* Instr Course Lect 1995;44:359-370.)*

sive approach), but long-term data regarding the efficacy of this procedure are not available.

The surgical treatment of these fractures typically is delayed 1 to 2 weeks to allow swelling to subside and lateral skin wrinkles to return. Initial enthusiasm for foot pumps to decrease swelling has subsided because of patient discomfort. Patients with Sanders types II and III intra-articular calcaneal fractures usually are initially placed in a bulky Jones type dressing, with the foot elevated, and do not bear weight until the swelling has resolved. The extensile lateral approach is used for anatomic reduction of the posterior facet and calcaneocuboid joint and correction of any varus or shortening of the calcaneus. Plating of the lateral calcaneus is the most popular method of fixation; separate screws can be used to maintain reduction of the posterior facet. Bone grafting is still controversial, and some studies have demonstrated no benefit from bone grafting when a lateral plate is used. Newer low-profile plates have locking screws that can be supplemented with small fragment screws placed in lag fashion across the posterior facet pieces.

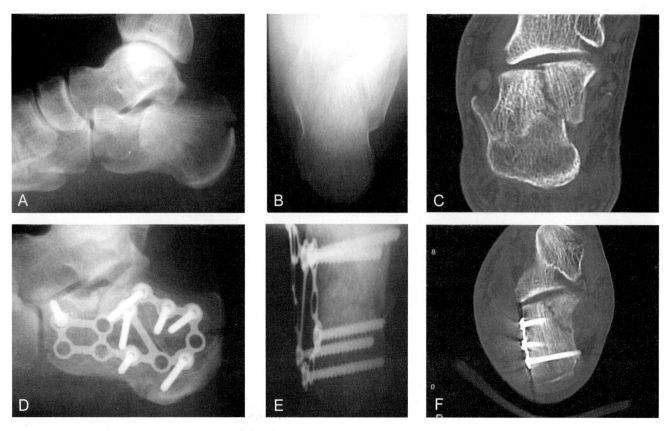

**Figure 4** **A,** Preoperative lateral radiograph showing depression of the posterior facet fragment within the body of calcaneus in a 35-year-old man who fell from a height of 8 feet. **B,** Preoperative axial radiograph of the same patient revealing shortening and varus malalignment of the posterior tuberosity. **C,** Preoperative coronal CT scan through posterior facet revealing a Sanders type IIB fracture with a displaced split in the midportion of the posterior facet. **D,** Postoperative lateral radiograph demonstrating a calcaneal perimeter plate in place. **E,** Harris axial view demonstrating the appropriate-length hardware and correction of varus malalignment. **F,** Postoperative CT scan demonstrating anatomic reduction of the posterior facet joint surface.

## Surgical Technique

Patients with a unilateral fracture can be placed in the lateral decubitus position, and patients with bilateral fractures are best treated prone. In general, an L-shaped, lateral extensile approach is used (Fig. 2). A no-touch technique with retraction pins placed in the fibula, talar neck, and cuboid minimizes trauma to the soft tissues during surgical reduction. A large Schanz or Steinmann pin placed in the posterior tuberosity of the calcaneus can be used for indirect reduction of the posterior tuberosity (Fig. 3). The anterior calcaneus and posterior facet are then reduced and held with provisional Kirschner wires, and appropriate low-profile hardware is placed to maintain the reduction (Fig. 4). Intraoperative direct visualization and fluoroscopic Broden's views can be helpful in assessing the reduction. A drain can minimize the risk of a large hematoma developing beneath the soft-tissue flap.

Postoperatively, a removable posterior splint is worn until the wound is healed and sutures are removed, usually at 3 weeks. Early range-of-motion exercise is initiated out of the splint within the first week, but weight bearing is delayed until 10 weeks after surgery. Patients gradually progress to full weight bearing without an assistive device by 12 weeks. Maximal medical improvement is seen by 18 months.

## Minimally Invasive Techniques

Recently, there has been renewed interest in minimally invasive treatment of certain calcaneal fractures. Forty-six patients with Sanders type IIC tongue-type fractures of the calcaneus were treated using a variation of a technique popularized by Essex-Lopresti in 1952. In these patients, a reduction spike and a guidewire for the 6.5-mm cannulated screws were placed in the tongue fragment. The reduction maneuver consisted of the following three components: (1) varus to unlock the tuberosity fragment, (2) plantar directed force on the forefoot and a reduction spike to improve the Böhler angle, and (3) valgus of the heel to correct varus of the tuberosity fragment. The cannulated screw guidewire was subsequently driven across the fracture to maintain reduction, and two 6.5-mm cannulated screws were inserted. Early range-of-motion exercise was initiated, and weight bearing was delayed 12 weeks. Good to excellent results were reported in 85% of patients at average follow-up of 3.4 years. Conversion to an open procedure because of lack of adequate reduction was required in five patients.

A sinus tarsi approach that uses an incision from the sinus tarsi to the posterior tuberosity also has been described for reduction of calcaneal fractures. In this technique, the peroneal sheath is entered, and the tendons are retracted plantarly. The posterior facet is then elevated and supported with bone graft. In addition, a limited lateral approach has been described in which a straight lateral approach is made, the peroneal tendons are retracted plantarly, the posterior facet is elevated, and the tuberosity fragment is reduced using a Schanz pin. The medial wall overlap and Böhler angle are corrected with this "closed" component of the procedure, and reduction is maintained by a cannulated screw. Lag screws and a bone graft are used to support the posterior facet. A subcutaneous plate can then be applied through this lateral approach to maintain reduction of the lateral wall; however, this increases the exposure.

Bone graft substitutes have been used in conjunction with minimally invasive techniques. Some bone substitutes, such as MIIG™ 115 (Wright Medical, Arlington, TN) allow hardware to be placed as soon as the injectable calcium sulfate graft hardens. Providing physicians with the ability to place screws across the hardened graft is an improvement over similar products.

### Primary Arthrodesis

Primary subtalar fusion is recommended only for some Sanders type IV comminuted intra-articular calcaneal fractures; however, most researchers report poor results with both nonsurgical and surgical treatment of this particular type of fracture. Sanders and associates reported only one good to excellent result in 11 type IV fractures treated with ORIF.

The technique for primary fusion includes reconstruction of the heel in a manner similar to that used for ORIF with restoration of anatomy and lateral wall plating. Cartilage is then removed from the undersurface of the talus and from any remnants of the posterior facet. Iliac crest bone graft or allograft is used, and the fusion is secured with a large, preferably fully-threaded, cannulated screw from the posterior tuberosity of the calcaneus into the talus. A bulky dressing and splint are worn until the sutures are removed and then a cast is worn until union occurs, which may take 16 weeks or longer. Results from this technically demanding procedure are encouraging even though options are limited and prognosis is guarded. It was noted in one study that 11 of 12 patients returned to work after primary fusion.

## Results and Complications

The literature on calcaneal fracture outcomes often is contradictory. Good results have been reported with both nonsurgical and surgical treatment of calcaneal fractures. There are several cohort studies and small prospective studies that seem to show a clear trend toward earlier return to work, better shape of the foot, and fewer problems with shoe wear after surgical treatment; however, there are few prospective, randomized studies comparing the results of nonsurgical to surgical treatment, and even these have had equivocal conclusions. A meta-analysis of treatment methods concluded that a trend was present for surgically treated patients to have better outcomes than nonsurgically treated patients but that the evidence for recommending surgical treatment is weak. Overall, displaced fractures seem to have a worse outcome than nondisplaced fractures; fractures with comminution and displacement of the posterior facet tend to produce worse outcomes than fractures with less involvement of the posterior facet. Tongue-type fractures have been reported to have better outcomes than joint depression-type fractures. Although posterior facet incongruity and degeneration, as measured by CT scanning, seem to be strong predictors of poor results, anatomic reduction of the posterior facet does not guarantee a good result. Long-term symptoms have been reported in most patients with displaced calcaneal fractures treated nonsurgically. Accurate clinical measurement of subtalar motion is difficult, but most studies describe an approximately 50% reduction in subtalar range of motion after surgical treatment. An analysis of prognostic factors determined that subtalar incongruity, talonavicular or ankle arthrosis, increased heel width, and fibulocalcaneal impingement are associated with poor outcome. In a recent prospective, randomized, controlled multicenter trial, the authors showed that surgical treatment as a whole provided no improvement over nonsurgical treatment; however, surgical treatment seemed more likely to produce good outcomes than nonsurgical treatment in specific types of patients: women and younger men; those with moderately lower Böhler angles, lighter workloads, and single, simple displaced intra-articular fractures; and those not receiving workers' compensation. One study found excellent or good results after surgical treatment of intra-articular calcaneal fractures in 88% of patients not receiving workers' compensation compared with 27% in patients receiving workers' compensation. Another study found that male gender, medium and heavy labor, workers' compensation support, and bilateral intra-articular fractures all were associated with poor results.

The most common and most potentially devastating problems after ORIF of calcaneal fractures are wound complications. Wound complications have been reported in 2% to 32% of patients, with most being superficial and treated with local measures. Rarely (< 1%), below-knee amputation is required. One recent study documented an 11% wound complication rate and 3.2% infection rate in 218 displaced articular fractures treated by ORIF through a lateral approach. In addition, there were six (2.8%) sural nerve problems, but only one of six was permanent. Subsequent procedures were required in 43.5% of patients, most of which (36%) were for hardware removal.

Although no nonunions were reported, 2% of fractures had varus malunions requiring osteotomy, and 2% underwent subtalar fusions.

Two studies documented risk factors associated with wound problems after ORIF for calcaneal fractures. One study of 64 fractures found single layer closure, obesity, extended time between injury and surgery (> 5 days), and smoking to be adverse risk factors. In the second study of 190 fractures, a 25% wound complication rate was reported, with 21% of wounds requiring some form of surgical treatment. Smoking, diabetes, and open fractures all increased the likelihood of wound complications.

## Posttraumatic Reconstruction

In addition to wound complications, varus malunion with a wide, short heel and posttraumatic osteoarthritis of the subtalar joint commonly occur after nonsurgical or surgical treatment of displaced articular fractures of the calcaneus. These two complications often are associated with other problems, including peroneal or calcaneofibular abutment with tendon (peroneal) and bony (calcaneal lateral wall [fibular malleolus]) pain, sinus tarsi pain, difficulty with shoe wear, decreased ankle dorsiflexion as a result of loss of the normal talar declination angle, decreased gastrocnemius-soleus complex lever arm and strength resulting from loss of the normal Böhler angle, heel pad pain, and sural nerve symptoms.

Malunion of the calcaneus is caused in part by the superior and lateral translation of the tuberosity along the primary fracture line. This causes loss of height, a widened heel, and lateral impingement. Dorsiflexion of the talus causes reduction of the talar declination angle (< 20°), which can lead to anterior impingement between the neck of the talus and the anterior tibia. The talar declination angle is measured by the intersection of a line drawn to the longitudinal axis of the talus and a line drawn parallel to the floor on a standing lateral view of the foot. This angle normally measures 20° or more; an angle of less than 10° is likely associated with symptomatic anterior ankle impingement.

CT has been used to classify calcaneal malunions. Type I includes lateral wall exostosis without subtalar arthrosis; type II includes a lateral wall exostosis with subtalar arthrosis; type III includes lateral wall exostosis, subtalar arthrosis, and varus malunion of the heel.

Initial treatment should begin with conservative care and may include shoe wear modification, molded insoles, or bracing. Bracing can consist of a molded plastic ankle-foot orthosis (AFO); a double upright metal brace with channels built into shoes with a locked ankle, rocker sole, and outside T-strap; or a weight-bearing AFO, consisting of molded material inside a leather casing with Velcro straps. The advantages of this latter type of brace are: it is molded to the subtalar joint and helps support it, and it

also decreases weight bearing through the ankle and subtalar joints by load transfer to the lower leg.

When nonsurgical treatment is not successful, there are surgical interventions for each type of malunion. Treatment of a type I malunion should consist of a generous lateral wall exostectomy. Some authors have cautioned against lateral exostectomy alone because of the frequent occurrence of subtalar arthritis in these patients. CT can aid in the evaluation of the degree of subtalar joint arthritis. A diagnostic local anesthetic injection into the subtalar joint may help differentiate subtalar pain from simple subfibular impingement pain, but inserting a needle into the joint can be difficult after an articular calcaneal fracture because of arthrofibrosis. Fluoroscopy can aid the accurate placement of the anesthetic in the subtalar joint. The position of the heel should be evaluated clinically and radiographically to determine the extent of varus deformity. Radiographic varus may not correlate directly with the extent of clinical varus when the patient is standing or prone with the ankle in dorsiflexion to neutral.

Type II malunions are treated with generous lateral exostectomy and in situ subtalar fusion. One or two large cannulated screws are placed across the subtalar joint, and bone graft is recommended. In one study, no difference in outcome between iliac crest bone graft or allograft to treat type II malunions was found.

The surgical treatment of type III malunions is controversial because there is currently no consensus regarding the method of subtalar fusion. Most authors recommend an osteotomy in conjunction with a subtalar fusion when ankle impingement is present along with varus malunion. However, other authors found no correlation between postoperative talar declination angle and American Orthopaedic Foot and Ankle Society (AOFAS) scores. Several procedures have been described for this condition, such as distraction bone block arthrodesis, osteotomy through the primary fracture line, and more recently, oblique sliding osteotomy. A variation of Carr's distraction bone block arthrodesis using a sinus tarsi approach has been described. A lateral closing wedge osteotomy, in addition to a lateral wall exostectomy and subtalar fusion, also has been recommended.

Distraction bone block arthrodesis has been criticized because of its tendency to fuse the subtalar joint in a varus position because of the tethering of the medial soft-tissue restraints when the joint is distracted. In addition, wound closure may be difficult after the subtalar joint is distracted. Osteotomy through the primary fracture line has been criticized because it is technically difficult to recreate the primary fracture line and because the risk this technique poses to the medial structures because of the anterolateral to posteromedial plane of osteotomy.

Currently, a lateral exostectomy and in situ fusion are preferred when possible. However, if an osteotomy is needed to correct varus malunion of the tuberosity fragment, a lateral closing wedge or an oblique sliding osteotomy is useful before subtalar joint arthrodesis. Postoperatively, the patient bears no weight for 8 to 12 weeks, but range-of-motion exercise of the ankle is started when the patient is comfortable, which usually is within the first 2 weeks.

There are not enough studies with an adequate number of patients to fully evaluate the results of these surgical techniques. However, most authors do not currently recommend an in situ triple arthrodesis for subtalar malunions accompanied by subtalar joint arthrosis, nor has any correlation been found between calcaneocuboid joint degenerative changes and patient symptoms or AOFAS scores.

## Anterior Process Fractures of the Calcaneus

A fracture of the anterior process of the calcaneus can cause chronic lateral hindfoot pain. The fracture is caused by an inversion and plantar flexion force, with avulsion of the bifurcate ligament and an anteromedial fragment from the anterior process of the calcaneus. The fragment usually is small and can be seen on lateral or oblique radiographs. These fractures should be treated with immobilization in a walking cast until the patient is symptom free, which may require 8 to 12 weeks. A symptomatic nonunion can be treated with excision of the fragment. A disturbing incidence of reflex sympathetic dystrophy has been reported in conjunction with these injuries, perhaps resulting from the difficulty in diagnosing these injuries and failure to immobilize the injured foot. A fragment larger than 1 cm that involves a significant portion of the calcaneocuboid joint should be treated by ORIF with a lateral approach.

## Avulsion Fractures of the Tuberosity

An avulsion fracture of the tuberosity may be an extraarticular or intra-articular fracture caused by a strong contraction of the gastrocnemius-soleus complex with a failure in tension. Frequently, it occurs in osteopenic bone, and maintaining reduction even after secure fixation may be difficult. Minimal displacement of these fractures is rare. More commonly, significant displacement caused by the pull of the Achilles musculotendinous unit requires ORIF. The fragment should be reduced as soon as reasonably possible because of the risk of pressure necrosis of the overlying skin. Occasionally, full-thickness skin necrosis occurs, requiring a local rotational flap or free-tissue transfer.

Small fragments can be excised, but larger fragments should be approached through a midline incision or just medial to the Achilles tendon and reduced and fixed with cannulated screws. However, fixation is often difficult because of comminution and osteopenic bone. Engaging the opposite cortex with the screw(s) may reduce the incidence of loss of reduction.

Although large fragments that include part of the posterior lip of the posterior facet can be approached and fixed through the longitudinal limb of an extensile lateral approach, an indirect reduction with an Essex-Lopresti maneuver can be tried first.

Postoperative care includes a splint or cast with the ankle in resting equinus position for 3 to 4 weeks. The ankle is brought to neutral position with serial casting over the next 2 to 3 weeks followed by gentle active range-of-motion exercise. Patients do not bear weight until fracture union is confirmed clinically and radiographically. Protected weight bearing to tolerance is continued in the removable boot cast until near-normal ankle motion returns.

## Summary

Intra-articular calcaneal fractures continue to be a challenging problem, but the role of surgery in the treatment of acute fractures and malunions is becoming clearer. The most widely used surgical technique for treating these fractures is lateral calcaneal plating through an extensile lateral approach; less invasive techniques also are applicable. Overall, the best results are achieved with anatomic restoration of the subtalar joint; however, even with a perfect surgical reduction, the long-term pain relief and function for these particularly troublesome fractures is guarded.

## Annotated Bibliography

*Mechanism of Injury*

Sanders R: Displaced intra-articular fractures of the calcaneus. *J Bone Joint Surg Am* 2000;82:225-250.

This excellent "current concepts review" covers the mechanism, treatment, and complications of calcaneal fractures.

*Treatment*

Chen YJ, Huang TJ, Hsu KY, Hsu RW, Chen CW: Subtalar distractional realignment arthrodesis with wedge bone grafting and lateral decompression for calcaneal malunion. *J Trauma* 1998;45:729-737.

Thirty-four patients who underwent a distraction bone block arthrodesis for calcaneal fracture malunion using a sinus tarsi approach were evaluated. At a mean follow-up of 64 months, solid fusion was reported in 32 of 34 patients, neutral to slight valgus in 26 of 32, and varus in 6 of 32. Good to excellent results were found in 26 of 32 patients.

Randle JA, Kreder HJ, Stephen D, Williams J, Jaglal S, Hu R: Should calcaneal fractures be treated surgically? A meta-analysis. *Clin Orthop* 2000;377:217-227.

In this meta-analysis, a Medline search was conducted looking for articles pertaining to calcaneal fractures that were published from 1980 to 1996. A total of 1,845 articles were found, but only six met the inclusion criteria comparing surgical and nonsurgical treatment. As a result of variability in reporting, no real conclusions could be drawn, but there was a trend for surgical results to be slightly better.

Sangeorzan BJ: Salvage procedures for calcaneus fractures. *Instr Course Lect* 1997;46:339-346.

This review article discusses the surgical treatment options used for the salvage of calcaneal fracture sequelae.

Thermann H, Krettek C, Hufner T, Schratt HE, Abrecht K, Tscherne H: Management of calcaneal fractures in adults: Conservative versus operative treatment. *Clin Orthop* 1998;353:107.

This review article discusses the surgical options for the treatment of displaced calcaneal fractures and surgical technique.

Tornetta P III: Percutaneous treatment of calcaneal fractures. *Clin Orthop* 2000;375:91-96.

This series report examines 46 patients with 41 successful closed reductions of 36 type IIC and 5 type IIB tongue-type fractures of the calcaneus. The surgical technique described is a modification of the original Essex-Lopresti maneuver. The Maryland Foot Score and radiographs were used to evaluate patients. At a mean follow-up of 3.4 years, 85% of patients reported good to excellent results; no poor results were reported.

### Results and Complications

Abidi NA, Dhawan S, Gruen GS, Vogt MT, Conti SF: Wound-healing risk factors after open reduction and internal fixation of calcaneal fractures. *Foot Ankle Int* 1998; 19:856-861.

This is a retrospective study of 63 calcaneal fractures treated by ORIF with an extensile lateral approach. Wound complications to varying degrees were found in 20 patients. Risk factors for wound problems included single layer closure, smoking, increased body mass index, and delay of treatment for more than 10 days. The use of a hemovac drain did not improve wound healing.

Aktuglu K, Aydogan U: The functional outcome of displaced intra-articular calcaneal fractures: A comparison between isolated cases and polytrauma patients. *Foot Ankle Int* 2002;23:314-318.

Thirty-seven calcaneal fractures in 28 patients were analyzed, including 17 fractures caused by polytrauma and 18 caused by isolated trauma. Treatment was either conservative (closed method) or surgical. Patients were evaluated using the Maryland Foot Score; overall, patients with isolated trauma fractures reported better functional outcome than those with polytrauma fractures.

Buckley R, Tough S, McCormack R, et al: Operative compared with nonoperative treatment of displaced intra-articluar calcaneal fractures: A prospective, randomized, controlled multicenter trial. *J Bone Joint Surg Am* 2002; 84:1733-1744.

Although overall outcomes were similar in surgically treated and nonsurgically treated fractures, surgical treatment produced significantly better results in specific patients: women, those not receiving workers' compensation, younger (< 29 years) men, and those with a lower Böhler angle (0° to 14°), a comminuted fracture, a light workload, or an anatomic reduction.

Coughlin MJ: Calcaneal fractures in the industrial patient. *Foot Ankle Int* 2000;21:896-905.

Cost analysis and time back to work were evaluated in 48 calcaneal fractures that occurred among workers' compensation patients.

Folk JW, Starr AJ, Early JS: Early wound complications of operative treatment of calcaneus fractures: Analysis of 190 fractures. *J Orthop Trauma* 1999;13:369-372.

One hundred ninety calcaneal fractures were studied retrospectively for wound complications following ORIF with an extensile lateral approach and using two layer closure and a drain. Wound complications were found in 25%. Smoking, diabetes, and open fractures all increased the risk of complications.

Geel CW, Flemister AS Jr: Standarized treatment of intra-articular calcaneal fractures using an oblique lateral incision and no bone graft. *J Trauma* 2001;50:1083-1089.

Although anatomic or near anatomic reductions were obtained in 97% of 33 fractures and all fractures healed uneventfully, outcomes were significantly different in nonworkers' compensation patients (88% good or excellent results) and workers' compensation patients (27% good or excellent results). Of those employed before injury, 92% returned to the workforce.

Harvey EJ, Grujic L, Early JS, Benirschke SK, Sangeorzan BJ: Morbidity associated with ORIF of intra-articular calcaneus fractures using a lateral approach. *Foot Ankle Int* 2001;22:868-873.

Two hundred eighteen displaced intra-articular calcaneal fractures were reviewed for wound complications following ORIF with an extensile lateral approach. Eleven percent required local wound care, and one deep infection resulted in amputation; 2.8% had sural nerve findings, and five patients subsequently underwent subtalar fusion, including two patients who were treated with distraction bone block arthrodesis.

Loucks C, Buckley R: Bohler's angle: Correlation with outcome in displaced intra-articular calcaneal fractures. *J Orthop Trauma* 1999;13:554-558.

Ninety-five fractures were evaluated using a visual analog scale and Short Form-36. Fractures with a Böhler angle of less than 0 had a poorer 2-year outcome regardless of the treatment used.

Tufescu TV, Buckley R: Age, gender, work capability, and worker's compensation in patients with displaced intraarticular calcaneal fracture. *J Orthop Trauma* 2001;15:275-279.

One hundred sixty-nine patients were randomly assigned to surgical or nonsurgical treatment for displaced intra-articular calcaneal fractures, and outcomes were measured using the Short Form 36 and work history. Poorer outcomes were found in men, heavy laborers, those receiving workers' compensation, and those with bilateral fractures. Patients who underwent surgical treatment returned to work faster (average 87 days) compared with those who received nonsurgical treatment.

### Posttraumatic Reconstruction

Chandler JT, Bonar SK, Anderson RB, Davis WH: Results of in situ subtalar arthrodesis for late sequelae of calcaneus fractures. *Foot Ankle Int* 1999;20:18-24.

This is a retrospective review of 19 feet with a mean follow-up of 27 months following in situ subtalar fusion for calcaneal fracture malunion. No correlation was found between AOFAS hindfoot scores and talar height or talar declination angle. Peroneal impingement, smoking, and sural nerve injury were associated with lower scores. Calcaneocuboid degenerative changes did not correlate with symptoms or scores.

Flemister AS Jr, Infante AF, Sanders RW, Walling AK: Subtalar arthrodesis for complications of intra-articular calcaneal fractures. *Foot Ankle Int* 2000;21:392-399.

Eighty-six subtalar fusions using a variety of techniques for either primary fusions for comminuted fractures or as a reconstructive procedure following failed ORIF or malunion were evaluated. AOFAS score was used to evaluate patients. Eighty-three of 86 fusions were successful. Four cases of malunion and four cases of osteomyelitis were found, and a significantly shorter hospital stay was associated with not using an iliac crest graft.

No correlation between postoperative talar declination angle and AOFAS scores could be made.

## Classic Bibliography

Benirschke SK, Sangeorzan BJ: Extensive intraarticular fractures of the foot: Surgical management of calcaneal fractures. *Clin Orthop* 1993;292:128-134.

Böhler L: Diagnosis, pathology, and treatment of fractures of the os calcis. *J Bone Joint Surg* 1931;13:75-89.

Broden B: Roentgen examination of the subtaloid joint in fractures of the calcaneus. *Acta Radiol* 1949;31:85-91.

Essex-Lopresti P: The mechanism, reduction technique, and results in fractures of the os calcis. *Br J Surg* 1952;39:395-419.

Gallie WE: Subastragalar arthrodesis in fractures of the os calcis. *J Bone Joint Surg* 1943;25:731-736.

Lindsay WRN, Dewar FP: Fractures of the os calcis. *Am J Surg* 1958;95:555-576.

Myerson M, Quill GE Jr: Late complications of fractures of the calcaneus. *J Bone Joint Surg Am* 1993;75:331-341.

Romash MM: Reconstructive osteotomy of the calcaneus with subtalar arthrodesis for malunited calcaneal fractures. *Clin Orthop* 1993;290:157-167.

Sanders R, Fortin P, DiPasquale T, Walling A: Operative treatment in 120 displaced intraarticular calcaneal fractures: Results using a prognostic computed tomography scan classification. *Clin Orthop* 1993;290:87-95.

Thordarson DB, Krieger LE: Operative vs. nonoperative treatment of intra-articular fractures of the calcaneus: A prospective randomized trial. *Foot Ankle Int* 1996;17:2-9.

# Chapter 6

# Fractures of the Midtarsals, Metatarsals, and Phalanges

C. Christopher Stroud, MD

## Introduction

Most fractures of the metatarsals and phalanges can be treated nonsurgically, unless they are severely comminuted or displaced. Fractures of the midfoot (navicular and tarsometatarsal joint complex) often require surgical stabilization. Lisfranc fracture-dislocations of the tarsometatarsal joint are infrequent injuries, but failure to recognize and appropriately treat them can lead to disabling degenerative changes in the joint.

## Navicular Fractures

Navicular fractures are uncommon foot injuries and include dorsal lip, tuberosity, and body fractures. Stress fractures of the navicular also occur occasionally in running athletes, causing chronic midfoot pain. The navicular is an important component of the midfoot at its articulation with the talus. It has a mobile talonavicular joint along its proximal edge and relatively immobile naviculocuneiform joints along its distal aspect. A watershed area of blood supply makes the central third of the navicular prone to stress fractures and osteonecrosis. Radiographic evaluation includes AP, lateral, and oblique views of the foot. Bone scanning, CT, and MRI can be useful in the diagnosis of stress fractures.

### Dorsal Lip Fractures

Avulsion fractures of the dorsal lip are the most common navicular fractures and usually are caused by excessive plantar flexion. They are characterized by associated ligamentous injury and usually respond well to conservative treatment with a short course of protected weight bearing. On occasion, nonunited fragments are persistently symptomatic and may require excision.

### Tuberosity Fractures

Fractures of the navicular tuberosity can occur with an avulsion mechanism of eversion of the foot. Most of these fractures are nondisplaced because of the complex and broad insertion of the posterior tibialis tendon and can be treated with a period of immobilization. A symptomatic nonunion usually can be treated with excision. De-

pending on the size of the fragment and the presence of displacement, screw fixation also may be used.

### Body Fractures

Navicular body fractures are rare, but they can have a devastating effect on hindfoot function. An incongruent talonavicular joint can lead to talonavicular arthritis, which will markedly impair all hindfoot motion. These fractures have been classified into three types. Type I body fractures have a fracture line that produces dorsal and plantar fragments (axial plane fractures), usually without associated deformity of the foot (Fig. 1). With any degree of displacement, type I body fractures should be treated with open reduction and internal fixation with interfragmentary lag screws. Type II body fractures are the most common type. They are caused by axial compression, which produces an oblique fracture from dorsal lateral to plantar medial (sagittal plane fracture line) and frequently an associated adduction deformity of the forefoot with subluxation of the talonavicular joint (Fig. 2). Some comminution may be present, making fracture reduction more difficult. Type II body fractures should be treated with fixation across the navicular when there is no significant comminution. If comminution is severe, the largest fracture fragments can be secured to the cuneiforms to avoid talonavicular pin fixation, which can lead to significant postoperative stiffness. Type III body fractures result from an axial load with central and/or lateral comminution of the navicular (Fig. 3). These have the poorest outcome because of the articular cartilage damage at the time of initial injury and difficulty in reestablishing articular congruity. These fractures should be treated with open reduction and internal fixation. Comminution often requires independent fixation of the large navicular fragments to the cuneiforms with no reduction of the comminuted segment and possibly bone grafting acutely.

### Stress Fractures

Stress fractures of the navicular are often easily overlooked. However, this fracture should be suspected in any athlete with chronic midfoot pain, particularly long-

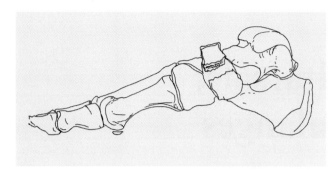

Figure 1    Lateral view of a type I navicular fracture (axial plane fracture line).

distance runners and basketball players. Results from the physical examination may be deceptively benign. Tenderness generally is localized to the midfoot along the mid-medial border. Plain radiographs frequently are nondiagnostic and in such cases, MRI can help establish the diagnosis. If a fracture plane is evident on plain radiographs, CT is more helpful in defining bony sclerosis and determining whether the fracture completely traverses the navicular.

Nondisplaced incomplete fractures can be treated with 6 to 8 weeks of cast immobilization without weight bearing followed by 6 weeks of gradually increasing activity level. In patients with persistent pain or in competitive athletes, primary screw fixation of these fractures with or without local bone grafting can maximize the

chances of primary healing. This is followed by non–weight-bearing cast immobilization until the fracture has healed.

## Cuboid and Cuneiform Injuries

Isolated injuries of the cuboid or cuneiforms are uncommon because these bones are all densely secured to the adjacent tarsal bones and metatarsals. The cuboid is most commonly injured as a component of a "nutcracker fracture," in which an abduction force results in a midfoot fracture medially (usually propagation of a medial and/or central Lisfranc injury) and compression of the cuboid along the lateral column of the foot. Shortening of the lateral column through the cuboid must be corrected as a component of the reduction of the Lisfranc injury (Fig. 4). Similarly, cuneiform injuries usually are a component of a Lisfranc variant in which there is a tarsometatarsal (TMT) injury with propagation through the intercuneiform and naviculocuneiform joints proximally. Any significant displacement of either the cuneiforms or cuboid should be treated with open reduction and internal fixation.

## Lisfranc Fractures

Fracture dislocations of the TMT joint complex are referred to as Lisfranc fractures, taking their name from the napoleonic-era surgeon who described amputations

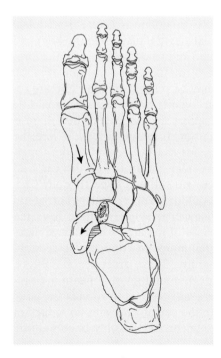

Figure 2    AP view of a type II navicular fracture (sagittal plane fracture line). The arrows indicate the direction of applied force. Note also subluxation of the talonavicular joint and proximal migration of the first ray, a common component of type II fractures.

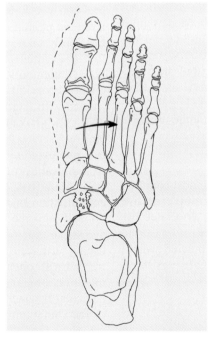

Figure 3    AP view of a type III navicular fracture. Note the comminution, displacement, and incongruity of the talonavicular and naviculocuneiform joints. Arrow indicates the direction of applied force.

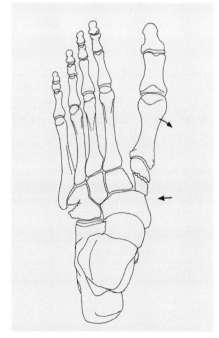

Figure 4    AP view of a Lisfranc variant fracture with an associated fracture of the navicular and a "nutcracker" fracture of the cuboid. The lateral wall of the cuboid is compressed and thereby shortened, which is difficult to depict in a one-dimensional figure. Arrows indicate the direction of applied force.

American Academy of Orthopaedic Surgeons

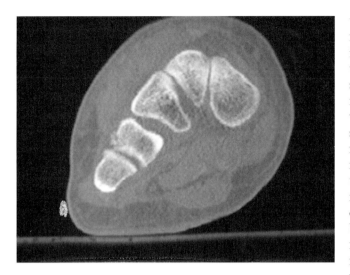

**Figure 5** Coronal CT scan demonstrating the arch configuration of the Lisfranc complex. Note the narrow plantar wedge of cuneiforms two and three and the narrow dorsal wedge of the first medial cuneiform. This bony anatomy is important for proper screw and pin placement.

about this level of the foot. Although these injuries represent only 0.2% of all fractures, if undetected and untreated, they can cause significant morbidity and disability. Significant trauma to the foot causes an obvious fracture, but an occult injury may produce only mild swelling and tenderness along the midfoot. A high degree of suspicion of injury to this area must be maintained when a patient reports midfoot pain following trauma.

### Anatomy

The stability of the TMT joint complex is maintained by the unique wedge-shaped anatomy of the metatarsal bases and their corresponding cuneiform articulations, which are arranged in an arch configuration (Fig. 5). The thick plantar capsular structures about the lesser TMT articulations and the recessed base of the second metatarsal effectively "lock" the metatarsals to the midfoot. Lisfranc's ligament is a thick structure composed of three portions running from the medial cuneiform to the base of the second metatarsal. The thickest and strongest part is the plantar portion of the ligament, which is the main stabilizing component of the first and second metatarsal interspace. Ten degrees to 20° of sagittal plane motion occurs at the fourth and fifth metatarsal cuboid junction, with progressively less motion about the remaining, more medial TMT joints.

### Mechanism

Injuries to the TMT joint can be caused by direct or indirect forces. Direct forces usually produce a crush injury with bony comminution and significant soft-tissue injury. The potential development or coexistence of a compartment syndrome must be considered with this type of injury. Indirect causes, such as bending or twisting moments applied to the midfoot, are more common. Bending or

twisting moments usually occur when the ankle is plantar flexed and the toes are dorsiflexed (extended) and an axial load (or longitudinal force) is applied to the heel. A tensile force is thus applied to the convexity of the dorsum of the TMT junction, disrupting the supporting ligaments. This type of injury can occur in horseback riders who fall from the horse while the forefoot is fixed in the stirrup. A pronation and abduction force is applied to the midfoot resulting in disruption of the supporting ligaments within the joint complex. More commonly, the patient will state that the foot was fixed and his or her body rolled or twisted over the midfoot, resulting in injury. The classic scenario for this type of injury occurs when a football player has the ankle flexed, toes extended, and forefoot fixed to the ground when another player lands directly on the heel, buckling the metatarsals at their base where the midfoot is fixed. Missing a step while descending stairs and axially loading the midfoot is another common mechanism of injury. Rotational forces applied to the midfoot can result in a variety of injury patterns.

An injury to this joint complex should be suspected when the patient gives a history consistent with a bending load applied to the midfoot. Patients with Lisfranc injuries typically report pain and swelling in the midfoot and have difficulty bearing weight on the affected extremity. The presence of plantar midfoot ecchymosis is indicative of severe soft-tissue disruption; frequently, this will be a TMT joint injury, even though plain radiographs may not show significant bony nonarticular abnormalities. Any midfoot "sprain" in which swelling, pain, and tenderness are more than the mechanism or severity of injury would indicate should be evaluated for a Lisfranc injury. An AP radiograph with partial weight bearing and the patient's foot flat on the cassette and/or CT may aid in making the diagnosis when plain radiographs are negative. An examination under anesthesia for instability of the metatarsaltarsal articulations may also be needed to rule out this injury with occult instability.

### Classification

Traditionally, injuries of the TMT articulation have been classified as total incongruity (type A), partial incongruity (type B), or divergent incongruity (type C) based on a three-column concept of the midfoot. The medial column consists of the first metatarsal, the medial cuneiform, and its navicular facet. The middle column consists of the second and third metatarsals and their corresponding cuneiform bones and the central and lateral facets of the navicular. The lateral column consists of the fourth and fifth metatarsals and their articulations with the cuboid. The importance of this classification system is that injury to one portion of a column usually indicates injury to other portions of that column; an awareness of this concept reduces the likelihood that propagation of a fracture through the cuneiform or navicular-cuboid-calcaneal articulations will be unrecognized (Fig. 4).

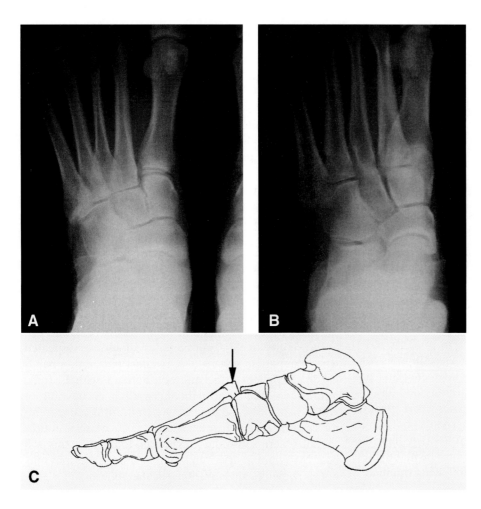

Figure 6 AP (**A**) and oblique (**B**) views of the foot denoting normal bone relationships. Note the medial border of the third metatarsal is contiguous with the medial border of the lateral cuneiform on the oblique view and the medial border of the second metatarsal is contiguous with the medial border of the second cuneiform on the AP view. There should not be more than 2 mm of "clear space" between the base of the second metatarsal and the adjacent border of the medial cuneiform on the AP view. **C**, Lateral view of the foot with a disrupted Lisfranc ligament. Note dorsal displacement of the second metatarsal (arrow).

## Treatment

Radiographs should be obtained when a midfoot injury is suspected. These views include AP, 30° medial oblique, and lateral views of the foot, and they should be at least partially weight bearing if the patient can bear weight. On the AP view (Fig. 6, *A*), the first TMT joint should be congruent with no "overhang" of the medial or lateral borders of the first metatarsal-medial cuneiform articulation. In addition, the medial aspect of the second metatarsal should be in continuity with the medial aspect of the middle cuneiform. On the oblique view (Fig. 6, *B*), the medial aspect of the fourth metatarsal should line up with the medial portion of the cuboid. On the lateral view (Fig. 6, *C*), there should be no dorsal subluxation of the metatarsals in relation to the cuneiforms, particularly the first and second metatarsals.

If symptoms persist in a patient who is unable to adequately bear weight during the initial examination, the patient should return in 10 to 14 days for another attempt at obtaining weight-bearing radiographs. A view of the contralateral foot also can be obtained when there is any question of abnormality on initial radiographs. Any subluxation of the metatarsals in relation to the cuneiforms should be interpreted as abnormal. When the injury is suspected but weight-bearing radiographs appear normal,

stress radiographs should be obtained with the patient under anesthesia. The forefoot is supinated and abducted and then pronated and adducted while the hindfoot is kept fixed, noting any abnormal widening or displacement of the TMT complex. Compression and distraction are applied to the metatarsals, particularly the first and second, to identify any displacement in the sagittal plane that may cause instability.

CT scanning can be helpful in preoperative planning for midfoot injuries with significant comminution or severe trauma. Axial cuts, which are reformatted in the sagittal and coronal planes, are used to determine the extent and degree of disruption to the joints of this complex (Fig. 7). Presence of the "fleck sign," an avulsion of bone off the base of the second metatarsal or medial cuneiform, should alert the physician that an injury to the ligamentous complex has occurred. MRI can accurately identify disruption of the Lisfranc ligament, but its usefulness is limited in acute injuries, and it does not replace radiography.

A dislocation or displaced fracture-dislocation of the TMT joint complex can be reduced and stabilized with an open or percutaneous technique. A percutaneous technique usually is easier when there is a pure dislocation and the midfoot can be easily reduced. In such instances,

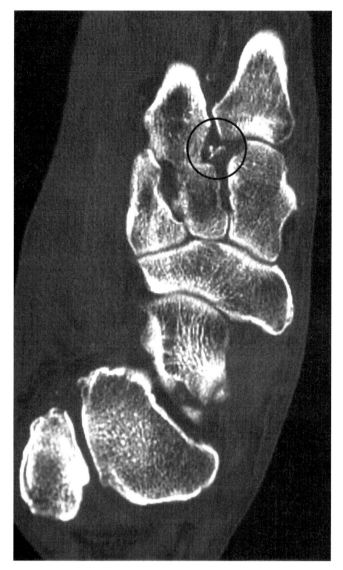

Figure 7   Note the presence of the "fleck sign," which is a bony fragment seen at the plantar medial base of the second metatarsal and represents a Lisfranc ligament avulsion (circle). Note also the subtle lateral subluxation of the second tarsometatarsal joint.

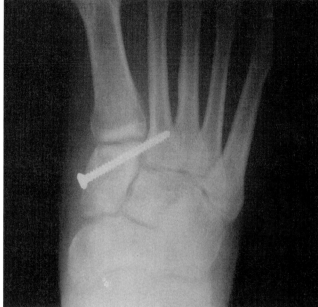

Figure 8   Percutaneously placed screw reducing the subluxation.

a reduction clamp is placed around either the second or third metatarsal base and about the medial cuneiform and is used for provisional fixation. After the anatomic reduction has been confirmed with fluoroscopy or radiography, cannulated screws are inserted percutaneously for fixation (Fig. 8).

Open reduction and fixation are indicated for articular comminution that prevents a reduction or an associated displaced fracture of the metatarsals that requires stabilization. The standard approach uses two longitudinal incisions on the dorsum of the foot (Fig. 9). The first incision is made over the first intermetatarsal space and extends proximal and distal to the TMT junction, allowing access to the first and second TMT joints. Care should be taken to protect the neurovascular structures, which lie immediately lateral to the incision. The second inci-

sion is made over the third intermetarsal space and permits access to the third and fourth TMT junction. Hematoma, clot debris, and nonosseous articular fragments that block reduction are removed from the joint space. A pointed reduction clamp is then placed around the second metatarsal base and medial cuneiform while the reduction is held and inspected radiographically. Once the reduction is acceptable, it is stabilized, preferably with screw fixation.

The use of Kirschner wires (K-wires) has been advocated in the past; however, there is a risk of loss of fixation if pin migration or breakage occurs and a risk of redisplacement after pin removal. Infection also is a concern with percutaneously placed wires. Screw fixation results in a more stable construct to allow ligamentous healing. Cortical screws (3.5 mm) can be placed in a noncompression ("set") mode for stabilization. The screws are placed across each unstable joint and from the medial cuneiform to the second metatarsal base, if possible. When the lateral metatarsal joint complex is involved, this column can be stabilized with smooth K-wires placed from the fourth and fifth metatarsals into the cuboid (Fig. 10). The K-wires are maintained for approximately 6 weeks and can be removed in an office setting. Another indication for the use of K-wires is severe comminution at the metatarsal bases that makes screw fixation impossible. Alternatively, a low-profile plate can be used to span the TMT joint with fixation from the metatarsal to the corresponding cuneiform.

Recently, bioabsorbable screws have been studied as an alternative method of fixation for these injuries. Bioabsorbable screws obviate the need for hardware removal, and the screw-holding strength and resistance to dis-

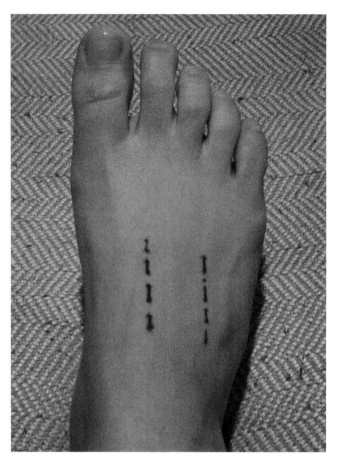

Figure 9  Two dorsal incisions may be used when an open approach is made.

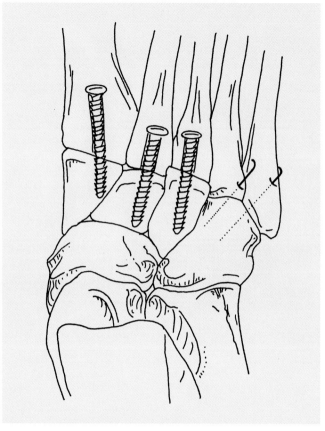

Figure 10  In situ fusion accomplished with individual screws placed across each affected joint.

placement appear to be equal to those of standard stainless steel screws. The disadvantage of bioabsorbable screws is that they may begin to degrade before ligamentous healing occurs.

Particular attention should be paid to the cuboid and lateral column, which may be injured when a significant abduction force is applied to the midfoot. This is best appreciated on a 30° medial oblique view of the foot. Congruity of the articular surface of the cuboid should be restored by elevating the articular fragments and restoring the "nutcracker" compressed cuboid with bone graft, if necessary. A cervical H-plate applied from either the calcaneus or cuboid to the metatarsals and spanning the cuboid-metatarsal junction can help maintain the length of the lateral column. However, this approach would necessitate hardware removal at a later date. Alternatively, a mini-external fixator can be applied, with half pins placed in the fifth metatarsal and calcaneus, and distraction applied to maintain length during the healing period.

As mentioned, a variety of segmental injury patterns can occur with injury to this complex, including disruption of the intercuneiform bones or the naviculocuneiform junction. The surgical approach should provide access to all of the injured joints of the foot. Articular disruption in this area can be treated with either stan-

dard internal fixation techniques or a spanning plate used as an internal distractor. Spanning plates must be removed after ligamentous and bony healing.

## Rehabilitation

Postoperatively, a splint is applied over a bulky soft dressing. The splint and dressing remain in place for 10 to 14 days. Subsequently, the splint is replaced by a short leg nonwalking cast, and the sutures are removed if appropriate. At 3 to 4 weeks, if the midfoot has been stabilized securely, a removable short leg boot cast can be applied, and range-of-motion exercises can be initiated. The patient should not bear weight for 6 to 8 weeks. At that time, protected weight bearing in a boot brace can begin, generally for an additional 6 weeks. The need for hardware removal is a subject of debate. However, it should be left in place for at least 4 months; in patients with purely ligamentous injury, 5 to 6 months of protected weight bearing is advised. Hardware removal is advocated for symptomatic individuals or those who hope to return to athletic activities.

## Outcome

There are few well-performed recent studies that document the long-term outcomes of treatment of injuries to the midtarsal joints. The prevalence of symptomatic degenerative changes after these injuries has been noted to be as high as 58%. The outcome following surgical intervention has been shown to be affected by the accuracy of reduction, with an anatomic reduction giving the best chance of a good or excellent result. Widening or displacement of more than 2 mm between the first and second metatarsal bases and more than 15° of malalignment about the TMT joints of the midfoot consistently result in a poor outcome for the patient. In contrast, factors such as age, injury pattern, the amount of trauma to the foot, and associated injuries have not been shown to affect treatment outcomes. Additionally, the results of one study suggest that purely ligamentous injuries have a worse outcome than osseous injuries, although this conclusion warrants further research.

## Neglected Midfoot Injuries and Failed Open Reduction and Internal Fixation

Given the relatively limited number of midfoot injuries and the varying degrees of severity (deformity may be very subtle), up to one third of these injuries may be missed and treatment neglected. Increased awareness of these injuries and their consequences should help reduce the number of missed or neglected midfoot injuries, and anatomic reduction and stabilization should be attempted. However, some patients develop degenerative changes about the midfoot despite appropriate reduction and fixation. If treatment is neglected, the risk of developing arthrosis is increased. Sequelae of midfoot injuries include painful degenerative changes about the midfoot, possibly associated with a flatfoot deformity.

When degenerative changes have developed, shoe modifications and orthotic treatment are appropriate for symptomatic individuals. Shoe modifications include a rocker-bottom shoe with a steel or fiberglass shank to limit the bending moment across the symptomatic joint complex. An accommodative orthotic device also can provide support and cushion the load that is applied to the midfoot during weight bearing.

Failure of conservative treatment may necessitate surgical intervention when symptoms persist. If the alignment of the TMT joint complex has been restored or has not been grossly disturbed, then an in situ fusion of the symptomatic joints is appropriate. In most cases, this involves the first, second, and/or third TMT joints and the respective intercuneiform articulations. Given the mobility of the lateral column, these joints rarely are symptomatic to the extent that orthotic and footwear modifications will not reduce symptoms to the patient's tolerance.

An in situ fusion of the symptomatic joints is performed through one or two dorsal longitudinal incisions strategically placed over the affected joints. The injured cartilaginous surfaces are removed, taking care not to resect too much bone. Individual screws are then placed across each affected joint. The most common technical error during fusion in this region is taking more bone dorsally than plantarly, thus resulting in metatarsals that are dorsally angulated after fixation. Angulation of the metatarsals should be avoided because it may result in lateral weight transfer with overload of the lateral column.

When the injury has been missed or neglected and the TMT joint complex is disorganized and displaced, a realignment arthrodesis should be done. Correction of the deformity has been shown to be the most important predictor of a successful outcome. Guidelines for the amount of displacement that requires this procedure are vague, but more than 15° of angulation of any joint articulation should be corrected. A preoperative CT scan in three planes can aid in the identification of the direction and magnitude of displacement of the metatarsals in relation to the cuneiforms and cuboid, as well as help assess the intercuneiform, navicular, and cuboid alignment.

Realignment can be achieved by (1) taking down the affected joints and repositioning them in an anatomic position (assuming the deformity and articular cartilage damage are minimal); (2) resecting a wedge of bone from each affected joint or from the entire midfoot/forefoot junction to create a reduction, which usually involves a biplanar joint osteotomy; and (3) inserting a tricortical iliac crest bone graft if there is significant shortening of the medial or lateral columns. To maximize improvement, it is essential that the alignment and length of the columns are restored.

Fixation of a midfoot arthrodesis or realignment can be obtained with individual screws in each joint or a plantar or medial plate. The fourth and fifth TMT joints are not commonly symptomatic after injury, given the significant motion at their articulations. If this area is symptomatic and surgical intervention is planned, it deserves special attention. Patients generally do not tolerate a fusion across the entire TMT joint complex. The symptomatic lateral column can be treated with resection hemiarthroplasty of the fourth and fifth TMT joints with or without tendon interposition.

## Metatarsal Fractures

### Isolated Metatarsal Fractures

Isolated metatarsal fractures usually are the result of an inversion injury, a direct blow, or repetitive stress. An isolated fifth metatarsal diaphyseal fracture, the so-called dancer's fracture, occurs when the ankle or hindfoot is inverted about the fixed forefoot. Isolated fractures of the remaining metatarsals are unusual with this mechanism, but a direct or crush injury may also be responsible for an isolated metatarsal fracture. In this case, attention must be paid to the soft tissues, and the presence of an underlying compartment syndrome must be ruled out. Stress fractures can occur in people who engage in repetitive weight-bearing exercises (for example, runners) or

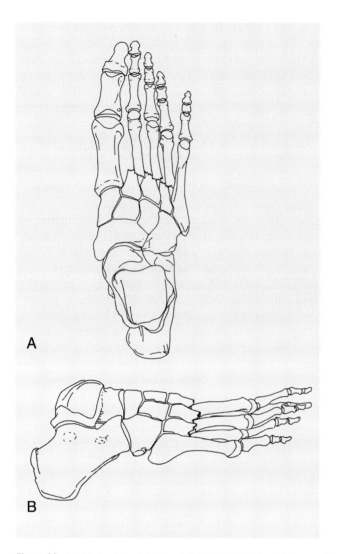

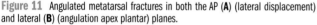

**Figure 11** Angulated metatarsal fractures in both the AP (**A**) (lateral displacement) and lateral (**B**) (angulation apex plantar) planes.

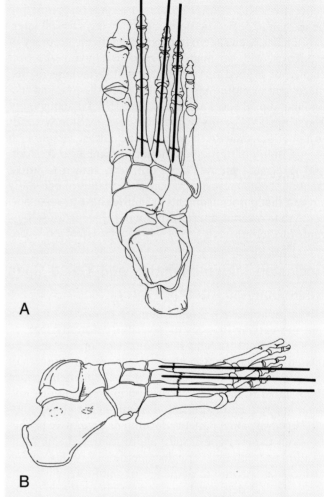

**Figure 12** Postfixation of displaced central metatarsals using Steinmann pins inserted retrograde distally and followed by proximal antegrade placement on AP (**A**) and lateral (**B**) views.

those who have an underlying loss of bone mineral density when the bone is repetitively overloaded and its ability to remodel has been exceeded.

Fractures of the metatarsals also can be categorized by location (ie, whether they occur at the metatarsal base, shaft, or neck). Nondisplaced fractures of the metatarsal base are treated with protected weight bearing and usually heal in 6 to 8 weeks. Fractures of the second or third metatarsal base with displacement of more than 3 to 4 mm should be treated with surgical intervention. This usually entails a closed reduction and pinning or an open approach if the reduction is inadequate. This fracture pattern should raise suspicion of an underlying injury to the TMT joint complex.

An isolated, nondisplaced, metatarsal shaft fracture usually is treated nonsurgically. If displaced, the degree of angulation, particularly in the sagittal plane, should be analyzed. Generally, angulation of less than 10° and displacement of no more than 3 to 4 mm is well tolerated

and successfully treated with protected weight bearing. The pull of the strong plantar flexors can result in displacement, particularly with more distal metatarsal fractures. Angulation in the sagittal plane should be inspected with medial and lateral oblique radiographs as well as AP and lateral orthogonal views (Fig. 11). Depending on the direction of angulation, displacement in the sagittal plane may result in either transfer metatarsalgia or increased plantar pressure beneath the head of the fractured metatarsal. If angulation exceeds these guidelines or the metatarsal head appears unduly prominent or impinges against an adjacent metatarsal head, reduction and stabilization are indicated. These fractures can be stabilized by antegrade advancement of a K-wire from the metatarsal head proximally across the fracture site with the toes held in dorsiflexion (Fig. 12). Alternatively, if an open incision is used, the pin can be advanced retrograde to exit under the proximal phalanx and then advanced antegrade across the fracture site. Most authors advocate passing the pin through a portion of the proximal phalangeal base during retrograde insertion of the pin and then advancing the K-wire as noted, which limits the degree of trauma and subsequent scarring of the plantar plate. However, a fracture of the first metatarsal should not be treated according to these guidelines because the first metatarsal carries approximately twice the load of the lesser metatarsals (one third of the body weight). As a result, any displacement can result in altered weight bearing and increased plantar pressures or transfer lesions. The unopposed pull of either the tibialis anterior or the peroneus longus tendon may cause late displacement if the base of the bone is fractured. During radiographic evaluation, malalignment of this metatarsal should be noted and fixation performed, if necessary.

Most isolated fractures of the metatarsal neck are treated nonsurgically, with surgical treatment reserved for fractures with significant angulation, particularly in the sagittal plane. Again, the pull of the plantar flexors acts as the main deforming force and can cause subsequent shortening and angulation.

Acute (ie, Jones) and stress fractures of the fifth metatarsal at the metaphyseal-diaphyseal junction can be particularly difficult fractures to treat. This area of the fifth metatarsal has a tenuous blood supply and is susceptible to delayed union and nonunion. Most authors recommend that patients do not bear weight for 6 to 8 weeks and frequent radiographs are obtained to assess healing progression. In high-performance athletes, percutaneous screw fixation for these fractures should be considered because they have a propensity for delayed union, nonunion, or recurrence.

### Multiple Metatarsal Fractures

Multiple metatarsal fractures imply instability and deformity and should be stabilized surgically (Fig. 12). Open reduction and internal fixation through a longitudinal incision over the affected metatarsals usually is required. Once length and angulation have been corrected, the fixation method depends on the degree of comminution and location of the fracture. Longitudinal K-wires can be used if there is minimal fragmentation of the metatarsal. A low-profile or mini-fragment plate can be used to maintain length.

## Phalangeal Fractures

Phalangeal fractures are the most common fractures of the forefoot and usually result from a crushing or axial load injury to the toe. An associated subungual hematoma may develop after this type of crush injury or after an object is dropped on the toe; if symptomatic, the hematoma should be evacuated through a small hole made in the toenail. These fractures should be examined for angulation or intra-articular involvement.

Proximal phalangeal fractures of the hallux, particularly at the metatarsophalangeal joint, should be careful-

ly assessed for any intra-articular involvement, and surgery performed if the fracture is displaced. A closed reduction can be attempted, and displaced fragments can be manipulated with a K-wire. If the reduction is adequate, the K-wire(s) can be used as definitive fixation. If necessary, a dorsal L-shaped incision can be made to expose the interphalangeal joint, taking care to remain proximal to the nail matrix. Fixation can include K-wires or mini-fragment screws to reduce the joint surface. Conversely, fractures involving the distal phalanx usually are treated conservatively with protected weight bearing as symptoms warrant. Joint incongruity and arthrofibrosis at the interphalangeal joint usually are well tolerated.

Fractures of the lesser toe phalanges usually are treated nonsurgically unless there is significant angulation or rotation. When there is a visible deformity, closed reduction with the patient under local anesthesia usually is successful. After reduction, the injured toe can be buddy-taped to the adjacent toe for 4 weeks.

## Summary

Avulsion fractures of the lip of the navicular usually can be treated conservatively, but displaced fractures of the tuberosity or body frequently require open reduction and screw fixation. Stress fractures of the navicular can be particularly difficult to diagnose and treat. Early recognition and treatment are essential for Lisfranc fracture-dislocations. Surgical reduction and stabilization, either percutaneous or open, often are required. Unrecognized and untreated midfoot injuries may require osteotomy or arthrodesis, or both, to realign the midfoot and hold it in position. Isolated metatarsal fractures usually can be treated nonsurgically, unless displacement is more than 3 to 4 mm and angulation in the sagittal plane is greater than 10°. Acute and stress fractures of the fifth metatarsal are prone to delayed union and nonunion, and percutaneous screw fixation may be indicated, especially in high-performance athletes. Fractures of the lesser toe phalanges generally can be treated with buddy-taping, and proximal phalangeal fractures of the hallux, if articular or grossly angulated, may require closed or open reduction and K-wire or mini-fragment screw fixation.

## Annotated Bibliography

### Navicular Fractures

Pinney SJ, Sangeorzan BJ: Fractures of the tarsal bones. *Orthop Clin North Am* 2001;32:21-33.
   A review of mechanisms of injury, evaluation, and treatment of cuboid, navicular, and cuneiform fractures is presented.

Richter M, Wippermann B, Krettek C, Schratt HE, Hufner T, Therman H: Fractures and fracture dislocations of the midfoot: Occurrence, causes and long-term results. *Foot Ankle Int* 2001;22:392-398.

Etiology and outcome of 155 patients with midfoot fractures were analyzed. Traffic accidents accounted for 72% of the injuries. Isolated midfoot fractures occurred in 35% of patients, Lisfranc fracture-dislocations in 31%, Chopart-Lisfranc dislocations in 17%, and Chopart fracture-dislocations in 16%. Regardless of age, gender, cause, time from injury to treatment, and method of treatment, the highest scores in all groups were those fractures treated with early open reduction and internal fixation.

## Cuboid and Cuneiform Injuries

Miller CM, Winter WB, Bucknell AC, Jonassen EA: Injuries to the midtarsal joint and lesser tarsal bones. *J Am Acad Orthop Surg* 1998;6:249-258.

A review of etiology, evaluation, and treatment of navicular, cuboid, and cuneiform fractures and dislocations is presented.

Weber M, Locher S: Reconstruction of the cuboid in compression fractures: Short to midterm results in 12 patients. *Foot Ankle Int* 2002;23:1008-1013.

In 12 patients with cuboid fractures, good results were obtained with open reduction using a distracting iliac external fixator and internal fixation. Symptoms after surgical treatment were caused primarily by associated midfoot injuries.

## Lisfranc Fractures

Chiodo CP, Myerson MS: Developments and advances in the diagnosis and treatment of injuries to the tarsometatarsal joint. *Orthop Clin North Am* 2001;32:11-20.

This article presents a review of the causes, classification, radiographic evaluation, and treatment of TMT joint injuries.

Mulier T, Reynders P, Dereymacker G, Broos P: Severe Lisfranc injuries: Primary arthrodesis or ORIF? *Foot Ankle Int* 2002;23:902-905.

Patients with severe, acute Lisfranc dislocations were treated with partial (5) or complete (6) arthrodesis or open reduction and internal fixation (16). The open reduction and internal fixation group and the partial arthrodesis group had less pain than those with complete arthrodesis. Stiffness of the forefoot, loss of metatarsal arch, and sympathetic dystrophy were more frequent in those with complete arthrodesis. Open reduction and internal fixation is recommended as the treatment of choice, with primary complete arthrodesis reserved as a salvage procedure.

Perugia D, Basile A, Battaglia A, Stopponi M, De Simeonibus AU: Fracture dislocations of Lisfranc's joint treated with closed reduction and percutaneous fixation. *Int Orthop* 2003;27:30-35.

At nearly 5-years follow-up of 42 patients, there were no significant differences in outcome scores between patients with perfect anatomic reductions and patients with near anatomic reductions; however, patients with combined fracture-dislocations had better scores than patients with pure dislocations.

Teng AL, Pinzur MS, Lomasney L, Mahoney L, Harvey R: Functional outcome following anatomic restoration of tarsal-metatarsal fracture dislocation. *Foot Ankle Int* 2002;23:922-926.

At 41-month follow-up of 11 patients with excellent radiographic results after surgical treatment of Lisfranc fracture-dislocations, objective measures of gait analysis were returned to normal but subjective patient outcomes were less than satisfactory.

Thordarson DB: Fractures of the midfoot and forefoot, in Myerson MS (ed): *Foot and Ankle Disorders*. Philadelphia, PA, WB Saunders, 2000, pp 1265-1296.

An in-depth discussion of evaluation, treatment, surgical technique, and outcomes of injuries to the midfoot and forefoot is presented.

Thordarson DB, Hurvitz G: PLA screw fixation of Lisfranc injuries. *Foot Ankle Int* 2002;23:1003-1007.

Lisfranc injuries in 14 patients were treated with open reduction and internal fixation with polylactic acid absorbable screws. No patient had a soft-tissue reaction to the screws, no osteolysis was seen on follow-up radiographs, and no loss of reduction occurred.

## Neglected Midfoot Injuries and Failed Open Reduction and Internal Fixation

Berlet GC, Anderson RB: Tendon arthroplasty for basal fourth and fifth metatarsal arthritis. *Foot Ankle Int* 2002; 23:440-446.

Of 12 patients requiring arthroplasty for painful arthrosis of the fourth and fifth metatarsal, arthrosis followed Lisfranc fractures in 6 and fractures of the base of the fifth metatarsal in 3. Intermediate-term results of this procedure showed high satisfaction rates and moderate pain relief.

Kuo RS, Tejwani NC, DiGiovanni CW, Holt SK, Benirschke SK, Hansen ST Jr: Outcome after open reduction and internal fixation of Lisfranc joint injuries. *J Bone Joint Surg Am* 2000;82:1609-1618.

At 52-month follow-up, 48 patients with purely ligamentous injuries had worse outcomes than those with ligamentous and osseous injuries. The major determinant of a good result was anatomic reduction.

## Metatarsal Fractures

Kelly IP, Glisson RR, Fink C, Easley ME, Nunley JA: Intramedullary screw fixation of Jones fractures. *Foot Ankle Int* 2001;22:585-589.

In this cadaver study, 6.5-mm screws used for stabilization of Jones fractures had significantly greater pull-out strength than 5-mm screws. Most fifth metatarsals can accommodate the larger screw.

Larson CM, Almekinders LC, Taft TN, Garret WE: Intramedullary screw fixation of Jones fractures: Analysis of failure. *Am J Sports Med* 2002;30:55-60.

Six failures occurred in 15 fractures (4 refractures and 2 symptomatic nonunions). More failures occurred in elite athletes who returned to full activity before complete radiographic union.

Shah SN, Knoblich GO, Lindsey DP, Dreshak J, Yerby SA, Chou LB: Intramedullary screw fixation of proximal fifth metatarsal fractures: A biomechanical study. *Foot Ankle Int* 2001;22:581-584.

This cadaver study found that initial failure loads and ultimate failure loads were not significantly different between fractures with 4.5-mm screws and those fixed with 5.5-mm screws.

Rosenberg GA, Sferra JJ: Treatment strategies for acute fractures and nonunions of the proximal fifth metatarsal. *J Am Acad Orthop Surg* 2000;8:332-338.

The rate of successful union of Jones fractures treated with non–weight-bearing cast immobilization is between 72% and 93%. Early intramedullary screw fixation is an accepted treatment option for high-performance athletes.

Wiener BD, Linder JF, Giattini JF: Treatment of fractures of the fifth metatarsal: A prospective study. *Foot Ankle Int* 1997;18:267-269.

Sixty avulsion fractures of the base of the fifth metatarsal were treated with a short leg cast or a soft (Jones) dressing. All fractures healed. The average length of recuperation was 33 days for those treated with a soft dressing and 46 days for those treated with a cast. The average modified foot score for those treated with a soft dressing was 92 (excellent) compared to 86 (good) for those treated with a short leg cast.

*Phalangeal Fractures*

Armagan OE, Shereff MJ: Injuries to the toes and metatarsals. *Orthop Clin North Am* 2001;32:1-9.

The review of etiology, evaluation, and treatment of metatarsal and phalangeal fractures are reviewed.

## Classic Bibliography

Arntz CT, Veith RG, Hansen ST: Fractures and fracture-dislocations of the tarsometatarsal joint. *J Bone Joint Surg Am* 1988;70:173-181.

DeLee JC, Evans JP, Julian J: Stress fracture of the fifth metatarsal. *Am J Sports Med* 1983;11:349-353.

Hardcastle PH, Reschauer R, Kutscha-Lissberg E, Schoffmann W: Injuries to the tarsometatarsal joint: Incidence, classification and treatment. *J Bone Joint Surg Br* 1982; 64:349-356.

Komenda GA, Myerson MS, Biddinger KR: Results of arthrodesis of the tarsometatarsal joint after traumatic injury. *J Bone Joint Surg Am* 1996;78:1665-1676.

Main BJ, Jowett RL: Injuries of the midtarsal joint. *J Bone Joint Surg Br* 1975;57:89-97.

Mann RA, Prieskorn D, Sobel M: Mid-tarsal and tarsometatarsal arthrodesis for primary degenerative osteoarthrosis or osteoarthrosis after trauma. *J Bone Joint Surg Am* 1996;78:1376-1385.

Myerson MS, Fisher RT, Burgess AR, Kenzora JE: Fracture dislocations of the tarsometatarsal joints: End results correlated with pathology and treatment. *Foot Ankle* 1986;6:225-242.

Sangeorzan BJ, Benirschke SK, Mosca V, Mayo K, Hansen ST Jr: Displaced intra-articular fractures of the tarsal navicular. *J Bone Joint Surg Am* 1989;71:1504-1510.

Sangeorzan BJ, Veith RG, Hansen ST Jr: Salvage of Lisfranc's tarsometatarsal joint by arthrodesis. *Foot Ankle* 1990;10:193-200.

Schenck RC Jr, Heckman JD: Fractures and dislocations of the forefoot: Operative and nonoperative treatment. *J Am Acad Orthop Surg* 1995;3:70-78.

Smith JW, Arnoczky SP, Herch A: The intraosseous blood supply of the fifth metatarsal: implications for proximal fracture healing. *Foot Ankle* 1992;13:143-152.

Torg JS, Balduini FC, Zelko RR, Pavlov H, Peff TC, Das M: Fractures of the base of the fifth metatarsal distal to the tuberosity: Classification and guidelines for nonsurgical and surgical management. *J Bone Joint Surg Am* 1984;66:209-214.

Torg JS, Pavlov H, Cooley LH, et al: Stress fractures of the tarsal navicular. *J Bone Joint Surg Am* 1982;64: 700-712.

# Section 3

# Reconstruction and Acquired Disorders

Section Editor:
Jeffrey E. Johnson, MD

## Chapter 7

# Lesser Toe Deformities, Freiberg's Infraction, and Bunionette Deformity

James J. Sferra, MD

## Introduction

Deformities of the lesser toes often are associated with deformities of the great toe, but many exist as isolated deformities. Although neuromuscular and congenital pathologies may contribute to lesser toe deformities, ill-fitting shoe wear coupled with the aging process is probably the leading cause.

## Lesser Toe Deformities

### Anatomy

The lesser toes contribute to balance and pressure distribution on the foot. Their positions and effectiveness depend on both passive and active stabilizers. Passive stabilizers include the plantar aponeurosis, plantar plate, joint capsule, and medial and lateral collateral ligaments. Active stabilizers include extrinsic muscles (extensor digitorum longus [EDL] and flexor digitorum longus [FDL]) and intrinsic muscles (flexor digitorum brevis [FDB], extensor digitorum brevis [EDB], interosseous, and lumbrical). The tibial nerve innervates the extrinsic flexor muscles, and the peroneal nerve innervates the extrinsic extensor muscles. The tibial nerve also innervates the intrinsic muscles through the medial and lateral plantar nerves.

On the dorsum of each toe, the EDL tendon forms three slips. The central slip inserts into the middle phalanx, and the other two merge into one tendon that inserts on the distal phalanx; the proximal phalanx has no significant direct tendon insertions. Through their pull on the extensor hood, the EDL and EDB tendons extend the metatarsophalangeal (MTP) joint, as well as the proximal interphalangeal (PIP) and distal interphalangeal (DIP) joints. On the plantar surface, the FDL courses deep to the FDB, which bifurcates and inserts into the middle phalanx. The FDL strongly flexes the DIP joint, while both the FDL and FDB flex the PIP and MTP joints. The lumbrical and interosseous tendons pass plantarly to the axis of motion of the MTP joint (thereby serv-

ing as plantar flexors of this joint) and via attachments to the extensor hood lie dorsal to the axis of motion of the PIP and DIP joints (thereby acting as extensors of these two joints). If this delicate balance between extrinsic and intrinsic forces is disrupted by weakness of either, deformities such as hammer toe or claw toe can result (Fig. 1).

A lesser toe deformity with a neurologic etiology is most often termed a claw toe deformity, with the primary pathology (hyperextension) being at the MTP joint and secondary deformity (flexion) at the PIP joint (Fig. 2). A repetitive PIP joint flexion deformity caused by a shoe that is too tight is called a hammer toe deformity (Fig. 3). Gradual attenuation of the plantar plate at the MTP joint or even a chronic tightness of the gastrocnemius-soleus complex with limitation of dorsiflexion at the ankle can exacerbate both hammer toe and claw toe deformities.

A mallet toe involves a contracture of the DIP joint in which the distal phalanx is flexed on the middle phalanx, with no deformity at the PIP or MTP joints (Fig. 4). This condition usually is caused by the attenuation of the terminal extensor tendons into the base of the distal phalanx with the unopposed FDL pulling the DIP joint into flexion.

### Physical Examination

Lesser toe deformities are typically symptomatic when the patient is wearing shoes. The flexed tips of the toes can develop painful corns (end corns) over the tuft of the distal phalanx just beneath the nail. The dorsal aspect of the PIP joint rubs against the toebox of the shoe, causing painful callosities or blisters. Any fixed extension contracture at the MTP joint can exacerbate symptoms; in patients with neuropathy, this can result in infection of soft tissues and bone. Hammer toes, claw toes, and mallet toes all begin as flexible deformities and with time can become rigid. During physical examination, the physician must assess the flexibility of the deformity to determine a treatment plan because surgical options vary based on whether the deformity is fixed or flexible (Fig. 5).

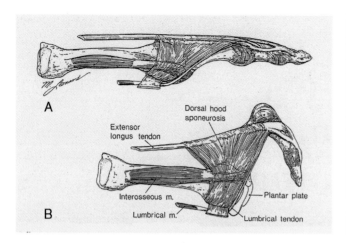

**Figure 1**  Anatomy of the intrinsic and extrinsic musculature in the normal foot (**A**) and in a foot with claw toe deformity (**B**). *(Reproduced with permission from Myerson M: Claw toes, crossover toe deformity, and instability of the second metatarsophalangeal joint, in Myerson M: Current Therapy in Foot and Ankle Surgery. St. Louis, MO, Mosby, 1993.)*

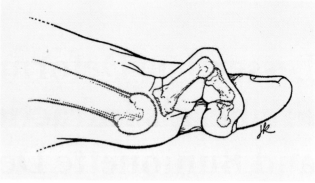

**Figure 2**  Claw toe deformity. *(Reproduced with permission from Alexander IJ: The Foot: Examination and Diagnosis, ed 2. New York, NY, Churchill Livingstone, 1997.)*

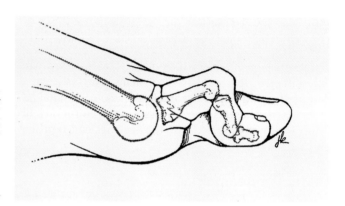

**Figure 3**  Hammer toe deformity. *(Reproduced with permission from Alexander IJ: The Foot: Examination and Diagnosis, ed 2. New York, NY, Churchill Livingstone, 1997.)*

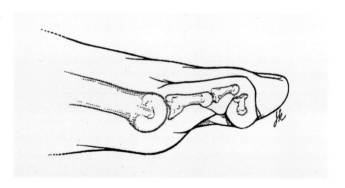

**Figure 4**  Mallet toe deformity. *(Reproduced with permission from Alexander IJ: The Foot: Examination and Diagnosis, ed 2. New York, NY, Churchill Livingstone, 1997.)*

In addition, it is important to determine whether a deformity of the first ray is present and, if so, which of the lesser toes is involved. With the patient bearing weight, a flexible deformity should correct at the MTP and PIP joints. Passive dorsiflexion of the ankle to a neutral position without the patient bearing weight should also lead to correction of a flexible deformity. If the deformity is rigid or fixed, bony resection and release of contracted tendons are required for correction. In flexible deformities, soft-tissue procedures alone may produce a satisfactory outcome. Bony procedures may be added to augment or stabilize the correction. The treatment alternatives vary with the primary and secondary causes of the deformity.

## Nonsurgical Treatment

Roomy, well-fitted shoes with a high toebox and a soft sole are the mainstay of first-line treatment. Shoes with high heels or pointed toes should be avoided. Crescent-shaped pads that loop around the toe and rest beneath the proximal phalanges of several toes help diminish toe-tip pressure. Foam or gel tubing applied to the end of the digit can provide a similar effect. Protective pads or sleeves over the dorsal aspect of the DIP or PIP joints diminish pressure from the toebox of the shoe. Metatarsal pads alone or with soft, accommodative custom inserts can apply forces to the plantar foot just proximal to the metatarsal heads. Pushing dorsally on the metatarsal (similar to the push-up test) helps relieve not only metatarsal head pain but also brings the proximal phalanx plantarward at the MTP joint, thereby reducing pressure on the metatarsal head. Manual stretching exercises can be used to treat flexible deformities and may also offer symptomatic improvement for small, fixed deformities. Nonetheless, the long-term effect of passive stretching remains unclear. Hammer toe slings attached to a metatar-sal pad and taping of the MTP joint toward a neutral position also can be beneficial.

The patient's age, activity level, occupation, and extent of deformity all contribute to the treatment plan. Many patients are unwilling to wear shoes that are wide with deep toeboxes. Others abandon the pads and corrective devices because they are too cumbersome or require shoes they find cosmetically unacceptable. Even with appropriate conservative treatment, surgical intervention may be required for deformity correction.

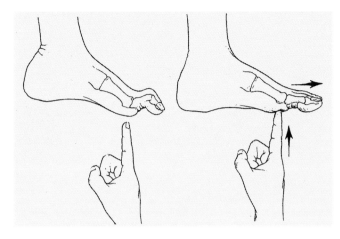

**Figure 5** "Push-up" test. With a flexible deformity, pushing up on the metatarsal heads straightens the toes. *(Reproduced with permission from Johnson KA: Surgery of the Foot and Ankle. New York, NY, Raven Press, 1989.)*

## Surgical Treatment

In general, surgical treatment of lesser toe deformities can produce satisfactory outcomes, but the potential for complications does exist and should be discussed with the patient at length preoperatively. The expectations of the patient and the surgeon, which often differ, must be clearly identified. Prolonged swelling and shortened, elongated, or stiff toes are common aftereffects of surgical treatment that may not be cosmetically acceptable to the patient. If a significant change in footwear is not made, deformities may recur.

Whether a deformity is flexible or fixed determines the extent of the surgical procedure; however, many surgeons do not see patients with lesser toe deformities until the deformities become rigid. Surgical correction requires a stepwise approach at each level of deformity. Postoperatively, the toe can be held in satisfactory position with a smooth Kirschner wire (K-wire) or with a dressing alone, depending on the surgeon's preference.

A flexible mallet toe, although rare, can be corrected by percutaneous release of the FDL. A rigid mallet toe, which is more common, can be corrected by release of the FDL tendon and removal of the distal condyles of the middle phalanx. The extensor tendon should also be repaired. If a K-wire is used to hold the toe in a satisfactory position, the K-wire should be removed 4 to 6 weeks after surgery.

Several surgical options are available to treat flexible hammer toe or claw toe deformities. Resection of a distal portion of the proximal phalanx and a tenotomy of the FDL tendon is one method. The tenotomy can be done percutaneously through a plantar approach or dorsally through the incision over the PIP joint. This technique usually allows a small amount of PIP joint motion and avoids a stiff, straight toe, which may drift in the frontal plane at the MTP joint and cause impingement symptoms on an adjacent toe. Another method, the Girdlestone-

Taylor transfer, involves transfer of the FDL tendon to the dorsum of the proximal phalanx to act as a checkrein to extension of the toe at the MTP joint. The FDL is percutaneously released from the distal phalanx and exposed at the plantar base of the toe. The tendon is then split into its medial and lateral segments along its raphe and each segment is tunneled along the medial and lateral sides of the proximal phalangeal base. On the dorsum of the phalanx, the two segments of the FDL are sutured to the extensor hood and to one another. The transferred FDL then acts as a plantar flexor of the MTP joint and an extensor of the PIP and DIP joints. As a result, the toe usually is straighter after surgery. Postoperative motion at the interphalangeal joints is minimal, but a functional degree of flexion and extension at the MTP joint usually is maintained. Modifications of the flexor-to-extensor transfer have been done, the most common of which combines the transfer with a PIP joint resection arthroplasty.

Rigid hammer toe and claw toe deformities require bony removal. The distal condyles of the proximal phalanx are resected just proximal to the metaphyseal flare but perpendicular to the shaft, and all sharp edges are smoothed. The FDL tendon is percutaneously released or is released through the resection site. A formal PIP fusion can be accomplished by removing cartilage and subchondral bone from the base of the middle phalanx and head of the proximal phalanx. Fusion of the PIP joint is most commonly used to correct severe deformity. A diaphysectomy of the proximal phalanx also can be used to treat severe deformity. The shortening of the phalanx functionally lengthens the taut tendons. On the other hand, resection of the proximal phalangeal base removes all intrinsic muscle and plantar plate stabilizing effect and often results in a shortened, unstable toe that is functionally and cosmetically unsatisfactory.

Correction of any MTP joint deformity should precede correction of PIP joint deformity. If correction of PIP joint deformity is done first, it often is difficult to grasp the digit when correcting the MTP joint deformity. Correcting MTP joint deformity first also allows for better assessment of which bony and soft-tissue procedure is required at the PIP joint. MTP joint deformity correction includes EDL Z-lengthening, EDB tenotomy, and dorsal capsulotomy. If the extension deformity has a fixed component with an intractable plantar keratosis (IPK), the medial and lateral collateral ligaments should be released. If a frank dislocation is present and still not reducible, a metatarsal head reshaping arthroplasty (DuVries arthroplasty) or a metatarsal shortening osteotomy should be done.

## Intractable Plantar Keratosis

An IPK is a painful callus on the sole of the foot caused by pressure of the metatarsal head on the plantar fat pad (Fig. 6). IPKs can be localized or diffuse. A diffuse IPK is caused by shear forces and is associated with systemic

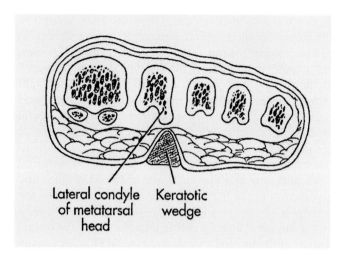

Figure 6   IPK can form under prominent lateral condyle of the metatarsal head. *(Reproduced with permission from Murphy GA: Lesser toe abnormalities, in Canale ST: Campbell's Operative Orthopaedics, ed 10. St. Louis, MO, Mosby, 2003.)*

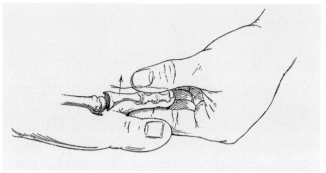

Figure 7   Test for instability of the MTP joint. Toe and metatarsal are stabilized and dorsal subluxation of the MTP joint is attempted. Normally minimal deviation is allowed, but with attenuation of the plantar plate little resistance to subluxation is present. *(Reproduced with permission from Myerson M: Claw toes, crossover toe deformity, and instability of the second metatarsophalangeal joint, in Myerson M: Current Therapy in Foot and Ankle Surgery. St. Louis, MO, Mosby, 1993.)*

diseases, biomechanical foot deformities, and fat pad atrophy. Initial treatment consists of callus shaving and the use of appropriate soft-soled flat shoes and inserts to cushion the area and alleviate stress. If satisfactory pain relief is not obtained, then surgery is indicated. When a discrete IPK lesion is present, a plantar exostectomy (removing bone mostly from the prominent plantar metatarsal condyle) is done. This can be added at the time of MTP release if there is an extension deformity at the MTP joint.

A diffuse IPK lesion is not caused by a prominent plantar condyle. Rather, the entire metatarsal head contributes to its formation as the result of an elongated metatarsal or a metatarsal in excessive plantar flexion. If nonsurgical treatment fails, DuVries arthroplasty or shortening and/or dorsiflexion osteotomies are most commonly recommended. In the DuVries arthroplasty, a portion of the distal articular surface is removed with an osteotome, and the head is reshaped with a rongeur and a rasp. Typically, this results in a painless, neutral MTP joint with a functional range of motion remaining (50% to 75%). The entire metatarsal head is never resected to prevent the development of transfer metatarsalgia. A variety of metatarsal osteotomies have been described, which can be done proximally, in the midshaft, or distally. Osteotomies result in shortening of the metatarsal, dorsiflexion of the distal weight-bearing segment, or both. DuVries arthroplasty and osteotomy both decrease plantar pressure, thus relieving IPK pain, but a transfer lesion may develop regardless of the success of the procedure for the symptomatic digits.

## Second Toe Abnormalities

Because of its position next to the hallux and the greater length and limited motion at the second tarsometatarsal joint, more patients report abnormalities of the second

toe both at the PIP and MTP joints than in the remaining three lesser toes. Many abnormalities of the second toe originate from the influence of the hallux, but other problems are caused by the greater stresses endured at this ray than the other lesser rays. An elongated second ray (Morton foot) combined with repetitive stresses at the second MTP joint induce a reactive synovitis. Repetitive injury of the plantar plate from buckling of the long second toe and chronic extension of the MTP attenuate the plantar plate. This attenuation of the plantar plate fosters deformity in the sagittal plane, and reactive synovitis with stretching of the capsuloligamentous apparatus of the MTP joint can cause frontal and axial plane deformities. Global instability of the second MTP joint may result with extension, medial deviation (crossover toe), and rotational components to the deformity. A pure sagittal plane deformity at this joint is less difficult to treat surgically than a multiplane deformity (crossover toe deformity). Instability of the plantar plate is evaluated by the drawer test applied in the sagittal plane (Fig. 7).

Activity modification usually is necessary to resolve synovitis. Avoiding shoes with a tight and narrow toebox is essential. Taping the second, third, and fourth toes together for 10 to 12 weeks, placing a metatarsal pad in the shoe to relieve pressure on the plantar plate, and wearing a shoe with a firm sole may prevent further synovitis and soft-tissue attenuation. Metatarsal bars on the soles of the shoes or a full-length rocker-bottom sole with a metal inlay are excellent means of relieving pressure at the second MTP joint, but these shoe modifications require the patient to wear sneakers or other laced shoes.

Dislocation of the second MTP joint most commonly occurs in association with long-standing hallux valgus, with the second toe crossing dorsal to the hallux (Fig. 8). Often the patient has a painful IPK beneath the second metatarsal head resulting from plantarly directed pressure applied by the dorsally dislocated proximal phalanx. A painful dorsal corn subsequently develops over the PIP

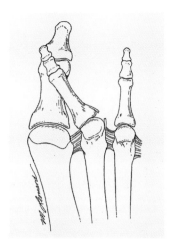

**Figure 8** Crossover toe deformity results from rupture of the lateral collateral ligament and volar plate and contracture of the medial collateral ligament. *(Reproduced with permission from Haddad SL, Sabbagh RC, Resch S, Myerson B, Myerson MS: Results of flexor-to-extensor and extensor brevis tendon transfer for correction of the crossover second toe deformity.* Foot Ankle Int *1999;20:781-788.)*

joint as a result of impingement on the toebox of the shoe. The nonsurgical treatments described for MTP subluxation, particularly use of a rocker-bottom sole, metalshank, or extra-depth shoe, are indicated initially but are generally not as successful in the treatment of dislocation as they are for subluxation.

If surgery is required and the MTP joint is not reducible, partial resection at the metatarsal head (DuVries arthroplasty) or a shortening osteotomy of the second metatarsal with relocation of the MTP joint is necessary. The short oblique distal metatarsal osteotomy is useful. The bony shortening relaxes the surrounding soft tissue, allowing reduction of the joint. This may, however, be associated with reduced MTP joint flexion. Deformities within the digit itself also are corrected with PIP resection arthroplasty, PIP fusion, or Girdlestone-Taylor tendon transfer. Vascular compromise of the digit can occur after correction of an MTP dislocation. After tourniquet release, reperfusion of the digit must be allowed. If vascular compromise persists, the K-wire from across the MTP joint is removed, along with the dressing, if necessary. If a tendon transfer was part of the procedure, this too may need to be released. Syndactylization of the second and third toes after resection of the head and neck of the proximal phalanx of the second toe may be done alternatively once the MTP joint is reduced. However, this procedure usually is reserved for revision surgery because it may result in third MTP joint subluxation or dislocation. In an elderly patient unable to find shoes to accommodate the deformity, a second toe amputation can achieve satisfactory results with faster recuperation.

When lateral or medial forces are applied to an irritated, unstable second MTP joint, a crossover toe results. If a hallux valgus deformity is already present, the crossover toe deformity proceeds rapidly. Conversely, a second digit subluxated and resting dorsal to a normally aligned hallux often is complicated by a rapidly developing hallux valgus deformity.

## Freiberg's Infraction

Freiberg's infraction or osteochondrosis of a lesser metatarsal head was first described in 1914. It typically involves the second metatarsal, but it can also involve the third or fourth metatarsals and most often occurs in teenage or young adult females. Frieberg's infraction initially was thought to develop secondary to trauma; however, many possible etiologies exist, including but not limited to microtrauma, hypercoagulability, increased intraosseous pressure, overload resulting from an elongated metatarsal, and forefoot surgery, all of which may predispose the subchondral bone to osteonecrosis and collapse.

A patient with Freiberg's infraction reports acute pain, swelling, and limitation of MTP joint motion. The pain is worse with weight-bearing activities. If osteonecrosis of the subchondral bone persists, secondary revascularization and repair occurs. The metatarsal head can collapse, become misshapen, and enlarge as the result of exostoses from both the metatarsal head and subsequently from the proximal phalanx base. Because it is not discernable from other causes of metatarsalgia early in the course of the disease and radiographs are generally normal at that time, Freiberg's infraction can be radiographically confirmed only later in the disease process.

Several radiographic classifications exist on which treatment modalities can be loosely based. Thompson and Hamilton described four stages of Freiberg's infraction based on the degree of vascular insult of the metatarsal head. In type I, no articular cartilage loss occurs, and the transient lesion heals. In type II, a large vascular insult is present, osteophytes develop, but the articular cartilage is preserved. Type III results in articular destruction along with proliferative degenerative changes. Type IV, a rare entity thought to be a form of epiphyseal dysplasia, also was included in their staging system. Katcherian devised a staging process for Freiberg's infraction that incorporates several previous classification systems, including that of Thompson and Hamilton. In Katcherian's classification, level A Freiberg's infraction exhibits a fissure developing through the epiphysis. Level B is a progression of the subchondral fracture and bone resorption. Level C demonstrates continued deformation with collapse of the central portion of the metatarsal head. Level D describes Freiberg's infraction when loose bodies around the head are present. Finally, level E represents the end stage of the disease. As the disease progresses with further metatarsal head involvement and collapse, greater deformity, stiffness, and exostoses develop.

In the acute phase, protective footwear with metatarsal pads or bars, anti-inflammatory medication, toe strapping, or possibly a steroid injection may alleviate symptoms. A walking cast that extends distal to the toes also may be helpful if worn for many weeks and followed by protective footwear for several months. If symptoms per-

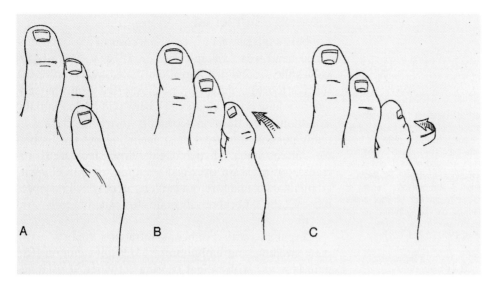

Figure 9 Rotational and angular deformities of the fifth toe. **A**, Congenital overlapping. **B**, Congenital underlapping. **C**, Primary rotary deformity. *(Reproduced with permission from Cooper PS: Disorders and deformities of the lesser toes, in Myerson MS: Foot and Ankle Disorders. Philadelphia, PA, WB Saunders, 2000.)*

sist and surgical intervention is required, MTP joint synovectomy and core decompression of the metatarsal head with a 0.045-inch K-wire are indicated if little or no deformity of the metatarsal head is present. However, if there is articular cartilage loss on the dorsum of the head and its overall shape remains intact, a dorsiflexion osteotomy at the metatarsal neck is done. If the metatarsal head is misshapen and joint motion is reduced, a synovectomy and metatarsal head cheilectomy are done. The cheilectomy incorporates removal of osteochondral fragments, débridement of areas of avascular bone, and resection of any osteophytes. The degeneration of articular cartilage and deformity of the metatarsal head may be so severe that partial resection of the metatarsal head is indicated (DuVries arthroplasty). If most of the deformity and degeneration are dorsal, a dorsiflexion osteotomy and removal of any dorsal osteophytes can be helpful. Basilar hemiphalangectomy results in an unstable MTP joint; therefore, this procedure should be avoided. Additionally, complete excision of the metatarsal head must not be done to avoid an unstable MTP joint and transfer metatarsalgia.

## Congenital Deformities of the Fifth Toe

Several unique deformities, such as underlapping, overlapping (varus fifth toe), and cock-up malpositions, occur in the fifth toe (Fig. 9). When the toe is dorsally subluxated at the fifth MTP joint, the digit does not participate in push-off during ambulation. This allows excessive pressure to be placed on the metatarsal head, resulting in a painful plantar metatarsal head callosity. When the fifth toe is in varus position and crossing under the fourth toe, it may also cause a painful callosity as well as a painful nail deformity over the tibial corner of the nail of the fifth toe. Two-boned fifth toes with no middle phalanx have a higher incidence of hard corn and hammer toe deformities at the only remaining interphalangeal joint.

An overlapping fifth toe in varus position and in extension at the MTP joint overrides the fourth toe and usually is familial and bilateral. Because the extensor tendons are short and there is a dorsomedial MTP capsular contracture, soft tissues are believed to play an important role in these deformities. In infancy, stretching and taping of the toe into a corrected position are attempted. If this fails, surgery is indicated. Surgery includes lengthening of the dorsal skin as well as the tendon of the EDL and release of the dorsal and medial MTP capsule. Lapidus described rerouting of the EDL tendon under the MTP joint to transfer it into the abductor digiti minimi for further restraint against recurrence. In older patients, bony resection is done in addition to the soft-tissue release and tendon lengthening and/or realignment.

Recurrence of the deformity to some degree is common, even with bony resection, Z-plasty of contracted skin, dermodesis of redundant skin, capsuloligamentous release, imbrication, and tendon lengthening and/or realignment. Syndactylization of the fifth toe or a Ruiz-Mora procedure can be used as salvage options.

Occasionally, the underlapping and overlapping toes may result from angular deformities within the phalanges themselves and not from soft-tissue tightness. This can be confirmed on radiographic evaluation. In a symptomatic adolescent patient, a closing wedge osteotomy through the offending phalanx can be done. After skeletal maturity is reached, resection arthroplasty at the PIP or DIP joint may be needed to correct the deformity. In a cock-up fifth toe, the deformity involves a rigid hammer toe and dorsiflexion at the MTP joint. This is primarily a uniplanar (sagittal plane) deformity. When mild to moderate, it is corrected as described previously for other lesser toes. If severe, the Ruiz-Mora procedure is used, which involves a total proximal phalangectomy through a plantar ellipse of skin. When the ellipse is closed, the dermodesis contributes to correction of the deformity. Re-

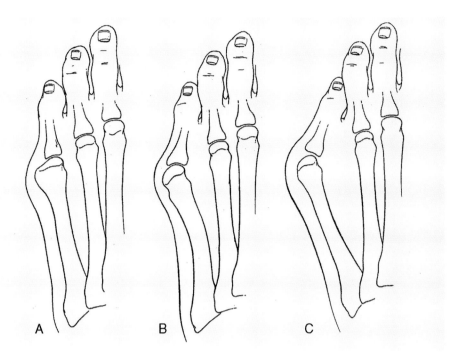

Figure 10 Types of bunionette deformities. **A**, Type I is associated with an enlarged head. **B**, Type II is associated with lateral bowing of the diaphysis. **C**, Type III is associated with increased lateral bowing of the diaphysis. *(Reproduced with permission from Cooper PS: Disorders and deformities of the lesser toes, in Myerson MS: Foot and Ankle Disorders. Philadelphia, PA, WB Saunders, 2000.)*

currence of the deformity, unsatisfactory cosmetic appearance, and even increased discomfort may result in the inability to convince patients that this procedure is justified.

## Bunionette Deformity

A bunionette or tailor's bunion is characterized by a prominence of the distal lateral aspect of the fifth metatarsal head. Most often, ill-fitting shoes compress the skin against the underlying bony prominence. Pain may result after chronic irritation of the overlying bursa or with the development of a hyperkeratosis, making shoe wear difficult.

Several anatomic variations of the fifth metatarsal have been documented and may lead to a bunionette deformity. The location of the deformity along the metatarsal often will dictate which treatment option is most appropriate. The deformity may be located at the metatarsal head or the metatarsal diaphysis or be the result of divergence of the fourth and fifth metatarsals. Bunionette deformities have been classified into three types based on anatomic variation (Fig. 10). Type 1 is an enlarged fifth metatarsal head, type 2 is a lateral bow within the fifth metatarsal, and type 3 is characterized by an abnormally wide 4-5 intermetatarsal angle (IMA) (a 4-5 IMA > 8° is abnormal). Most deformities include some degree of medial deviation of the fifth toes. The MTP-5 angle determines the degree of this deviation, which normally is less than 10°. When hallux valgus and an increased intermetatarsal 1-2 angle coexist, a splayfoot results.

The indication for treatment of a bunionette deformity is pain over the lateral condylar process of the fifth metatarsal. The prominent lateral process also may be associated with bursitis and intractable plantar, lateral, or plantar-lateral keratosis causing difficulty wearing most shoes. The initial treatment should be conservative, including the use of properly fitting shoes with a wider toebox and padding over the prominent metatarsal head. A metatarsal pad or custom orthotic also may be beneficial if the bunionette keratosis is plantar or is associated with pronation of the foot or pes planus (flatfoot). Conservative treatment is effective in most patients; however, failure to provide pain relief is an indication for surgical intervention.

Weight-bearing AP, lateral, and oblique radiographs of the foot should be obtained to determine the location of the deformity, to assess for arthrosis of the MTP joint, to determine the 4-5 IMA and MTP-5 angles and any subluxation of the fifth MTP joint. In symptomatic bunionettes, the 4-5 IMA and MTP-5 angle average greater than 10° and 16°, respectively.

Multiple surgical procedures have been described for treating bunionette deformity, including lateral metatarsal head condylectomy, distal metatarsal osteotomy, proximal osteotomy, diaphyseal osteotomy, and metatarsal head resection. The procedure chosen should be based on the anatomic and radiographic deformity. Proximal osteotomies can be used to treat bunionette deformity, but they are not recommended because the tenuous blood supply of the proximal metaphyseal-diaphyseal junction can lead to problems with delayed union or nonunion.

Lateral condylectomy alone is indicated when the deformity is caused by an enlarged lateral eminence and reactive bursa without a significant increase in the 4-5 IMA or lateral metatarsal bowing. This procedure has limited use but may be helpful in treating mild, localized deformities. The resection is done at the lateral margin of the articular surface parallel to the lateral border of the foot. Capsular reefing is necessary to prevent varus instability of the fifth toe. If the fifth toe deviates medially and passive alignment does not occur, then a medial capsular release through the MTP joint is required.

For longer-standing lateral eminence enlargement and soft-tissue irritation, resection of the prominent lateral process in conjunction with distal chevron osteotomy are indicated. A distal chevron osteotomy also is indicated for treatment of lateral bowing of the fifth metatarsal or a mild increase in the 4-5 IMA (< 12°). Because of the narrowness of the metatarsal head, stabilizing these osteotomies can be difficult; the medial shift of the fifth metatarsal head usually is limited to 2 or 3 mm, and the lateral overhanging of the proximal fragment can only be resected flush with the fifth metatarsal shaft. The osteotomy is held with a 0.045-inch K-wire for 4 to 6 weeks.

When a wide 4-5 IMA (> 12°) is present, a diaphyseal shaft osteotomy is indicated, which can correct larger deformities than can a distal osteotomy. If an IPK is associated with the deformity, the angle of the blade can be directed from a lateral-plantar direction to a medial-dorsal direction, which causes slight dorsiflexion of the metatarsal head as the distal fragment is displaced medially and internally fixed. A short leg cast is used for up to 6 weeks postoperatively, during part of which the patient should not bear weight, depending on the stability of the osteotomy after fixation.

Fifth metatarsal head resection is associated with an unacceptably high complication rate, including fifth toe retraction, transfer lesions, and malalignment of the fifth toe. Therefore, this procedure is rarely recommended. Head resection should be reserved as a salvage procedure for severe deformity, infection, and for patients with rheumatoid arthritis in whom multiple metatarsal heads are resected.

Complications associated with any procedures to correct lesser toe deformities are not uncommon and include delayed union, nonunion, malunion, MTP joint subluxation, transfer metatarsalgia, and recurrence of the deformity. These complications can be minimized by using careful preoperative planning and patient selection.

## Summary

Deformities of the lesser toes can cause significant pain and discomfort. They may be caused by several intrinsic or extrinsic factors, including inflammatory arthritis, trauma, congenital abnormalities, neuromuscular disorders, and poorly fitting shoes. Goals of treatment of lesser toe deformities are to restore function, alleviate pain, and allow a reasonable variety of footwear. Surgical treatment may require a combination of bony and soft-tissue procedures.

## Annotated Bibliography

### Lesser Toe Deformities

Coughlin MJ: Lesser toe abnormalities. *Instr Course Lect* 2003;52:421-444.
Identification of the etiology of the lesser toe deformity is necessary to determine whether conservative or surgical treatment is warranted and possibly halt progression of the deformity.

Edwards WHB, Beischer AD: Interphalangeal joint arthrodesis of the lesser toes. *Foot Ankle Clin North Am* 2002;7:43-48.
Interphalangeal joint fusion is used to treat lesser toe deformities including claw toe, hammer toe, and mallet toe. Using this procedure alone with consideration of the complete foot deformity and muscle imbalance can compromise the outcome of surgery. Alternative or adjunctive procedures that should be considered include flexor-to-extensor tendon transfer, MTP joint release, and metatarsal shortening or realignment osteotomy.

Femino JE, Mueller K: Complications of lesser toe surgery. *Clin Orthop* 2001;391:72-78.
Complications associated with lesser toe surgery include recurrence of the deformity, malunion and nonunion of osteotomies and arthrodeses, and stiffness and limitation of motion. Common complications are discussed, and recommendations are given for avoiding complications.

Marks RM: Anatomy and pathophysiology of lesser toe deformities. *Foot Ankle Clin* 1998;3:199-214.
This article describes normal and abnormal lesser toe anatomy, the effect of contributing causes, and the pathophysiologic changes they entail.

Richardson EG: Lesser toe deformities: An overview. *Foot Ankle Clin* 1998;3:195-198.
The goals of treatment of lesser toe deformities are to restore function to the lesser toes, alleviate pain, and allow a reasonable variety of footwear. Careful evaluation and treatment choices make these goals obtainable in most patients.

### Second Toe Abnormalities

Coughlin MJ, Dorris J, Polk E: Operative repair of the fixed hammertoe deformity. *Foot Ankle Int* 2000;21:94-104.
At an average 61-month follow-up of PIP resection arthroplasty for fixed hammer toe deformity, 86% of 118 toes were subjectively rated as being in acceptable alignment and 79% had good radiographic alignment, 92% of patients reported pain relief, and 84% were satisfied with their results.

Deland JT, Sung IH: The medial crossover toe: A cadaveric dissection. *Foot Ankle Int* 2000;21:375-378.
Dissection revealed medial displacement of the flexor tendons and plantar plate along with deformity of the plate itself,

in addition to contracture of the medial collateral ligaments and rupture of the lateral collateral ligaments. These findings help explain the difficulty in obtaining long-term correction with a soft-tissue procedure alone.

Dhukaram V, Hossain S, Sampath J, Barrie JL: Correction of hammer toe with an extended release of the metatarsophalangel joint. *J Bone Joint Surg Br* 2002;84:986-990.

MTP soft-tissue release and PIP arthroplasty were used to treat 84 patients (179 toes) with hammer toe deformities. At an average follow-up of 28 months, 87% were satisfied with their results and 17% were dissatisfied. Pain at the MTP joint was the most common cause of dissatisfaction; 14% had moderate or severe pain.

Feeney MS, Williams RL, Stephens MM: Selective lengthening of the proximal flexor tendon in the management of acquired claw toes. *J Bone Joint Surg Br* 2001;83:335-338.

Acquired claw toe deformities in 10 adults were successfully corrected by lengthening of the flexor hallucis longus and flexor digitorum longus alone or in combination.

Haddad SL, Sabbagh RC, Resch S, Myerson B, Myerson MS: Results of flexor-to-extensor and extensor brevis tendon transfer for correction of the crossover second toe deformity. *Foot Ankle Int* 1999;20:781-788.

After review of treatment of 35 feet with crossover toe deformities, the authors concluded that extensor brevis tendon transfer is appropriate for stages 1 and 2 and flexible stage 3 deformities, whereas flexor-to-extensor transfer is appropriate for rigid stage 3 and stage 4 deformities and all patients with symptomatic neuromas of the second web space.

Murphy GA: Mallet toe deformity. *Foot Ankle Clin* 1998; 3:279-292.

The anatomy, cause, epidemiology, and treatment of this problem are explored, and practical conservative techniques and a variety of surgical procedures are described.

Padanilam TG: The flexible hammer toe: Flexor-to-extensor transfer. *Foot Ankle Clin* 1998;3:259-268.

This article discusses the use of the flexor tendon-to-extensor transfer for the treatment of flexible hammer toe deformity. The surgical technique and a review of the literature are included.

Sands AK, Byck DC: Idiopathic clawed toes. *Foot Ankle Clin* 1998;3:245-258.

Toe deformity often leads to skin compromise with resultant pain, ulcers, infection, and amputation. Correction involves straightening the toes and changing the forces acting on them.

Weinfeld SB: Evaluation and management of crossover second toe deformity. *Foot Ankle Clin* 1998;3:215-228.

Surgical treatment often is necessary for crossover second toe deformity and consists of correction of the PIP joint contracture, as well as release of the tight dorsomedial structures and reefing of the lateral side of the MTP joint.

## Freiberg's Infraction

Chao KH, Lee CH, Lin LC: Surgery for symptomatic Freiberg's disease: Extraarticular dorsal closing-wedge osteotomy in 13 patients followed for 2-4 years. *Acta Orthop Scand* 1999;7:483-486.

Thirteen patients with Freiberg's disease were treated with débridement and dorsal closing wedge osteotomy of the metatarsal neck. The lesion was located in the second metatarsal head in 10 patients and in the third metatarsal head in three patients. After osteotomy, the lesion was away from the joint, so that the smooth and healthy articular cartilage of the metatarsal head faced the phalangeal cartilage. The average follow-up period was 40 months (range, 28 to 54 months). The subjective outcome was good or excellent in 11 patients, fair in one, and poor in one. MRI was useful in determining the extent of the lesion when planning correction.

Katcherian DA: Treatment of Freiberg's disease. *Foot Ankle Clin* 1998;3:323-344.

Dorsiflexion osteotomy of the metatarsal head is presented as a technique that is simple, reliable, and capable of obtaining good results regardless of the stage of the disease.

## Congenital Deformities of the Fifth Toe

Denore LT: The congenital, overlapping fifth toe. *Foot Ankle Clin* 1998;3:313-322.

This article describes the anatomy, epidemiology, and surgical and nonsurgical treatments of this condition.

de Palma L, Zanoli G: Zanoli's procedure for overlapping fifth toe: Retrospective study of 18 cases followed for 4-17 years. *Acta Orthop Scand* 1998;69:505-507.

In 16 patients (23 feet) treated with Zanoli's procedure (tenodesis using the extensor tendon of the fifth toe), pain relief was achieved in all patients. Although three toes were overcorrected as the result of technical errors and were considered unsatisfactory by objective criteria, all patients were satisfied with the results and would advise other patients to undergo the same operation.

Dyal CM, Davis WH, Thompson FM, Elonar SK: Clinical evaluation of the Ruiz-Mora procedure: Long-term follow-up. *Foot Ankle Int* 1997;18:94-97.

In 12 patients in whom the Ruiz-Mora procedure was done, most were satisfied with the results of the procedure. Unacceptable cosmesis was the primary complaint of all dissatisfied patients. Assessment of preoperative and postoperative symptoms indicated an improvement in symptoms as well as maintenance of stability and function at 4-year follow-up. Because of patient dissatisfaction with cosmesis, consideration should be given to showing patients postoperative photographs of the procedure before surgery and reserving this procedure for salvage of iatrogenic cock-up deformities, recalcitrant hard corns, and congenital cock-up deformities.

Thordarson DB: Congenital crossover fifth toe correction with soft tissue release and cutaneous Z-plasty. *Foot Ankle Int* 2001;22:511-512.

The results of three patients treated with MTP capsular release dorsally and medially, oblique lengthening of the extensor tendon, and Z-plasty of the skin are reported. At an average 33-month follow-up, no recurrences were noted with this simple procedure.

### Bunionette Deformity

Koti M, Maffulli N: Bunionette. *J Bone Joint Surg Am* 2001;83:1076-1082.

Surgical management to decrease the width of the foot and the osseous prominence is indicated when nonsurgical treatment does not control symptoms and when the patient has special demands, particularly in sports. A proximal osteotomy is able to correct most deformities. A distal osteotomy is recommended if medial translation of the head for one third of the width of the metatarsal shaft produces a normal 4-5 IMA.

Okuda R, Kinoshita M, Morikawa J, Jotoku T, Abe M: Proximal dome-shaped osteotomy for symptomatic bunionette. *Clin Orthop* 2002;396:173-178.

At an average follow-up of 30 months after proximal dome-shaped osteotomy in 10 feet with symptomatic bunionette deformities, all eight patients reported pain relief and satisfaction with the results of their surgery. The overall results were good in all 10 feet, although three had delayed union of the osteotomy.

## Classic Bibliography

Conklin MJ, Smith RW: Treatment of atypical lesser toe deformity with basal hemiphalangectomy. *Foot Ankle Int* 1994;14:585-594.

Coughlin MJ: Crossover second toe deformity. *Foot Ankle* 1987;8:29-39.

Coughlin MJ: Operative repair of the mallet toe deformity. *Foot Ankle Int* 1995;16:109-116.

Fortin PT, Myerson MS: Second metatarsophalangeal joint instability. *Foot Ankle Int* 1994;16:306-313.

Freiberg A: Infraction of the second metatarsal bone: A typical injury. *Surg Gynecol Obstet* 1914;19:191-193.

Katcherian DA: Treatment of Freiberg's disease. *Orthop Clin North Am* 1994;25:69-81.

Kinnard P, Lirette R: Freiberg's disease and dorsiflexion osteotomy. *J Bone Joint Surg Br* 1991;73:864-865.

Kitaoka HB, Holiday AD Jr, Campbell DC II: Distal chevron metatarsal osteotomy for bunionette. *Foot Ankle* 1991;12:80-85.

Kitaoka HB, Holiday AD Jr, Campbell DC II: Metatarsal head resection for bunionette: Long-term follow-up. *Foot Ankle* 1991;11:345-349.

Lapidus PW: Transplantation of extensor tendon for correction of overlapping fifth toe. *J Bone Joint Surg* 1942;24:555-560.

Lehman D, Smith R: Treatment of symptomatic hammertoe with a proximal interphalangeal joint arthrodesis. *Foot Ankle Int* 1995;16:535-541.

Mizel MS, Yodlowski ML: Disorders of the lesser metatarsophalangeal joints. *J Am Acad Orthop Surg* 1995;3:166-173.

Myerson M, Shereff M: The pathologic anatomy of claw and hammertoes. *J Bone Joint Surg Am* 1989;71:45-49.

Newman RJ, Fitton JM: An evaluation of operative procedures in the treatment of hammer toe. *Acta Orthop Scand* 1979;50:709-712.

Ruiz-Mora J: Plastic correction of overriding fifth toe. *Orthop Letter Club* 1954;6:6.

Sarrafin SK: Correction of fixed hammer toe deformity with resection of the head of the proximal phalanx and extensor tendon tenodesis. *Foot Ankle Int* 1995;16:447-451.

Thompson F, Hamilton W: Problems of the second metatarsophalangeal joint. *Orthopedics* 1987;10:83-89.

# Chapter 8

# Acute and Chronic Tendon Injury

Christopher P. Chiodo, MD

## Introduction

Although the foot is sometimes referred to as a pedestal, even the most cursory review of its complex articulations proves this to be an understatement. The graceful motion these articulations allow is controlled largely by the tendons that cross the ankle. Not surprisingly, an injury to one of these tendons can be debilitating. Optimal treatment begins with a firm grasp of relevant anatomy and the establishment of an accurate diagnosis. Tendon injuries in the foot and ankle can also be classified as acute or chronic. This further aids in defining the nature and appropriate treatment of each particular injury. Beyond this, one must remain abreast of treatment advances and refinements, especially with regard to surgical technique.

## Peroneal Tendons

Originating primarily from the lateral fibula, the peroneus brevis (PB) and peroneus longus (PL) muscles are the main evertors of the hindfoot and help to dynamically maintain the alignment of both the heel and medial longitudinal arch. In the lower leg, the peroneal tendons descend first laterally and then posteriorly to the fibula. At the level of the ankle joint, the posterior fibula usually becomes concave and forms a retromalleolar sulcus in which the peroneal tendons travel. This sulcus, also referred to as the fibular groove, plays an important role in stabilizing the tendons and is further deepened by a fibrocartilaginous rim on the posterolateral ridge of the fibula. In 18% to 28% of individuals, the posterior fibula is flat or convex. The superior peroneal retinaculum (SPR) covers the fibular groove and is equally important to the stability of the tendons. The SPR originates from the posterolateral ridge of the fibula and inserts onto the lateral calcaneus and/or the anterior sheath of the Achilles tendon. It can vary significantly in size, shape, and tissue quality.

Distal to the fibula, the peroneal tendons course over the lateral calcaneus and are usually separated by the peroneal tubercle. The PB tendon inserts onto the base of the fifth metatarsal. The PL tendon, however, has a more tortuous course. In the region of the calcaneocuboid joint,

the PL tendon makes nearly a 90° turn toward the medial aspect of the foot. In this region, a fibrocartilaginous or osseous sesamoid is present within the substance of the tendon. When calcified (5% to 20%), this structure is referred to as an os peroneum. The PL tendon then crosses the plantar surface of the foot to insert onto the first metatarsal base and medial cuneiform.

Two clinically significant variations in the normal anatomy of the peroneal tendons are worth noting. An anomalous peroneus quartus muscle has an incidence of 10% to 20% and most commonly originates from the PB muscle. Distally, it can crowd the fibro-osseous tunnel through which the peroneal tendons travel and thereby cause pain, attenuation of the SPR, and tendon subluxation. A peroneus quartus tendon can also be confused with split tears of the PB tendon. Another important anatomic variation of the peroneal musculature is the presence of a low-lying PB muscle belly, which may also crowd the fibular groove and result in tendon instability.

### Acute Injury

Complete traumatic ruptures of the peroneal tendons are rare, and most probably occur in tendons with degeneration or inflammation. Traumatic ruptures have been reported in healthy athletes, in whom successful results have been obtained with primary repair.

Many acute peroneal tendon injuries, however, are subluxations or dislocations rather than ruptures. Because these injuries can occur alone or in combination with lateral ligament sprains, acute peroneal tendon subluxation can mimic lateral ligament sprains and may be initially misdiagnosed.

The mechanism of acute peroneal tendon subluxation is usually a violent, reflexive contraction of the tendons. This creates an anteriorly directed force that commonly causes an avulsion of the SPR from its anterior attachment on the lateral fibula or, in rare instances, a rupture of the SPR itself. The types of injury associated with the position of the foot at the time of injury (ie, inverted or everted) are controversial, but dorsiflexion of the ankle is constant. The frequency of peroneal tendon subluxations in skiers (that is, when the tips of the skis dig into

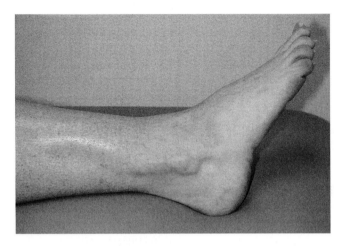

**Figure 1** Persistent anterior displacement of the peroneal tendons following an ankle injury.

the snow) supports the role of sudden ankle dorsiflexion as a mechanism of injury on the fixed, inverted or everted foot. Regardless of the position of the ankle or hindfoot, forceful contraction of the tendons seems to be necessary for subluxation or dislocation to occur.

Clinically, patients feel or hear a pop in the injured ankle and are usually unable to continue with physical activity. Some patients may even report the sensation of tendon dislocation followed by spontaneous reduction. Lateral ankle swelling and ecchymosis are present. In some patients, the tendons can be detected anterior to the fibula (Fig. 1); however, in most patients, spontaneous reduction of the tendons will have occurred. The diagnosis of acute peroneal tendon subluxation or dislocation is difficult and often missed. Strength testing may be painful, but results are usually good to excellent. Two provocative maneuvers can be used to elicit subluxation of the peroneal tendons. In one, the patient everts and then actively dorsiflexes the ankle from a plantar flexed position. In the other, the examiner holds one finger over the tendons at the level of the fibular groove and asks the patient to roll the ankle in a circular motion. With both maneuvers, the contralateral ankle should always be examined because subtle subluxation may be present normally.

Eckert and Davis developed a classification system for acute peroneal dislocations. In grade I injuries, the anterior attachment of the SPR, along with a cuff of periosteum, is avulsed from the fibula. In grade II injuries, the fibrocartilaginous rim that lines the posterolateral fibula is avulsed along with the SPR. In grade III injuries, a small fragment of bone is also avulsed. This is known as the fleck sign and is highly suggestive of peroneal tendon subluxation or dislocation.

Nonsurgical management of acute peroneal instability has had limited success. With both compressive dressings and cast immobilization, the success rate in most published series has not exceeded 50%. For this reason,

closed management of these injuries should probably be reserved for patients with low functional demands and those opposed to or unable to tolerate surgery.

Given the unreliable results of closed management, the surgical repair of acute peroneal tendon dislocations is now generally recommended, especially for active individuals who wish to return to their preinjury level of function. The surgical procedure is tailored to the nature of the pathology encountered at the time of surgery. If the SPR is avulsed alone without a rim of cartilage or bone, it can be incised and imbricated either to itself or to the fibula through drill holes. Similarly, an avulsed rim of fibrocartilage can be attached with drill holes through the fibula. An avulsed rim of fibular bone usually can be reduced and fixed using sutures.

### Chronic Injury

Chronic injuries of the peroneal tendons most often involve the PB tendon and can be classified as tendinosis, longitudinal split tears, or chronic instability. These conditions may exist in isolation but usually form a continuum. Cadaveric and imaging studies have indicated that chronic tears of the PB tendon begin with attenuation and incompetence of the SPR. This, in turn, leads to subluxation of the ribbon-like PB tendon over the sharp, posterolateral ridge of the fibula. When combined with the repetitive compressive forces exerted by the PL tendon, tendinosis or longitudinal split tears of the PB tendon develop. This sequence of events is thought to be more likely with a shallow or convex fibular groove. A recent clinical series, the largest to date, also supports this pathophysiologic mechanism. Of 20 patients who underwent surgery for chronic PB tendon tears, 19 had demonstrable peroneal tendon subluxation intraoperatively. Eight patients also had deficient fibular grooves.

Vascular supply may also play a role in the development of chronic peroneal tendon injuries. Although a perfusion study using India ink injections failed to demonstrate a hypovascular region in the peroneal tendons, a more recent immunohistochemical study using antilaminin antibodies suggested that there is an avascular zone in the PB tendon at the level of the fibular groove.

Clinically, the peroneal tunnel compression test may be useful to distinguish PB tendon split tears from other causes of lateral ankle pain. With this test, the patient sits with the knee bent over the edge of the examination table while the examiner's thumb is held firmly over the SPR. The patient then actively moves the foot from a plantar flexed inverted position to a dorsiflexed everted position. Reproduction of the patient's pain is considered a positive test result.

MRI evaluation of chronic peroneal tendon injuries has become increasingly useful in establishing an accurate diagnosis in patients with lateral ankle pain. Typically, split tears are seen as linear clefts and irregularities of the tendon contour. In addition, the PB tendon often

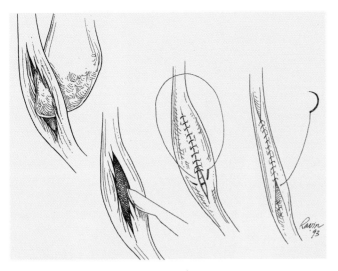

**Figure 2**  Technique for surgical débridement and repair of longitudinal split tears of the PB tendon.

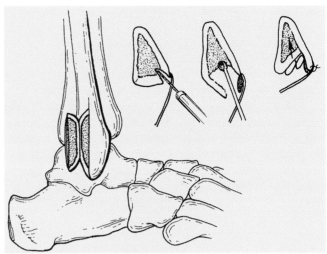

**Figure 3**  Technique for peroneal groove deepening through decancellization of the fibula.

can be seen wrapping around the PL tendon. Signal change within the tendon is best seen on proton density-weighted and T2-weighted images. MRI is also useful for detecting pathologic conditions associated with peroneal tears and other intra-articular or extra-articular pathology. In a recent study, a flat or irregular fibular groove was seen in 15 of 31 MRI scans of patients with PB tendon tears.

Nonsurgical therapy remains the first line of treatment for chronic peroneal tendinosis and split tears. Beneficial modalities include anti-inflammatory medications, braces, physical therapy, rest, and immobilization. If symptoms persist, surgical exploration is recommended. At exploration, both the PB and PL tendons should be closely inspected. Split tears of the PL tendon, although less common than PB tendon tears, should be débrided or repaired. Tears of the PB tendon are almost always longitudinal split tears. When the tear is centrally located in the tendon, the frayed edges of the tear should be débrided and the remaining tendon tubularized with an absorbable suture of 3-0 or 4-0 density. If the tear is peripheral, up to 50% of the outer tendon can be resected. Finally, if severe fraying involves most of the tendon, the degenerative segment can be excised and the proximal and distal ends tenodesed to the PL tendon (Fig. 2).

Given the recent advances in understanding the pathophysiology of chronic peroneal tendon tears, it is now recommended that any underlying anatomic anomalies be corrected at the time of surgery. The concept of tendon stability should remain paramount. The SPR must be closely inspected, and, if attenuated, imbricated either in a pants-over-vest fashion or through drill holes in the posterolateral fibula. A peroneus quartus should be excised; a low-lying PB muscle should be reduced in size. Finally, a flat or convex fibular groove should be deepened.

Three methods for deepening the fibular groove have been described. In the sliding bone-block technique, an osteotomy is used to translate or rotate a segment of the lateral fibula posteriorly over the peroneal tendons. This technique, however, is technically demanding. One series reported a 31% complication rate, including fractures of the graft and malleolus and intra-articular screw placement, and more than 42% of patients complained of painful hardware. The fibular groove can also be deepened by decancellization of the fibula. With this technique, an osteotome or small saw is used to create a rectangular corticotomy in the posterior fibula. A trapdoor is then elevated on a posteromedial hinge and the underlying cancellous bone is excised with either a burr or curet. The trapdoor is then replaced and recessed into the resulting defect, thus deepening the groove (Fig. 3). When using a decancellization technique to deepen the fibular groove, two technical considerations should be kept in mind. First, the groove should not be excessively deepened because this can result in cortical irregularities that can irritate the tendons. Second, the posteromedial hinge can fracture if not accurately cut and gently handled. A recently described technique for deepening the fibular groove involves the use of a 4.5- to 5.0-mm drill bit to decancellize the fibula and then impact the posterior surface into the defect in the fibula.

In addition to a shallow fibular groove, malalignment of the hindfoot and forefoot may contribute to the development of chronic peroneal tendon pathology. In some patients, hindfoot varus may need to be corrected with either a lateral displacement or closing wedge calcaneal osteotomy. Similarly, a plantar flexed first ray associated with hindfoot varus can be corrected with a dorsiflexion osteotomy of the first metatarsal.

Ankle instability should also be considered and, if necessary, surgically addressed in patients with chronic peroneal tendon injuries. One recent series reported 18 instances in which split lesions of the PB tendon were associated with chronic ankle instability. The authors speculated that ankle laxity may contribute to such lesions and warned that residual pain after ligamentous repair may be caused by an untreated peroneal injury.

Although peroneal instability and split tears of the PB tendon often coexist, a subset of patients have chronic instability in the absence of split tears. These are frequently patients with traumatic subluxations or dislocations that were either undiagnosed or treated with closed management. In these patients, surgery is necessary to reduce and stabilize the tendons, and the attenuated SPR must be imbricated, if possible. Additionally, if shallow, the fibular groove should also be deepened. If imbrication of the SPR is not possible, the tendons can be stabilized using a rerouting procedure. With such a procedure, the tendons are passed deep to the calcaneofibular ligament. As with the treatment of chronic split tears of the peroneal tendons, the fibular groove should be closely inspected and, if flat or convex, surgically deepened in those patients with chronic peroneal tendon instability.

## Anterior Tibial Tendon

The anterior tibial tendon (ATT) is the main dorsiflexor of the ankle joint. Originating primarily from the anterolateral tibia, concentric contraction of this muscle allows the foot to clear the ground during the swing phase of the gait cycle. After heel-strike, eccentric contraction results in a gradual and controlled return of the foot to the ground. In the lower leg, the ATT passes under the superior extensor retinaculum, sometimes in its own tunnel. Distally, after crossing the ankle, the ATT passes beneath the inferior extensor retinaculum and then inserts onto the base of the first metatarsal and medial cuneiform.

### Acute Injury

Acute ATT injuries have three general etiologies: open lacerations, closed contusions, and closed ruptures. Closed ruptures have been subdivided into two distinct clinical presentations. The first is atraumatic rupture in elderly, less active patients. In these patients, the tendon is probably weakened by attrition, local steroid injections, or systemic diseases such as diabetes mellitus and inflammatory arthropathy. The second presentation is traumatic rupture, which can be a high-energy injury caused by a forceful eccentric tendon contraction in young patients. More commonly, however, traumatic rupture is a low-energy injury in older but active patients. Despite their age, these patients are often still active in sports. As with atraumatic ruptures, tendon attrition, local steroid injections, and systemic disease may be factors in these low-energy injuries.

Patients with closed injuries usually report anterior ankle or lower leg pain. The pain is often transient and

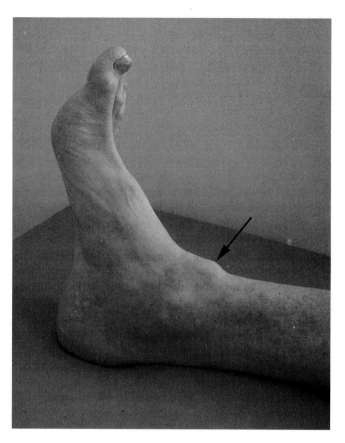

**Figure 4** ATT rupture with typical appearance of the lower leg mass formed by the retracted proximal segment (arrow).

resolves quickly. Many patients have either a painless mass or gait abnormality. The normal contour of the ATT is absent, which is especially apparent with resisted ankle dorsiflexion. Palpation reveals a gap in the tendon and at times a discreet mass formed by the retracted proximal stump (Fig. 4). Ankle dorsiflexion strength usually is diminished, and the patient everts the forefoot as a result of using the toe extensors to dorsiflex the ankle. Finally, gait analysis may reveal a steppage pattern during swing phase and a foot-slap pattern during early stance phase. Secondary recruitment of the extensor hallucis longus (EHL) and extensor digitorum longus (EDL) tendons to dorsiflex the ankle cause the forefoot to rotate into pronation and abduction (Fig. 5).

Too often, there is a delay in the diagnosis of ATT injuries. One reason for this is that ankle dorsiflexion is still possible because of the remaining extensor tendons that cross the front of the joint. In addition, the pain associated with ATT injuries is often minimal and abates quickly. In elderly patients, the injury can be painless and the resulting gait abnormality subtle. Finally, the proximal tendon segment may retract behind the superior extensor retinaculum, making accurate diagnosis difficult.

In young patients, closed treatment can be used for open lacerations involving only a small portion of the tendon and closed contusions in which the tendon is strong

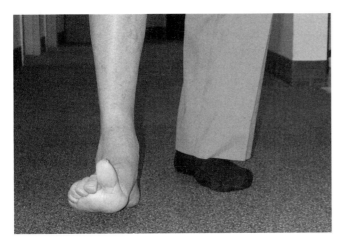

Figure 5 Secondary recruitment of the EHL and EDL tendons during swing phase in a patient with an ATT rupture.

and in continuity. With closed management, it is paramount that the foot adequately clears the ground during the swing phase and that there is no evidence of foot-slap during the stance phase. If these criteria are met, temporary immobilization in a fracture boot or walking cast followed by physical therapy should result in the return of normal function.

Closed management is also acceptable for atraumatic ruptures in low-functioning, elderly patients. In these patients, even complete ruptures can be treated with an ankle-foot orthosis or double upright brace. Some patients who function well may not need any type of supportive device.

Complete lacerations and closed ruptures of the ATT should be surgically repaired in both young patients and active older patients who wish to maintain a high level of function. If it is possible to approximate healthy tissue, various techniques can be used to primarily repair the tendon, including a Bunnell stitch and a Kessler suture technique. However, a locking stitch, such as that described by Krakow, is nonstrangulating and offers superior pull-out strength. At the time of repair, an attempt should be made to repair the extensor retinaculum and prevent bowstringing of the tendon across the anterior ankle.

Often, tendon retraction and degeneration at its insertion make the direct apposition of healthy tendon impossible. In these cases, several augmentation techniques, including sliding or VY ATT grafts, EHL tendon transfer, and the use of an interposition graft, have been used. Various donor sites for grafts have been described, including the EDL, plantaris, and PB tendons. No study has demonstrated the superiority of one technique over the others, and the decision regarding which technique to use should be made on an individual basis.

### Chronic Injury

Chronic injuries of the ATT occur primarily in middle-aged and elderly patients, who usually have chronic ten-

dinosis or acute-on-chronic tears of a tendon weakened by attrition or systemic disease. As with the peroneal tendons, it was initially believed that there was no hypovascular zone in the ATT, but a recent study using antilaminin antibodies suggested that there is an avascular zone in the anterior half of the tendon proximal to the ankle joint.

The treatment of chronic ATT injury depends on the preinjury level of function. In less active patients, the use of an ankle-foot orthosis may be adequate treatment. In more active patients who wish to maintain a high level of function, surgical repair should be considered. Tendon degeneration or retraction may necessitate the use of one of the augmentation techniques mentioned previously.

## Flexor Hallucis Longus Tendon

The flexor hallucis longus (FHL) muscle originates from the posterior tibia and fibula inferior to the soleal line. In the lower leg, the FHL tendon passes deep to the flexor retinaculum along with the other flexor tendons and neurovascular bundle. Posterior to the ankle joint, the tendon travels through a strong fibro-osseous tunnel located between the medial and lateral tubercles of the posterior process of the talus. It passes inferior to the sustentaculum tali and then crosses the flexor digitorum longus tendon at the knot of Henry. In this region, multiple intertendinous connections may exist between the FHL and flexor digitorum longus tendons. This complex anatomy rigidly stabilizes the FHL tendon and predisposes it to chronic disorders, such as stenosing tenosynovitis and degenerative tears.

### Acute Injury

Most acute FHL tendon injuries are lacerations. Patients typically have wounds in the region of the metatarsal head, and the flexor hallucis brevis (FHB) tendon and digital nerves must be carefully evaluated for concomitant injury. If both the FHL and FHB tendons have been lacerated, surgical repair generally is recommended to preserve hallux function. In the absence of an FHB tendon injury, however, the need to repair an isolated FHL tendon laceration is controversial. In one series of 10 FHL tendon lacerations in young athletes, four were not repaired. Although active interphalangeal joint flexion of the hallux was lost in these four patients, all had full function and were able to return to sports. Similarly, in another small series, no functional disability was noted in patients in whom surgical repair failed. Because a large series has yet to be conducted that compares closed and open treatment of FHL tendon lacerations, the optimal treatment of these injuries remains undecided.

Although rare, both traumatic and atraumatic closed ruptures of the FHL tendon have been reported. Anatomically, these injuries have occurred anywhere from the sustentaculum tali to the knot of Henry. Despite the equivocal results noted with repair of FHL tendon lacerations, satisfactory results have been reported with surgical treatment of closed ruptures by either direct repair or débridement and tenodesis to an adjacent tendon.

### Chronic Injury

Chronic injury of the FHL tendon is typically caused by tendinitis and stenosing tenosynovitis as the tendon passes through its fibro-osseous tunnel posterior to the talus. With long-standing injuries, a distinct nodule may form on the tendon, causing triggering and eventually stenosing tenosynovitis. These conditions are seen primarily in gymnasts and dancers (particularly those who dance on the toes) who place excessive and repetitive loads on the tendon. Nevertheless, in a recent series describing one surgeon's experience treating chronic FHL tendon injuries over 16 years, one half of the patients were not dancers.

Patients with chronic FHL tendon injuries are typically young athletes with posteromedial ankle pain exacerbated by physical activity. In dancers, the pain is worse with the demi-pointe and full-pointe positions. In addition to pain, crepitus and triggering of the hallux may be noted. Tenderness is present over the sheath of the FHL tendon at the posteromedial ankle, and both locking and crepitus may be noted.

Clinically, it is important to distinguish FHL tenosynovitis from posterior ankle impingement caused by either an os trigonum or an enlarged posterior tubercle. This can be difficult because both disorders often coexist, especially in dancers, and both disorders result in posterior ankle pain. The pain and tenderness associated with FHL tenosynovitis are typically posteromedial, whereas posterior ankle bony impingement occurs posterolaterally. Additionally, with FHL tendinitis, pain or triggering occurs with motion of the hallux. With posterior impingement, pain is noted with terminal plantar flexion of the ankle. MRI or bone scanning may be helpful in establishing an accurate diagnosis. Even with a thorough physical examination and appropriate radiographic and imaging studies, however, posterior ankle symptoms are often difficult to diagnose.

The initial treatment of FHL tendinitis and stenosing tenosynovitis is nonsurgical. In addition to anti-inflammatory medications, icing, and physical therapy, rest and modified training or modified dance routines are helpful. The demi-pointe and full-pointe positions should particularly be avoided by dancers with FHL tendinitis and stenosing tenosynovitis. If symptoms persist, surgery may be necessary. A posteromedial approach will allow access to the FHL tendon and, if necessary, a symptomatic os trigonum or trigonal process. The sheath of the tendon should be opened longitudinally and a careful tenolysis done. Any nodules should be excised and any partial tears repaired. The tendon sheath is left open at the end of the procedure.

In the recent series describing the treatment of chronic FHL tendon injuries over 16 years, surgery produced good or excellent results in 14 of 15 patients who were dancers and in 9 of 11 patients who were not dancers. The authors concluded that chronic FHL tendon injury is not rare and should be carefully considered in all patients with posterior ankle pain. Surgical intervention is recommended for those who fail to respond to 3 to 6 months of nonsurgical therapy. The authors also emphasized that surgery should be tailored to the specific pathology present. A tenosynovectomy should be performed if any significant inflammation is encountered. Chronic longitudinal tears should be débrided and repaired with a running suture. When a pseudocyst or nodular thickening of the tendon is present, the tendon should be débrided and thinned to the diameter of the normal tendon. Finally, a triagonal process or os trigonum should be excised if posterior ankle impingement is suspected.

## Extensor Hallucis Longus Tendon

The EHL tendon is the main dorsiflexor of the hallux. It travels superficially across the anterior ankle and dorsum of the foot and is stabilized by the superior and inferior extensor retinaculum. Distally, the EHL tendon inserts onto the extensor hood and base of the distal phalanx.

### EHL Tendon Laceration

Most acute injuries of the EHL tendon are lacerations. Hallux dorsiflexion strength is diminished or absent, and the tendon is not palpable. Associated injuries of the EHB tendon, peripheral nerves, and dorsalis pedis artery may also be present. Diagnosis of an EHL tendon laceration can be delayed by an inadequate physical examination and excessive focus on the treatment of an open wound.

There is no consensus regarding the closed or open treatment of EHL tendon lacerations. Satisfactory results have been reported with primary repair. The level of the injury should play a role in determining the need for surgery. Function is usually regained with closed management of lacerations within the extensor hood at or distal to the base of the proximal phalanx because there is little tendon retraction at this level. The extensor hood tethers the proximal portion of the lacerated tendon, preventing all but a few millimeters of retraction. The hallux is taped in dorsiflexion, and a short leg walking cast extending distal to the toes is applied for 6 to 8 weeks.

With both primary and delayed repair, a second incision may be necessary to retrieve the retracted proximal end of the tendon, which is often trapped at the level of the inferior or superior extensor retinaculum. If direct apposition of the tendon ends is possible, a grasping stitch should be used. If apposition of the tendon ends is not possible, other techniques can be used, including a tendon turndown or augmentation with an autologous graft, such as a strip of the PB tendon or one of the EDL tendons (Fig. 6).

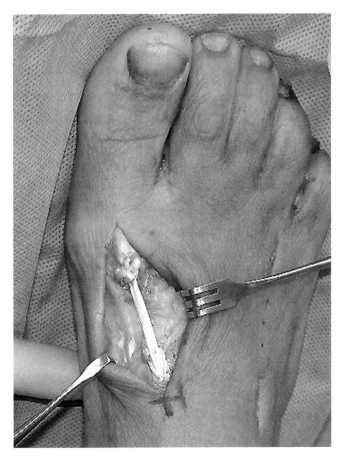

**Figure 6** Intercalated autologous EDL tendon graft in a patient in whom direct repair of a lacerated EHL tendon was not possible.

## EHL Tendon Rupture

Spontaneous rupture of the EHL tendon is extremely rare, with only five instances described in the literature. In three young patients, the mechanism of injury was active extension against resistance. In two middle-aged patients, the proposed mechanisms of injury were steroid injections and repetitive microtrauma. The location of the rupture has ranged from the musculotendinous junction to the metatarsophalangeal joint. In all patients, surgery was done because of pain or deformity. In two patients, primary repair was not possible and either a tendon graft or transfer was required. Satisfactory results were reported in all patients.

## Extensor Digitorum Longus Tendon

The EDL tendon is the main dorsiflexor of the lesser toes. It also serves to dorsiflex and evert the ankle. The EDL tendon originates from several structures in the anterior compartment of the leg. Deep to the extensor retinaculum, it first divides into two separate tendons, each of which then further subdivides distally in the forefoot. At the level of the metatarsophalangeal joints, each of the four individual tendons of the EDL is anchored by a dorsal aponeurosis. Distal to this, the tendons split into three

terminal slips that insert onto the middle and distal phalanges.

EDL tendon injuries predominantly (if not exclusively) consist of acute lacerations. Although the literature on these injuries is sparse, proponents of both surgical repair and closed management can be found. The main arguments in favor of repair are preservation of normal function and avoidance of a future claw toe deformity. Opponents of surgery cite painful dorsal scars and satisfactory function with closed management. Generally, most recent authors recommend surgical repair. Nevertheless, closed management remains a reasonable alternative in certain patients, especially older and less active individuals.

## Summary

Tendon injuries of the foot and ankle are complex and understanding of them continues to evolve. Appropriate treatment varies not only by the tendon involved, but also by such critical factors as the nature of the injury, the activity level of the patient, and the presence of coexisting pathoanatomy.

## Annotated Bibliography

### Peroneal Tendons

Bonnin M, Tavernier T, Bouysset M: Split lesions of the peroneus brevis tendon in chronic ankle laxity. *Am J Sports Med* 1997;25:699-703.

Eighteen patients with concomitant split lesions of the PB tendon and chronic ankle instability were assessed. The authors speculate that ankle laxity may contribute to PB splits and warn that residual pain after ligamentous repair can be caused by untreated peroneal injury.

Bruce WD, Christofersen MR, Phillips DL: Stenosing tenosynovitis and impingement of the peroneal tendons associated with hypertrophy of the peroneal tubercle. *Foot Ankle Int* 1999;20:464-467.

This article describes three patients with stenosing tenosynovitis of the PL tendons associated with an enlarged peroneal tubercle. All patients were asymptomatic following tendon débridement and excision of the tubercle.

Kollias SL, Ferkel RD: Fibular grooving for recurrent peroneal tendon subluxation. *Am J Sports Med* 1997;25:329-335.

Twelve ankles in 11 consecutive patients with recurrent peroneal tendon dislocations were studied after undergoing a fibular groove deepening procedure. In five instances, the PB tendon was also débrided and repaired, and in three instances, a concomitant reefing of the anterior talofibular ligament was done. In all patients, pain relief and functional improvement were excellent.

Krause JO, Brodsky JW: Peroneus brevis tendon tears: Pathophysiology, surgical reconstruction, and clinical results. *Foot Ankle Int* 1998;20:464-467.

This article evaluates the clinical results of surgical reconstruction for chronic PB tendon tears. Débridement and repair are recommended when there is damage to less than 50% of the cross-sectional area of the tendon. Excision of the damaged segment and tenodesis to the PL tendon are recommended when there is destruction of greater than 50% of the tendon.

Major NM, Helms CA, Fritz RC, Speer KP: The MR imaging appearance of longitudinal split tears of the peroneus brevis tendon. *Foot Ankle Int* 2000;21:514-519.

MRIs of 22 patients with split tears of the PB tendon were reviewed. Statistically significant associated findings included a chevron-shaped tendon, flattening of the peroneal grove, a lateral fibular spur, and abnormalities of the lateral ankle ligaments.

Petersen W, Bobka T, Stein V, Tillmann B: Blood supply of the peroneal tendons: Injection and immunohistochemical studies of cadaver tendons. *Acta Orthop Scand* 2000;71:168-174.

The authors used antilaminin antibodies to study the vascular supply of the peroneal tendons. A single hypovascular region was demonstrated in the PB tendon as it passes through the fibular groove. Two hypovascular regions were demonstrated in the PL tendon: one at the tip of the lateral malleolus and the other where the tendon changes direction at the level of the cuboid bone.

Rosenberg ZS, Beltran J, Cheung YY, Colon E, Herraiz F: MR features of longitudinal tears of the peroneus brevis tendon. *Am J Roentgenol* 1997;168:141-147.

The characteristic MR features of peroneal tendon injuries are described in this series of 31 patients. The authors also describe the pathologic conditions and normal variants associated with these tears.

### Anterior Tibial Tendon

Petersen W, Stein V, Tillmann B: Blood supply of the tibialis anterior tendon. *Arch Orthop Trauma Surg* 1999;119:371-375.

Immunohistochemical methods and antilaminin antibodies were used to study the vascular supply of the anterior tibial tendon. An avascular zone was demonstrated in the anterior half of the tendon. This zone ranged from 45 to 67 mm in length and, according to the authors, correlated with the region in which spontaneous ruptures of the tendon commonly occur.

### Flexor Hallucis Longus Tendon

Sammarco GJ, Cooper PS: Flexor hallucis longus tendon injury in dancers and nondancers. *Foot Ankle Int* 1998;19:356-362.

The authors retrospectively reviewed 31 FHL tendon injuries in both dancers and nondancers. Surgical correction of teno-

synovitis, pseudocyst, and tendon tear yielded good or excellent results in most patients.

Wei SY, Kneeland JB, Okereke E: Complete atraumatic rupture of the flexor hallucis longus tendon: A case report and review of the literature. *Foot Ankle Int* 1998;19:472-474.

This is the second case report of complete atraumatic rupture of the FHL tendon to appear in the medical literature. The article also reviews the literature and discusses the indications for surgical repair of this injury.

### Extensor Hallucis Longus Tendon

Kass JC, Palumbo F: Extensor hallucis longus tendon injury: An in-depth analysis and treatment protocol. *J Foot Ankle Surg* 1997;36:24-27.

The authors present an in-depth discussion of whether to repair a lacerated EHL tendon. A comprehensive literature review is presented and a detailed treatment protocol recommended.

Scaduto AA, Cracchiolo A: Lacerations and ruptures of the flexor or extensor hallucis longus tendons. *Foot Ankle Clin* 2000;5:725-736.

In this article, the nature of FHL and EHL tendon injuries is described and the medical literature is reviewed. Specific treatment plans are recommended based both on published articles and the authors' personal experience.

## Classic Bibliography

Earle AS, Moritz JR, Tapper EM: Dislocation of the peroneal tendons at the ankle: An analysis of 25 ski injuries. *Northwest Med* 1972;71:108-110.

Eckert WR, Davis EA: Acute rupture of the peroneal retinaculum. *J Bone Joint Surg Am* 1976;58:670-673.

Escales F, Figueras J, Merino J: Dislocation of the peroneal tendons: Long-term results of surgical management. *J Bone Joint Surg Am* 1980;62:451-453.

Floyd DW, Heckman JD, Rockwood CA Jr: Tendon lacerations in the foot. *Foot Ankle Int* 1983;4:8-14.

Frenette JP, Jackson DW: Lacerations of the flexor hallucis longus in the young athlete. *J Bone Joint Surg Am* 1977;59:673-676.

Griffiths JC: Tendon injuries around the ankle. *J Bone Joint Surg Br* 1965;47:686-689.

Hamilton WG, Geppert MJ, Thompson FM: Pain in the posterior aspect of the ankle in dancers: Differential diagnosis and operative treatment. *J Bone Joint Surg Am* 1996;78:1491-1500.

Kolettis GJ, Micheli LJ, Klein JD: Release of the flexor hallucis longus tendon in ballet dancers. *J Bone Joint Surg Am* 1996;78:1386-1390.

American Academy of Orthopaedic Surgeons

Larsen E, Flink-Olsen M, Seerup K: Surgery for recurrent dislocations of the peroneal tendons. *Acta Orthop Scand* 1984;55:554-555.

Lipscomb P, Kelly P: Injuries of the extensor tendons in the distal part of the leg and in the ankle. *J Bone Joint Surg Am* 1955;37:1206-1213.

Ouzounian TJ, Anderson R: Anterior tibial tendon rupture. *Foot Ankle Int* 1995;16:406-410.

Sarrafian SK: *Anatomy of the Foot and Ankle: Descriptive, Topographic, Functional,* ed 2. Philadelphia, PA, JB Lippincott, 1993.

Sobel M, DiCarlo EF, Bohne WH, Collins L: Longitudinal attrition of the peroneus brevis tendon in the fibular groove: An anatomic and histologic study of cadaveric material. *Foot Ankle Int* 1991;12:165-170.

Sobel M, Geppert MJ, Olson EJ, Bohne WH, Arnoczky SP: The dynamics of peroneus brevis tendon splits: A proposed mechanism, technique of diagnosis, and classification of injury. *Foot Ankle Int* 1992;13:413-422.

# Chapter 9

# Achilles Tendon Injuries: Acute and Chronic

William C. McGarvey, MD

## Introduction

Because of its unique anatomic structure, the Achilles tendon can be affected by both inflammatory and degenerative processes, alone or in combination. Determining the exact pathology present is essential to proper treatment. Thorough clinical examination usually allows diagnosis, but radiography, MRI, and sonography can provide information about the location and extent of tendon involvement. Achilles tendon disorders are common in athletes, and in this population, overuse microtrauma may be the basic etiology. In older individuals, tendon degeneration is a major contributing factor.

## Anatomy, Biomechanics, and Vascularity

### Anatomy

The Achilles tendon is the largest tendon in the body. The muscles of the superficial compartment of the leg and the two heads of the gastrocnemius and the soleus coalesce as they travel distally to form tendinous fibers, which ultimately insert into the middle third of the posterior tuberosity of the calcaneus. As the tendon fibers migrate distally, they spiral 90° such that the medial gastrocnemius tendinous fibers of insertion come to lie posterior to the tendinous fibers of the soleus, which originate anteriorly and at insertion are medial. The insertion of the tendon, or enthesis, expands to encase the entire distal tuberosity of the calcaneus. It is sandwiched between two bursae: the superficial or adventitious bursa (located posteriorly between the skin and tendon) and the retrocalcaneal bursa (located anterior to the tendon), which separates it from the posterolateral prominence of the calcaneus. The retrocalcaneal bursa communicates with the tendon anteriorly and lubricates it, thereby reducing friction between the Achilles tendon and the variably sized posterolateral prominence of the calcaneal tuberosity.

Unlike other tendons, the Achilles tendon has no synovial lining and is surrounded by a paratenon, which is divided into two layers: visceral and parietal. The two layers are connected by an interposed mesotenon. The enveloping layer of paratenon, which is loose and flexible, is able to stretch 2 to 3 cm and facilitates smooth tendon gliding within.

Histologically, the Achilles tendon is composed of mature, differentiated fibroblasts or tenocytes, which lie in an extracellular matrix of collagen, elastin, and proteoglycans. Within this milieu, compact bundles of connective tissue are produced and aligned by tension in a very specific construction. Five collagen molecules form a microfibril. Microfibrils group into subfibrils, which ultimately group into collagen fibrils. Multiple collagen fibrils and extracellular matrix form fascicles, which are surrounded by the endotenon (a loose connective tissue layer of elastin). The endotenon contains lymphatics, nerves, and vessels and is surrounded by an investing layer of epitenon that is in direct contact with the paratenon. Collectively, the surrounding layers of tissue are referred to as the peritendon.

### Biomechanics

The chief function of the Achilles tendon is plantar flexion of the foot and ankle. In addition, because of the orientation of its insertion, the Achilles tendon acts as a heel invertor, provided there is no bony or periarticular fixed deformity in the ankle or hindfoot. The gastrocnemius-soleus complex is also a weak knee flexor. Because of its asymmetric insertion on the heel, the Achilles tendon is subject to uneven forces during running or jumping, and these activities may predispose it to acute or chronic injury. Depending on the activity, the Achilles tendon may sustain anywhere from 2,000 to 7,000 N of force during a single leg stance. This translates into forces that are roughly 6 to 10 times the body weight in one cycle of single leg stance during running.

The Achilles tendon, like most tendons, is a viscoelastic structure. Under load, it elongates 7% to 15% of its length. Elongation depends not only on the amount of load but also on the rate applied. Cyclical stresses reduce stiffness, and increased rates of strain and the speed of elongation increase stiffness of the tendon. The ultimate tensile strength of the Achilles tendon is approximately 70% that of bone.

### Vascularity

Vascular supply to the Achilles tendon is derived from anterior muscular branches and osseous and periosteal vessels nearer the insertion, where there are limited but consistent intratendinous and peritendinous vascular contributors. The Achilles tendon is richly vascularized proximally and distally by the gastrocnemius-soleus musculotendinous vessels and the abundant calcaneo-Achilles network, respectively. The calcaneal plexus, particularly from the medial and (to a lesser degree) lateral calcaneal arteries, supplies the enthesis. A segment of the tendon beginning 2 to 3 cm from its insertion on the calcaneus and extending to 6 cm proximally remains poorly vascularized. Injection and nuclear imaging studies have shown this segment to have markedly reduced numbers of intratendinous and extratendinous vessels. What little vascularity is present is supplied by the paratenon via the mesotenal vessels. Superficial and deep plexi arise from anterior mesenteric branches that flow across the retro-Achilles fat pad anterior to the tendon and are evenly distributed throughout its length. These are transverse vincular attachments through which small vessels may reach the tendon directly. Disruption of these vessels may be critical in devascularizing the already hypovascular zone or watershed area.

### Classification

Several classification systems have been proposed to differentiate Achilles tendon pathologies. Traditionally, pathologies were classified as arising from the investing layers, specific to the tendon itself, or arising from both the investing layers and Achilles tendon and described as peritendinitis, tendinitis, or pure tendinosis. This classification system took into account the acuity and the prevailing tissue structures involved. More recently, consideration has been given to anatomic origin by including entities arising from the insertion as well. Consequently, no universally accepted system for classifying Achilles tendon pathologies currently exists.

Currently, standardized terminology revolves around dividing tendon inflammation and degeneration into three categories: paratenonitis, paratenonitis and tendinosis, and tendinosis. Paratenonitis is an inflammatory process limited to the investing layer of the Achilles tendon. No tendinous disease is present. Paratenon tissues are thickened and adhere to the tendon. Typical histologic signs of inflammatory change are present, including capillary proliferation, neovascularization, and acute inflammatory cells.

Paratenonitis and tendinosis include elements of the previously described pathology along with focal intratendinous degeneration. Macroscopically, tendinosis appears as thickened yellowish discoloration, implying xanthomatous degeneration. Normal tendon sheen and striation are lost. Microscopically, there is a disorganization of the normal structure of collagen, hypocellularity, and avascularity, with areas of necrosis and/or calcification. Tendinosis is a noninflammatory phenomenon that is more pathophysiologically in keeping with chronic degenerative processes.

Pure tendinosis reflects not only degeneration of tendon but also age-related changes in tissue. A decrease in cellularity and in extracellular matrix is evident. Fewer organelles exist within tenocytes, and the surrounding mucopolysaccharide and glycoprotein levels are reduced. The individual collagen fibrils are diminished in number and size.

### Diagnostic Imaging

MRI is universally considered the best and most comprehensive diagnostic imaging modality for Achilles tendon injuries. It is unparalleled in detailing incomplete tendon ruptures, the extent of degeneration, the infiltration of peritendinous tissues with inflammatory changes, and retrocalcaneal pathologies such as bursitis or calcaneal impingement. Additionally, sequential MRIs can aid in determining the progress and extent of healing of a tendon. Another advantage of MRI is its large field of view, which can typically include the entire hindfoot, ankle, and distal leg. As the most comprehensive screening study available, it is also helpful for defining less common pathologies (eg, ganglions and neoplasms). Its disadvantages include cost, inconvenience to the patient, and its relative oversensitivity in identifying areas of inflammatory change.

Sonography has gained popularity recently for its detail of the Achilles tendon and surrounding structures. Hypoechoic densities clearly reflect areas of tendon damage and/or disruption. Additionally, sonography can be used for dynamic evaluation of tendon function. Other advantages include the relative ease of use, convenience to the patient, and low cost. Less clear is the diagnosis of tendinosis, which appears as focal thickening and irregularity of the tendon. Because sonography is operator-dependent and clinical experience is gained by performing frequent examinations, lack of individual familiarity with the technique and interpretation by both radiologists and orthopaedic surgeons are the major limitations to the widespread use of sonography for imaging musculoskeletal conditions.

Plain radiographic studies can help evaluate insertional disorders. A lateral radiograph will disclose the presence or absence of calcium deposition at the Achilles tendon insertion. The presence of ossification at the insertion is an indicator of the chronicity of the disease (Fig. 1). A large amount of bone in the tendon insertion or indistinct, "fuzzy" borders of the ectopic bone may indicate conditions such as diffuse idiopathic sclerosing hyperostosis or one of the inflammatory seronegative spondyloarthropathies (eg, ankylosing spondylitis, Reiter's syndrome, and psoriatic arthritis). Additionally, a large

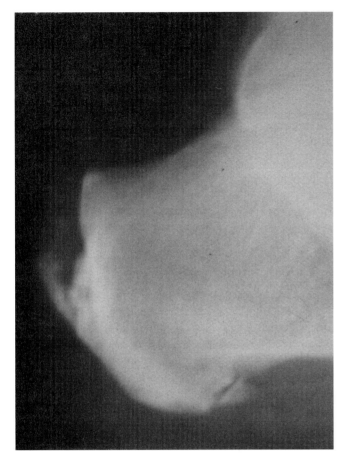

**Figure 1** Radiograph showing insertional Achilles tendon enthesopathy.

posterior tuberosity of the calcaneus may be present radiographically on this lateral view. Radiographic measurements can be made and compared with established criteria for abnormal calcaneal pitch angles or parallel pitch lines suggestive of Haglund's deformity, but consistent standard values are difficult to reproduce and correlate with clinical findings. Plain radiographs can also help identify bony sources of calcaneal pain, such as stress fractures, tumors, and Haglund's deformity (prominent posterior calcaneal tuberosity.)

## Types of Achilles Tendon Injuries

### Paratenonitis

Achilles tendinitis is a misnomer because sparse blood supply to the Achilles tendon and the absence of a synovial lining prohibit the generation of a true inflammatory response. Achilles tendinitis is in fact an acute inflammation of the relatively better vascularized surrounding layer of paratenon and is therefore more appropriately termed paratenonitis. This is typically a condition of overuse. A direct correlation exists between the incidence of Achilles paratenonitis and the intensity of training for running or jumping activities. Distance runners have a predilection for Achilles paratenonitis, with

up to 10% reporting symptoms at one point during their careers; however, this condition is not limited to these athletes because it also occurs frequently in those involved in pushing off or cutting activities, such as basketball, volleyball, tennis, soccer, and ballet. Many athletes with Achilles paratenonitis report a change in the frequency or duration of training habits, but onset may also be related to changes in running surfaces or even shoe wear.

Patients with Achilles paratenonitis describe burning pain and swelling after activity. There is usually fusiform swelling, warmth, and tenderness throughout active and passive range of motion. Pain can be exacerbated by creating friction along the paratenon between the thumb and forefinger. The diagnosis is typically clinical. Treatment is uniformly conservative because symptoms will resolve with rest. For most patients with Achilles paratenonitis (90% to 95%), nonsteroidal anti-inflammatory drugs, ice, stretching, modification of training surfaces and/or shoe wear, and using heel lifts or cushioned shock absorbers are effective.

Those individuals whose symptoms do not subside after more than 3 months require more aggressive treatment. Implementation of a formal physical therapy program, including modalities such as electrical stimulation, ultrasound, and iontophoresis, may reduce symptoms, albeit unpredictably. Discontinuation of sport-specific activity and cross-training along with gradual, scheduled reintroduction to sport-specific activity is the most predictable method of treatment for prolonged symptomatology. Brief periods of immobilization may also be used.

Chronic symptoms may lead to tendon thickening, an adhesion between the paratenon and tendon, or even crepitus when palpating the moving tendon. This crepitus does not move when dorsiflexing or plantar flexing the ankle as opposed to a tendinosis, which does move. More invasive measures may be indicated for patients with these symptoms. Brisement, for example, is a local injection procedure that involves inserting a needle between the paratenon and tendon and rapidly infusing 5 to 15 mL of saline or local anesthetic into the peritendinous space to mechanically lyse adhesions. Sonography can facilitate accurate needle placement. Prompt institution of physical therapy and range-of-motion exercises is crucial to prevent recurrence. Approximately one third of patients who undergo brisement improve. Steroid injections or infusions are not recommended for the treatment of Achilles tendon pathology because a local bolus of medication can lead to tendon necrosis and precipitate a rupture. Immobilization using a short leg walking cast or prefabricated walker boot for 4 to 8 weeks followed by a night splint that holds the ankle and foot at 90° to the leg until symptoms have subsided completely may preclude the need for surgical treatment.

Surgery for chronic paratenonitis is indicated for individuals who do not respond well to conservative measures. Thickened, scarred paratenon is débrided or excised through a single-layer medial incision. Care is taken to ensure full-thickness skin flaps and to avoid the anterior portion of the paratenon and its critical mesotenal vessels. Skin, subcutaneous tissue, and paratenon should all be raised as a thick, single layer if possible to avoid soft-tissue compromise. The tendon is inspected for split tears, and intratendinous repair is performed as needed. In this case, some degree of tendinosis may also be present. Closure is done by approximating the deep, investing fascia to prevent rescarring to subcutaneous tissues. Reinstitution of motion is immediate and weight bearing should follow when pain and swelling allow, usually within 1 week. Return to sports-specific activity usually takes between 6 and 12 weeks and return to competitive activity 3 to 6 months. Success rates are reported to be 70% to 100%.

## Tendinosis

Tendinosis of the Achilles tendon is typically a degenerative phenomenon, although it may be aggravated by repetitive heavy work or athletic activity. Intratendinous degradative lesions usually do not elicit pain; however, pain may occur with concomitant paratenonal inflammation. Patients with tendinosis are usually older than patients with paratenonitis, and variable degrees of activity and symptomatology occur, ranging from painless stiffness to severe, restricted, painful weight bearing (which typically represents a partial rupture). Examination often discloses palpable nodular thickening of the tendon beginning 6 to 8 cm proximal to the insertion and visible asymmetry in the width of the Achilles tendon when compared with the contralateral tendon. Weakness in plantar flexion is frequently present as well as a loss of push-off strength as the result of pain and often secondary calf atrophy. Tendon excursion may be limited because of fibrosis. In addition, traumatic partial tears in an already diseased Achilles tendon may allow elongation and increase passive dorsiflexion. Imaging modalities, either MRI or sonography, are helpful in determining the extent of tendon involvement and identifying continuity in clinical presentation suspicious for rupture.

Initial treatment for tendinosis is similar to that for paratenonitis. However, if advanced stages or partial tendon rupture is suspected or confirmed, more restrictive treatments are implemented. A walking boot with a rocker-bottom sole is frequently used with either a 1-inch heel lift or the ankle of the boot locked in 15° to 30° of equinus to unload the tendon. Physical therapy, including electrical stimulation, ultrasound, and particularly iontophoresis (as outlined previously), is then introduced until the acute symptoms have abated. Emphasis is placed on eccentric load activity to strengthen the calf and promote revascularization.

For symptoms resistant to treatment with conservative measures that have been implemented for 3 to 6

months or longer, surgical treatment is an option. In patients undergoing surgical repair, MRI is helpful in identifying the location and extent of the degenerative areas. Traditional surgical intervention includes an approach similar to that used to treat paratenonitis. Using a medial approach, full-thickness skin flaps are developed, and the paratenon is evaluated for thickening or adhesions and excised as necessary. More typically, the paratenon layer is minimally involved and is incised for inspection of the tendon itself. Areas of nodularity, fibrosis, and calcification of the tendon are identified, and rents, cleavage, or frank tears are repaired with small absorbable suture as atraumatically as possible. The diseased tendon often lies in the central core, and the peripheral tendon is more normal in appearance and function. Abnormal tissue is excised until tissue with normal sheen and striation is visible. The remainder of the normal tendon should be repaired longitudinally by tubularizing the remnants as atraumatically as possible using small (3-0 or 4-0) absorbable suture. It is not uncommon to find extensive disease requiring near-complete tendon excision. In these instances, augmentation or reconstruction must be included. If more than 50% of the tendon is abnormal, augmentation should be considered (techniques are described in the section on chronic Achilles tendon rupture).

Rehabilitation is cautious but progressive and allows for early weight bearing in equinus. Boot protection is used for 2 to 4 weeks, depending on the extent of disease. Range-of-motion exercises are also begun early and advanced quickly once the wound is healed. Success rates for this treatment vary widely, ranging from 36% to 100%, and good functional outcomes are related to the timing of the surgical intervention, the extent of tendon involvement, whether augmentation was required, the age of the patient, and patient expectations. Delayed diagnosis and treatment result in a slower recovery for the patient, prolonged weakness, and less predictable success.

Less invasive techniques have recently been suggested for the treatment of Achilles tendinosis. In patients with less significant tendon involvement as documented by sonography or MRI, multiple percutaneous vertical tenotomies can be done to, in theory, help revascularize the tendon and reduce, halt, or reverse the progress of disease. Five-stab incisions (proximal, distal, medial, lateral, and central) are made using intraoperative sonography as a guide to the degenerative tendon lesions. A No. 15 blade is inserted into the tendon through each incision, and the ankle is plantar flexed and dorsiflexed to create a 1-cm tenotomy with each introduction of the knife. Because there is no real compromise to the tendon integrity, weight bearing, range-of-motion exercise, and return to sport activity can be instituted earlier. In one study, initial results were successful using this technique, with good functional outcome reported in 77%; however, patients in this study were middle- or long-distance runners and therefore in ideal health otherwise. Results in the general population may not be as positive.

### Insertional Tendinopathy

Insertional Achilles tendinosis as an isolated component of Achilles tendinopathy has gained recognition over the past decade. Although this condition was once referred to as retrocalcaneal bursitis, it is quite distinct from the less commonly encountered isolated bursal inflammation. The histopathology of insertional tendinopathy suggests a degenerative condition in the area of tendon insertion, with occasional acute inflammatory changes occurring in the contiguous retrocalcaneal bursa and paratenon layers.

Insertional tendinopathy, like other Achilles tendon disorders, is usually caused by overuse and occurs most commonly among runners and individuals involved in athletic activities (such as basketball, volleyball, and soccer) requiring short bursts or push-offs. The highest incidence of insertional tendinopathy, however, clearly occurs among younger, more athletic individuals and older, more sedentary patients with comorbidities. This bimodal distribution is reinforced by the average age of patients on presentation, which is 44 years for those with insertional tendinopathy compared to 33 years for those with noninsertional tendinopathy. Although Achilles tendon pathology in athletes is fairly common and is present in 6% to 8% of all runners, insertional tendinopathy is less frequently identified in athletes with Achilles tendon disorders (10% to 20%). This may account for its relative obscurity until more recent reports and descriptions in the literature called attention to its bimodal distribution.

Symptoms arising from insertional tendinopathy occur at the bone-tendon interface (enthesis). Patients frequently report that their pain is worse after activity but gradually becomes constant. Pain may be aggravated by running on hills or hard surfaces or sudden changes in training intensity, frequency, or mileage. One reproducible sign of insertional tendinopathy is focal tenderness over the posterior or occasionally posterolateral portion of the enthesis. The examiner should look for palpable defects within the substance of the tendon, the presence of thickening or nodularity at the insertion, and the amount of dorsiflexion compared with that of the contralateral leg (which may be limited in many patients). A thorough medical history is important to determine the presence of contributory conditions, such as seronegative inflammatory disease (such as psoriasis and Reiter's syndrome), spondyloarthropathies, gout, familial hyperlipidemia, sarcoidosis, diffuse idiopathic skeletal hyperostosis, or the use of systemic medications (such as corticosteroids and fluoroquinolones) that are associated with an increased risk of Achilles tendon degeneration. It is particularly important to note contributory conditions in patients with bilateral involvement.

Radiographs are not necessary for diagnosis; however, approximately 60% of patients demonstrate a calcific deposit within the insertion of the tendon. This is helpful prognostically because these patients usually do not respond well to conservative treatment and take almost twice the expected time to recover. Radiographs may also suggest the presence of a Haglund's prominence, which can cause mechanical irritation of the tendon insertion. This bony deformity has been reported in 60% of all patients with chronic insertional Achilles tendinopathy.

Although sonography has been used in the diagnosis of degenerative tendinopathy and progressive healing, MRI is the imaging modality that is most helpful in determining the extent of degeneration and identifying other factors contributing to posterior heel pain, such as bursal inflammation or calcaneal impingement.

Conservative treatment for insertional tendinopathy is successful in most patients, particularly when the diagnosis is made before the condition has caused extensive change in the tendon and other retrocalcaneal structures. Liberal use of nonsteroidal anti-inflammatory drugs, heel lifts, stretching, and shoe modifications (eg, wider, softer counter) are initially helpful. Should these fail, more formal orthoses, night splinting, and therapy modalities, especially ice, contrast baths, and iontophoresis, are helpful. Ultimately, immobilization with gradual reintroduction to cross-training before return to activity is usually successful. As with noninsertional disorders, steroid injections into this region of the tendon are discouraged for fear of causing an insertional rupture, which is a difficult condition to manage (Figs. 2 and 3).

Surgery is indicated for the small subset of patients who do not respond to 6 to 12 months of appropriate nonsurgical treatment. The goals of surgery are to débride the diseased tendon insertion, decompress any bony impingement, remove all inflammatory bursal tissue, release the contracture of the gastrocnemius-soleus complex, and ensure functional quality of the tendon anchor (Fig. 4). Younger, healthier patients without comorbidities usually respond well to this type of treatment.

Surgery may be carried out through a number of approaches. Central tendon splitting or an isolated lateral approach seems to result in the most reliable outcomes and fewest complications. The presence of an intratendinous spur is an ominous finding because it suggests advanced degeneration. Patients with extensive calcific disease should be counseled that their recovery may be lengthier and less predictable and that it may take up to 2 years to maximize outcomes. This is particularly true if the entire tendon insertion must be removed in the repair (Fig. 5).

Patients older than 55 years, those with tissue compromise of more than 50% of the tendon insertion, or those with comorbidities recover more slowly and should undergo débridement supplemented with Achilles tendon reinforcement by a tendon transfer. These patients are treated as being Achilles tendon–deficient (discussed in the section on chronic ruptures). Tendon transfer options

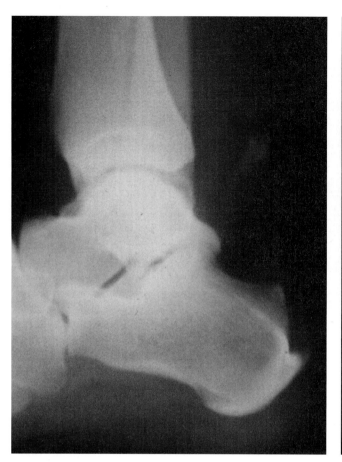

Figure 2  Radiographic evidence of insertional Achilles tendon avulsion.

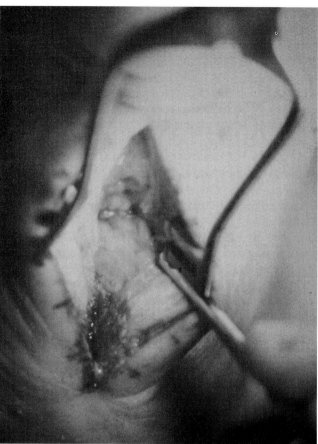

Figure 4  Central tendon splitting technique for débridement of insertional tendinosis. Note the inflammatory and degenerative changes at the Achilles tendon insertion.

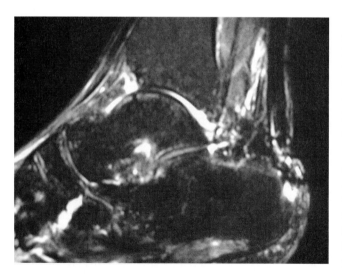

Figure 3  T2-weighted MRI demonstrating a subacute insertional tear.

include use of the flexor hallucis longus (FHL), flexor digitorum longus, peroneus brevis, or plantaris, if present. For anatomic reasons, the FHL tendon transfer seems to be the most advantageous and popular method.

Recovery from simple débridement requires 2 weeks in an equinus splint to allow wound healing. Weight bear-

ing is begun in an equinus boot once the wound is stabilized, and range-of-motion activity is instituted at that time. Eccentric resistance exercises are introduced at 4 weeks, and return to sport or activity usually occurs between 8 and 12 weeks. It should be noted that nonathletic, older, sedentary patients may require 1 year or longer for complete recovery.

### Acute Ruptures

Acute ruptures of the Achilles tendon are common and typically occur during athletic activity. The preponderance of acute Achilles tendon ruptures occur in men (reported male to female ratio is anywhere from 2:1 to 19:1) between age 30 and 40 years. Although roughly 75% of these injuries occur during athletic activity, careful analysis reveals that most injuries occur in poorly conditioned or episodic athletes, so-called weekend warriors. Up to 15% report prodromal symptoms of antecedent pain, swelling, or stiffness, but most are asymptomatic before a single event. Typically, patients relate a history of pushing off or landing on a plantarflexed foot and experiencing a palpable/audible pop or kick to the back of the leg while engaging in sprinting, running, or jumping activities. They may also describe resultant weakness and the inability to

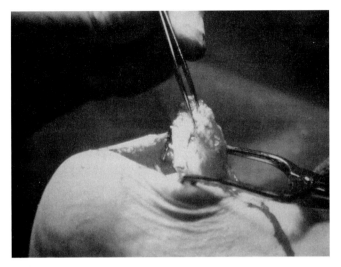

Figure 5   Removal of entire tendinous insertion in a patient with extensive degenerative disease.

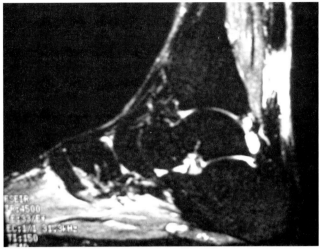

Figure 6   T2-weighted MRI demonstrating a complete Achilles tendon rupture.

push off. Pain ratings are variable and not reliable.

Physiologically, tendon degeneration occurs over time and is thought to be secondary to repetitive, incompletely resolved microtrauma. Regeneration is impeded by the repetition of the aggravating activity and compounded by the underlying hypovascular nature of the Achilles tendon as evidenced by the fact that most ruptures occur in the zone 4 to 6 cm from the calcaneal insertion. This degeneration, when combined with sudden, excessive load, ultimately leads to failure. Histopathologic evidence reveals variable degrees of hypoxic degeneration, mucoid degeneration, and calcific tendinopathy in acute ruptures. Associated conditions include rheumatoid arthritis, inflammatory arthropathies, collagen vascular diseases, and diabetes mellitus; the use of certain medications, especially corticosteroids (particularly by injection) and fluoroquinolone antibiotics can also be associated with acute Achilles tendon ruptures.

Diagnosis is usually clinical, although reports suggest that up to 25% of these injuries are initially missed in the emergency setting. Patients demonstrate marked weakness of plantar flexion, abnormal gait pattern, and an inability to perform a heel rise on the affected limb. A palpable and occasionally visible defect is often present 2 to 6 cm from the calcaneus, but this is sometimes obscured by acute swelling. Ecchymosis is variable. Active plantar flexion is usually present because the deep posterior compartment musculature remains intact. Results of the provocative Thompson test are frequently positive, which helps distinguish superficial from deep compartment contribution to plantar flexion. This test is performed with the patient prone and with the knee flexed while the examiner squeezes the calf. The loss of plantar flexion of the foot is considered a positive finding. The loss of resting equinus tone of the foot compared to the uninjured side with the patient prone with the knees flexed provides further clinical evidence of acute rupture.

Diagnostic imaging is typically not necessary unless a rupture is questionable, a patient has delayed seeking medical care, or nonsurgical treatment is being considered. Sonography and MRI are the best imaging modalities available for assessing these injuries (Fig. 6). Sonography has the distinct advantage of being able to dynamically determine whether tendon ends are reapposable.

Treatment of acute Achilles tendon ruptures has been controversial. Historically, studies have suggested that surgical treatment with early primary repair is more effective in restoring strength (10% to 20% stronger) and can minimize the incidence of rerupture (0% to 2% surgical versus 8% to 39% nonsurgical). Proponents of surgical intervention for the treatment of acute Achilles tendon ruptures also cite a more rapid return of patients to sport or activity. Advocates of the nonsurgical management of these injuries cite the lack of wound infection, skin necrosis, and neurologic (sural) complications as advantages. Regardless of treatment preference, nonsurgical management certainly plays a role in the treatment of this condition. It is typically reserved for the elderly, the sedentary, those affected by multiple medical comorbidities, patients undergoing long-term corticosteroid therapy, and patients not desirous of surgery. It is clear that functional rehabilitation with early return to weight bearing has a positive effect on tendon healing and ultimately strength and return to activity. Patients who are treated nonsurgically are placed in a gravity equinus boot or cast and the ankle position is gradually returned to neutral over 8 to 10 weeks. A heel lift in the shoe is maintained from 3 to 6 months when physical therapy is introduced. Ideally, patients undergoing nonsurgical treatment are seen immediately so as to properly position the foot. Sonography should be used to verify tendon end apposition at the site of rupture and also to follow the healing of the tendon throughout this process.

Surgical treatment may be done in several ways, but the goals are the same: to restore the muscle-tendon unit relationship and ensure appropriate tension. Surgery typically takes place within the first week after the injury. However, reports suggest that primary repair is successful up to 3 months after the injury has been detected. Posterior or posteromedial incisions are used to allow direct examination of the tendon remnants. Tendon ends are often frayed, resembling a horse's tail, in which case repair may require a specialized suturing technique (eg, Kessler, Bunnell, or Krakow suture) or require the separation of portions of each remnant into bundles for reattachment. The key to the repair is the reestablishment of the proper tension on the tendon. Therefore, it is important to compare resting equinus position to that of the unaffected limb by including this leg in the sterile field. An overstretching of the muscle-tendon unit results in residual equinus, whereas poor tendon apposition yields a limb that lacks push-off and balance, potentially leading to an altered gait pattern with the possibility of degenerative joint changes.

Whether to use absorbable or nonabsorbable suture material in the surgical repair of acute Achilles tendon ruptures is still being debated. Nonabsorbable suture is stronger and more reliable but tends to be heavier, more irritating, and may lead to sterile abscess formation. Absorbable sutures, such as polydioxanone surgical suture, are less reactive but are also weaker. Tendon repair may be augmented by cross-bridging of the plantaris tendon or turn down of the gastrocnemius aponeurosis. Alternatively, some have advocated minimally invasive percutaneous suture repairs. Although popular in Europe, these techniques have not met with enthusiasm in the United States because of the risks of sural nerve entrapment, skin adherence, unreliable tendon apposition, and the lack of strength of repair leading to higher re-rupture rates.

Early return to weight bearing and range-of-motion activity is crucial for a successful outcome after surgery. Prolonged cast immobilization after surgical repair or as primary treatment has been shown to have deleterious effects, including muscle atrophy, joint stiffness, cartilage atrophy, adhesion formation, and deep venous thrombosis. In addition, isokinetic testing has suggested that deficits in strength may be permanent as a result of prolonged cast immobilization. Histologically, early mobilization demonstrates increased fiber polymerization to collagen and organization of collagen at the repair site, resulting in increased strength at a faster rate. Early mobilization also has been shown to result in the presence of a greater number of spindle type cells and earlier reorganization of young collagen fibrils, which is indicative of more mature collagen. Theoretically, earlier stretching leads to a plastic deformation of neocollagen that promotes rapid turnover and maturation. This enhances the mechanical and tensile properties of the tendon sooner, thus providing a stronger tension repair in a shorter time.

In a properly repaired Achilles tendon, partial weight bearing may begin in a protective device with the foot in equinus position immediately after surgery. Range of motion is restricted until the wound is stable. Active motion is subsequently instituted, often within 2 weeks. Full weight bearing and range-of-motion activity are not allowed for 4 to 6 weeks postoperatively. By 3 to 4 weeks, however, most patients can perform some bicycling motion, therapy band exercises, or swimming. At 6 weeks, resistive eccentric loading exercises are begun. Patients are allowed to jog by 3 months and return to full sports activities by 6 months, although it is not unusual for them to take as long as 1 year. Criteria for return are a pain-free limb with full range of motion and 75% to 80% isokinetic strength compared to the unaffected extremity. Complications of surgery are reportedly as high as 20% and include skin necrosis, wound infection, sural neuroma, skin adhesion, stiffness, loss of strength, and re-rupture.

### Chronic Ruptures

Achilles ruptures that have not been treated as acute injuries are called chronic, neglected, or missed ruptures. Although successful outcomes may be obtained using primary repair techniques up to 3 months from the time of injury, isokinetic and isometric testing suggests that function can be compromised if repair is delayed 3 months or longer because strength testing at that time is notably weaker. After 6 weeks, cellular reorganization and collagen realignment is less predictable, and the void between torn remnants of tendon tends to fill with scar tissue (the tensile properties of scar tissue are much less than those of normal tendon tissue).

Findings on physical examination in patients with chronic ruptures are similar to those in patients with acute injuries, but they are frequently more subtle. Scar tissue fills the gap between the tendon ends, suggesting tendon continuity. Often, when compared to the contralateral side, the foot has greater passive dorsiflexion and less resting equinus tone with the patient prone with the knees flexed and usually even with the knees extended. Patients almost uniformly experience thickening of the tendon, calf atrophy, and gait abnormality. Results of the Thompson's test are equivocal; although sometimes a single leg heel rise is possible, repetitive rises on the injured side are impossible. Careful examination reveals that push-off results in a dynamic clawing of the toes, which is the result of substituting deep compartmental musculature for absent or ineffective function of the gastrocnemius-soleus complex. MRI is helpful in determining the size of the defect, the quality of the tissue, and the location of the gap.

Surgical treatment depends on the patient's functional status and the amount of pain experienced. Surgical repair of a chronic Achilles tendon rupture requires extensive dissection, and therefore surgical risks are in-

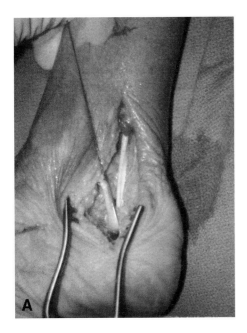
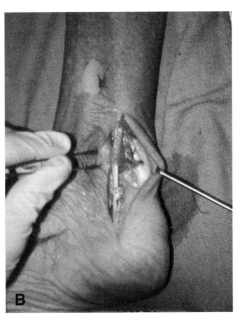

**Figure 7  A** and **B,** Flexor hallucis longus tendon transfer through traditional two-tunnel technique.

creased. As a result, careful consideration is needed for patients who may not tolerate extensive surgical dissection or prolonged recovery. Individuals with systemic disease, documented infectious or wound-healing problems, chronic arterial or venous disease, or heavy tobacco use should be counseled and probably encouraged to consider nonsurgical treatment. Nonsurgical treatment for Achilles deficiency consists of using an ankle-foot orthosis, which may be hinged, if necessary. In some patients, therapy to strengthen the deep compartment musculature may enhance push-off and promote more normal gait patterns.

Surgical treatment of neglected Achilles tendon ruptures tends to be complex, and the choice of procedures depends on the quality of the residual tissue and the size of the defect. Many procedures have been proposed using various forms of tissue augmentation. Free-tissue grafts use fascia lata; tendon transfers use ankle plantar flexors, including the FHL, flexor digitorum longus, peroneus brevis, and, if present and undamaged, the plantaris. Reconstruction of the damaged Achilles tendon with lengthening can be achieved using a V-Y advancement or a turndown procedure. On occasion, some of these procedures are used in combination. Allografts, synthetic materials such as Dacron, and more recently biologic inductive materials have also been used; however, because no reports on large, long-term series have been published, these procedures are currently considered to be experimental.

Defects measuring 1 to 2 cm that remain after a thorough débridement of the tendon ends to more viable tissue may be reparable by end-to-end anatomic repair. Because tissue loss is frequently underestimated, care must be taken to avoid overtightening. Should there be any concern about overtightening, a reconstructive procedure should be done.

For defects measuring 2 to 5 cm, a V-Y myotendinous lengthening, a tendon transfer, or both can be done. The choice of procedure may be dictated by the residual Achilles excursion. When the tendon is mobile, a V-Y lengthening can be done. An inverted V is made in the gastrocnemius fascia only so as not to disrupt the underlying gastrocnemius muscle. The arms of the V should be made twice the length of the defect. Attempting this procedure for defects greater than 5 cm may lead to complete detachment of the muscular portion of the gastrocnemius. Results demonstrate a loss in peak torque anywhere from 2% to 25% compared to the normal gastrocnemius-soleus Achilles muscle-tendon unit.

For individuals in whom the Achilles tendon is scarified and completely adherent, a tendon transfer is a good treatment option. The FHL tendon is used preferentially based on its relative strength of 30% of the gastrocnemius-soleus complex, anatomic proximity, axis of contraction, and phase synchronicity. This procedure can be done through one or two incisions, depending on the length of tendon needed. The transferred FHL tendon is anchored into the calcaneus just anterior to the Achilles insertion and may be tenodesed with the Achilles remnant to augment power if any excursion is left. Anchoring to the bone can be done using bone tunnels, suture anchors, or interference screw fixation (Fig. 7). Patients usually respond well and recover quickly. Occasionally, a loss of hallux push-off strength results, but this adverse effect is considered negligible and acceptable.

For defects longer than 5 cm, a turndown procedure with or without tendon transfer is indicated. A 1-cm wide strip of Achilles tendon is needed that is long enough to span the defect and overlap 2 cm proximally and 2 cm distally. This procedure usually requires a massive incision of skin and tendon. The turndown junction usually results in a large bulk of residual tissue with a tendency to adhere; therefore, early activity is critical to the success of this procedure. Strength is acceptable in noncompetitive athletes or older patients. Combining this with an FHL tendon transfer augments devitalized tendon tissue and promotes earlier return to activity.

Complications following procedures used to surgically repair chronic ruptures are similar to those after acute rupture repair, but they tend to be more severe, particularly as the size of the defect increases. Wound complications, which are the most common, are also potentially the most devastating. Local wound management may be successful, but plastic surgery consultation is recommended to provide early flap coverage that can reduce the risk of infection (which would require débriding the repair). Early skin coverage also allows the resumption of motion to promote tendon glide.

### Lacerations

Achilles tendon lacerations are uncommon. They are most often caused by shattered glass fragments or occur as a result of a stabbing. Infrequently, recreational (boat propeller) or industrial (fan blade) accidents lead to multilevel Achilles tendon lacerations or even tissue loss. As with any environmentally induced wound, appropriate emergency treatment includes tetanus prophylaxis, institution of antibiotics, and removal of foreign material. Surgical intervention is indicated and consists of débridement of devitalized tissue skin flaps and tendon edges, removal of all debris, repair of the tendon, and closure, if possible. In anticipation of a delay in surgical repair, which is best done within 48 to 72 hours, irrigation and débridement of the wound can be done in the emergency department with the patient under local anesthesia. For contaminated wounds or those recognized later, repeated débridements may be needed until tissue sterility is ensured.

Repair consists of end-to-end suturing of any lacerated tissue. Although strength is not affected until more than 50% of the tendon integrity is violated, direct repair reduces volume and risk of fibrotic nodules and adhesions by allowing the tendon to glide more freely. For tissue defects and multilevel injuries, augmentation should be done using the methods described for chronic Achilles tendon deficiency.

## Summary

Many disorders of the Achilles tendon, such as paratenonitis and insertional tendinopathy, can be effectively treated with rest or immobilization, nonsteroidal anti-inflammatory drugs, and physical therapy modalities. Tendinosis may be associated with partial or complete tendon ruptures that require surgical repair or excision and reconstruction. Acute ruptures in young, active individuals generally are better treated by primary repair than by nonsurgical methods, which may be appropriate in older,

more sedentary patients. Surgical treatment of chronic ruptures can be difficult and may require tendon lengthening, free-tissue grafts, tendon transfers, or combinations of these techniques.

## Annotated Bibliography

### Anatomy, Biomechanics, and Vascularity

Chao W, Deland JT, Bates JE, Kenneally SM: Achilles tendon insertion: An anatomic in vitro study. *Foot Ankle Int* 1997;18:81-84.

This cadaveric study demonstrates the configuration of the Achilles tendon attachment at the bone-tendon interface, showing a greater length of tendon inserted medially. The tendon insertion was shown to end at the posterior edges of the calcaneus and not wrap around the sides or extend past the borders.

Jozsa L, Kannus P: Histopathologic findings in spontaneous tendon ruptures. *Scand J Med Sci Sports* 1997;7:113-118.

This review of the natural evolution of the incidence of Achilles tendon ruptures identifies a paucity of reported injuries prior to the 1950s and a continual dearth of reports from developing countries. The authors also evaluate the histopathologic changes that occur as a result of these injuries.

Romanelli DA, Mandelbaum BR, Almekinders LC: Achilles ruptures in the athlete: Current science and treatment. *Sports Med Arthrosc Rev* 2000;8:377-386.

This excellent article on the pathophysiology, anatomy, biomechanics, and management of Achilles ruptures explores the rationale of more aggressive rehabilitation.

### Classification

Nehrer S, Breitenseher M, Brodner W, et al: Clinical and sonographic evaluation of the risk of rupture in the Achilles tendon. *Arch Orthop Trauma Surg* 1997;116:14-18.

Thirty-six patients were followed sonographically for achillodynia and graded based on thickening of the tendons. Thickening occurred in 33 of 72 tendons, and pain or localized swelling occurred in 48. Seven tendons ruptured spontaneously during the 5-year follow-up. All tendons had some thickening revealed sonographically. The authors concluded that sonography was a valuable assessment tool in patients with chronic Achilles tendon pain, with predictive value based on tendon thickening and circumscribed lesions with echotexture.

### Diagnostic Imaging

Marks RM: Achilles tendinopathy, peritendinitis, pantendinitis, and insertional disorders. *Foot Ankle Clin* 1999;4:789-810.

The authors present a new, comprehensive classification system that calls attention to historical misnomers and poor nomenclature surrounding diseases of the Achilles tendon, including disorders of the insertion. Condition-specific treatment protocols are also presented.

## Types of Achilles Tendon Injuries

Kann JN, Myerson MS: Surgical management of chronic ruptures of the Achilles tendon. *Foot Ankle Clin* 1997;2: 535-545.

This is an excellent review of the management of chronic ruptures of the Achilles tendon that also includes treatment algorithms for different length tendon deficits and techniques for V-Y lengthening and turndown procedures.

Maffulli N, Testa V, Capasso G, Bifulco G, Binfield PM: Results of percutaneous longitudinal tenotomy for Achilles tendinopathy in middle and long distance runners. *Am J Sports Med* 1997;25:835-840.

The authors reviewed the results of 48 patients who underwent percutaneous tenotomy for chronic tendinitis that failed conservative treatment, and 37 good or excellent, 7 fair, and 4 poor outcomes were reported. Complications were limited to four subcutaneous hematomas, three sensitive incisions, and one superficial infection; patient satisfaction was high. The authors recommend this as treatment for chronic recalcitrant Achilles tendinitis.

McGarvey WC, Palumbo RC, Baxter DE, Leibman BD: Insertional Achilles tendinitis: Surgical treatment through a central tendon splitting approach. *Foot Ankle Int* 2002; 23:19-25.

Twenty-two patients underwent tendon débridement using a new central approach. Sixty percent of the patients had concomitant Haglund's deformity. Twenty of 22 returned to work or sports activity in 3 months, but only 13 of 22 were pain free. Younger patients healed more reliably. Overall, an 82% satisfaction rate was reported with this procedure.

Myerson MS: Achilles tendon ruptures. *Instr Course Lect* 1999;48:219-230.

This comprehensive review of the diagnosis, pathogenesis, and management of Achilles tendon ruptures includes algorithms for the treatment of the neglected rupture.

Myerson MS, McGarvey WC: Disorders of the Achilles tendon insertion and Achilles tendinitis. *Instr Course Lect* 1999;48:211-218.

In the second installment of this comprehensive review of the diagnosis, pathogenesis, and management of Achilles tendon disorders, the authors focus on insertional problems and highlight the diagnostic dilemmas that arise when differentiating the retrocalcaneal pathologies. Insertional tendinopathy, retrocalcaneal bursitis, Haglund's deformity, and surgical options are discussed as well as the historic difficulty in treating Achilles tendon disorders and the lack of reliable results.

Porter DA, Mannarino FP, Snead D, Gabel SJ, Ostrowski M: Primary repair without augmentation for early neglected Achilles tendon ruptures in the recreational athlete. *Foot Ankle Int* 1997;18:557-564.

In this retrospective review, 11 patients with Achilles tendon ruptures underwent repair using primary end-to-end anastomoses between 4 and 12 weeks from injury. Aggressive rehabilitation was then instituted. Patients returned to preinjury levels of activity in an average of 5.8 months. No complications were reported, and no differences were noted in strength, range of motion, or pain compared with patients who underwent acute repair by the same surgeon.

Thermann H: Treatment of Achilles tendon ruptures. *Foot Ankle Clin* 1999;4:773-787.

The author challenges traditional treatment of acute ruptures by proposing the use of sonography as an adjunctive, dynamic measure of Achilles tendon injury and healing. The author also proposes using functional, nonsurgical management as the treatment of choice based on different patient demands.

Watson AD, Anderson RB, Davis WH: Comparison of results of retrocalcaneal decompression for retrocalcaneal bursitis and insertional Achilles tedinosis with calcific spur. *Foot Ankle Int* 2000;21:638-642.

The authors compared two groups of patients with retrocalcaneal pain; one group was identified as having retrocalcaneal bursitis and the other as having calcific insertional tendinitis. All were treated surgically. The group with calcific insertional tendinitis was older, took twice as long to reach maximum symptom improvement, was less satisfied with the outcome, and had more pain and shoe-wear problems than the group without radiographic evidence of calcific disease.

Wilcox DK, Bohay DR, Anderson JG: Treatment of chronic Achilles tendon disorders with FHL tendon transfer/augmentation. *Foot Ankle Int* 2000;21:1004-1010.

In this review of 20 patients undergoing FHL tendon transfer for chronic Achilles deficiency, patients were rated on Medical Outcomes Study 36-Item Short Form and American Orthopaedic Foot and Ankle Society scores and Cybex and range-of-motion testing. No reruptures, recurrences of tendinopathy symptoms, or wound complications were reported. The authors suggest this as a viable reconstruction procedure for chronic Achilles tendon deficiency.

## Classic Bibliography

Bosworth DM: Repair of defects in the tendo Achilles. *J Bone Joint Surg Am* 1956;38:111-114.

Carr AJ, Norris SH: Blood supply of the calcaneal tendon. *J Bone Joint Surg Br* 1989;71:100-101.

Cetti R, Christensen SE, Ejsted R, Jensen NM, Jorgensen U: Operative versus non-operative treatment of Achilles tendon rupture: A prospective randomized study and review of the literature. *Am J Sports Med* 1993;21:791-799.

Clain MR, Baxter DE: Achilles tendonitis. *Foot Ankle Int* 1992;13:482-487.

Fiamengo SA, Warren RF, Marshall JL, Vigorita VT, Hersch A: Posterior heel pain associated with a calcaneal step and Achilles tendon calcification. *Clin Orthop* 1982; 167:203-211.

Gerken AP, McGarvey WC, Baxter DE: Insertional achilles tendinitis. *Foot Ankle Clin N Am* 1996;1:237-248.

Keck SW, Kelly PJ: Bursitis of the posterior part of the heel: Evaluation of the surgical treatment of eighteen patients. *J Bone Joint Surg Am* 1965;47:467-471.

Kvist H, Kvist M: The operative treatment of chronic Achilles paratendinitis. *J Bone Joint Surg Br* 1980;62:353-357.

Lagergren C, Lindholm A: Vascular distribution in the Achilles tendon. *Acta Chir Scand* 1959;116:491-495.

Lynn TA: Repair of the torn Achilles tendon using the plantaris tendon as a reinforcing membrane. *J Bone Joint Surg Am* 1966;48:268-272.

Ma GW, Griffith TG: Percutaneous repair of acute closed ruptured Achilles tendon: A new technique. *Clin Orthop* 1977;128:247-249.

Mahler F, Fritschy D: Partial and complete ruptures of the Achilles tendon and local corticosteroid injections. *Br J Sports Med* 1992;26:7-14.

Nistor L: Surgical and non-surgical treatment of the Achilles tendon rupture: A prospective randomized study. *J Bone Joint Surg Am* 1981;63:394-399.

Puddu G, Ippolito E, Postacchini F: A classification of Achilles tendon disease. *Am J Sports Med* 1976;4:145-150.

Rufai A, Ralphs JR, Benjamin M: Structure and histopathology of the insertional region of the human Achilles tendon. *J Orthop Res* 1995;13:585-593.

Thermann H, Zwipp H, Tscherne H: Functional treatment concept of acute rupture of the Achilles tendon: 2 year results of a prospective randomized study. *Unfallchirurg* 1995;98:21-32.

Wapner KL, Pavlock GS, Hecht PJ, Naselli F, Walther R: Repair of chronic Achilles tendon rupture with flexor hallucis longus tendon transfer. *Foot Ankle Int* 1993;14:443-449.

# Chapter 10

# Chronic Ankle Instability

Gregory P. Guyton, MD

## Introduction

Ankle sprains remain among the most common of musculoskeletal injuries. Although only a small fraction of patients with ankle sprains develop chronic ankle instability, this disorder presents unique treatment challenges. This chapter discusses the anatomy, pathomechanics, and diagnosis of chronic ankle instability as well as nonsurgical and surgical treatment.

## Anatomy

Although the ankle is considered a simple rolling hinge joint, it has more complex aspects. The dome of the talus is not cylindrical but more closely approximates the surface of a cone with the apex on the medial side. This bony relationship causes the talus to rotate internally when the ankle is brought into plantar flexion and externally when it is brought into dorsiflexion. The deep fibers of the deltoid ligament (the portion of the deltoid that runs from the medial malleolus to the talus) also help guide the talus into internal rotation in plantar flexion and help restrict external rotation in dorsiflexion.

Because the talus rotates internally and externally within the mortise as ankle motion occurs, a single simple ligament on the lateral side of the ankle joint cannot maintain an isometric position. Instead, there are three separate ligaments, each tensioned in a different arc of motion and slack during another segment of the arc of ankle motion.

The anterior talofibular ligament (ATFL) blends with the capsule of the ankle joint and runs from the anteroinferior margin of the fibula to the lateral margin of the body of the talus, inserting at the junction of talar body and neck (Fig. 1). In a normal ankle, this thickened band measures approximately 7 mm in width and 1.2 to 1.7 cm in length. Well-defined ATFL margins can be difficult to discern in patients who have had multiple ankle sprains. The ATFL becomes progressively tighter when the ankle is brought into plantar flexion and restricts inversion when the ankle is in that position. In a neutral position, the ATFL also restricts anterior translation and internal rotation of the talus in the mortise.

The calcaneofibular ligament (CFL) originates along the inferior margin of the fibula distal to the origin of the ATFL attachment. It then courses deep to the peroneal tendons both inferiorly and posteriorly to insert on the lateral tubercle of the calcaneus. The CFL is contiguous with the ankle capsule, but it is usually a well-defined band of tissue that can be easily isolated. The angle that the CFL makes with the fibula varies from 113° to 150°, averaging 133° with the ankle in a neutral position. The CFL becomes progressively tighter when the ankle is brought into dorsiflexion and resists inversion in that position. The CFL crosses the subtalar joint and the ankle and plays an important role in stabilizing that joint.

The posterior talofibular ligament (PTFL) is a thickening of the capsule that runs from the posterior margin of the fibula to the lateral process of the posterior tubercle of the talus. When the other primary ligaments are intact, it contributes to limiting the end point of ankle dorsiflexion. Serial sectioning studies have demonstrated that the short fibers of the PTFL become important in restricting internal rotation after the ATFL has been torn. These studies also demonstrate that the PTFL restricts inversion with the ankle in a dorsiflexed position after the CFL has been lost.

## Pathomechanics

The position of the ankle at the time of an injury largely determines which structures are injured. An inversion in-

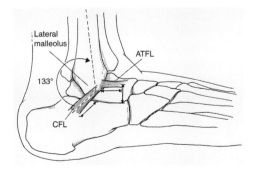

**Figure 1**   Lateral view of the ankle showing basic anatomy. ATFL = anterior talofibular ligament. CFL = calcaneofibular ligament. *(Reproduced from Colville MR: Surgical treatment of the unstable ankle. J Am Acad Orthop Surg 1998;6:368-377.)*

jury on a plantar flexed foot is most likely to result in an isolated injury to the ATFL, which is taut in that position, whereas the CFL is lax in that position and is often spared injury.

Inversion injuries in dorsiflexion almost invariably tear both the CFL and the ATFL. Biomechanical studies have found it essentially impossible to produce isolated tears of the CFL without injuring the ATFL, and large clinical series of ankle ligament repairs have consistently demonstrated that the ATFL is almost always torn with or without the involvement of the CFL. The broad, flat morphology of the ATFL makes it more susceptible to injury than the CFL, and the CFL has a maximal load to failure of almost three times that of the ATFL.

The peroneal muscles also provide critical dynamic support to the ankle when an inversion stress is applied. The peroneal musculotendinous unit reflexively contracts in response to sudden inversion movements of the ankle and subtalar joint. Investigators have found that electrical activity in the peroneal muscles begins between 50 to 65 ms after an unexpected applied inversion moment to the ankle. Some studies providing contrary findings exist, but many investigators have documented an increase in this reaction time in patients with chronic lateral ankle instability. It is not yet known whether patients with naturally prolonged reaction times are predisposed to ankle sprains or whether the sprain injures the mechanoreceptors involved in the reflex arc. It takes approximately 70 ms for the electrical signals arriving at the peroneal musculature to translate into muscle contraction. Thus, it takes more than one tenth of a second for the peroneal muscles to exert a dynamic protective force when the ankle is unexpectedly inverted. The time needed for the peroneal muscles to contract can be dramatically shorter if the muscles are preactivated (proprioceptively conditioned) before the inversion force is applied.

The position of the hindfoot plays a role if the calcaneus rests in varus while standing, which dramatically increases inversion forces on the lateral ankle. The same result is found in patients with an imbalance between the tibialis posterior and the peroneal muscles, which leads to dynamic hindfoot varus during gait.

Subtalar joint motion involves translation and rotation and cannot be defined by a single axis. The closest approximation of a simple axis of motion runs from a distal, medial, and slightly dorsal location to a posterior, lateral, and slightly inferior location. When the joint moves, this line describes a portion of the surface of a cone with an apex at the posterior margin of the calcaneus.

Both the tip of the fibula and the site of insertion of the CFL lie on the surface of this theoretical cone defining subtalar motion. The CFL that connects these two points is displaced over the surface of this cone when subtalar motion occurs. The CFL provides restraint for the ankle while permitting normal inversion and eversion.

Any ligament reconstruction that connects the fibula and the calcaneus in a course other than that of the normal CFL will restrict subtalar motion.

## Diagnosis
### History and Physical Examination
The clinical diagnosis of lateral ankle instability involves the assessment of mechanical and functional instability. Mechanical instability simply means that laxity of the ankle ligaments can be detected by an examiner. Functional ankle instability, however, implies that a patient has a history of major clinical instability episodes. Many patients with lax ankles on manual testing (ie, mechanical instability) have no clinical symptoms because the peroneal tendons provide more than enough supportive restraint for ordinary gait. The ankle ligaments can be considered the restraint of last resort for most activities. A patient's activity level, gait pattern, and hindfoot alignment all play a role in determining whether deficient lateral ankle ligaments cause clinically significant instability.

There is no agreement regarding the threshold of magnitude or frequency of symptoms that constitutes functional instability. A patient's history should specifically include whether the instability episodes include the inability to bear weight; the audible or palpable sensation of a pop, snap, or tear; the rapid onset of ecchymosis; and swelling as a result of the magnitude of soft-tissue disruption.

Manual testing is fundamental for the diagnosis of mechanical ankle instability. The anterior drawer test should demonstrate excessive anterior (sagittal plane) translation because the ATFL is always affected in these injuries. To perform this test, with the patient in the sitting position, the legs hanging freely, and the foot in 25° of plantar flexion, the examiner stabilizes the tibia with one hand while grasping the heel with the other. The foot is then pulled anteriorly and allowed to rotate internally as it translates. In thinner individuals, a dimple or suction sign will appear over the anterolateral corner of the joint.

The ankle is also tested for varus instability. To isolate CFL function, the foot is placed in a neutral position within the ankle mortise while an inversion stress is applied. The motion of the heel is a composite of varus tilt of the tibiotalar joint and normal subtalar joint motion. In the rare case of subtalar instability, abnormal motion at the subtalar joint can be difficult to distinguish from abnormal motion at the ankle. Occasionally, the lateral process of the talus can be palpated to help determine where the motion originates.

Test results for lateral ankle instability are difficult to quantify. Devices used to radiographically measure displacement of the talus indicate that up to 11 mm of displacement is normal with a force applied in a straight anterior-to-posterior direction. However, the deep fibers of the deltoid on the medial side are usually not attenuated, and the talus will translate anteriorly and rotate internally. The extent of laxity may be underestimated if internal rotation of the talus is not allowed during testing.

### Radiographic Evaluation

Stress views can be taken using a calibrated jig to apply a defined displacement force or by manual manipulation. For manual stressing, both the anterior drawer test and inversion of the ankle (talar tilt) should be done. As with manual testing, the results of stress views vary dramatically with changes in ankle position. The use of jigs allows more standardized positioning of the ankle, but the jigs do not account for the internal rotation of the talus in the mortise with failure of the ATFL.

The use of stress views has met with mixed clinical success. The sensitivity of stress radiography is approximately 57%. In addition, the results of anterior drawer and talar tilt stress views vary widely for healthy patients with no history of ankle ligament injury and for those with variations related to age and gender. Although grossly abnormal stress views can indicate severe mechanical instability, they do not offer a substantial advantage over a manual physical examination in most patients.

### Other Imaging Modalities

MRI has been used to evaluate the lateral ankle ligaments with variable success. The thin, broad ATFL is difficult to evaluate with MRI. This is particularly true in patients with chronic ankle instability in whom the ligament is often attenuated and lengthened. There is no basis for the use of MRI to predict whether a proposed ligament repair will be successful without augmentation.

In magnetic resonance arthrography, MRI is performed after the injection of a contrast agent into the ankle joint. Magnetic resonance arthrography can demonstrate the relative thickness of the ATFL and shows considerably more diagnostic promise than MRI. Nevertheless, because no standards have been developed, this technique has no clear diagnostic advantage over physical examination.

### Associated Injuries and Differential Diagnosis

Chronic laxity of the ankle is associated with abnormalities of other structures about the lateral side of the ankle, most commonly synovitis of the ankle joint. In addition to ligament and/or synovitic abnormalities, osteochondral lesions of the talus are identified in approximately 15% to 25% of patients and loose bodies in approximately 20%. Synovitis in the peroneal sheath and longitudinal tears of the peroneal tendons are common findings. Some series report rates of reparable peroneus brevis tendon tears as high as 25% in patients with severe ankle sprains.

Concurrent injury to the deltoid ligament as a component of global ankle laxity is not well defined. Manual

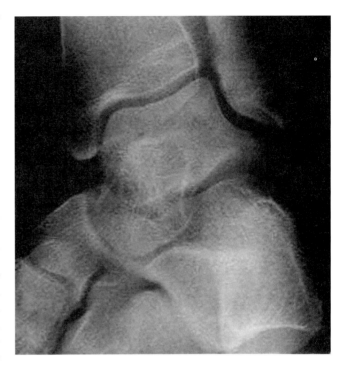

**Figure 2** Radiograph showing subtalar instability versus ankle instability on stress view.

testing for attenuation of the deltoid ligament is likely insensitive, but direct arthroscopic examination of the deltoid has found rates of injury as high as 40%. Some investigators believe that arthroscopically diagnosed deltoid injuries are almost universally associated with chondral injuries. However, no clear standards exist for making the diagnosis of deltoid ligament injury.

These associated injuries can cause symptoms similar to functional ankle instability even in patients without mechanical instability. Patients with osteochondral lesions of the talus or loose bodies may report the sensation of catching or giving way in the ankle. Isolated tears of the peroneus brevis or the superior peroneal retinaculum can cause similar symptoms and are associated with significant peroneal weakness. Pain from synovitis of the ankle or the peroneal sheath can be interpreted as an instability episode.

Injuries that result in isolated pathology of the subtalar joint are more difficult to diagnose. Tears of the interosseous ligament of the subtalar joint can cause pain in the region of the sinus tarsi and, in more severe cases, instability of the subtalar joint. Subtalar instability is uncommon, but it can occur with or without concurrent instability of the ankle. Distinguishing between the two entities can be very difficult on a manual examination of talar tilt unless the patient is thin. Talar tilt stress radiographs show the subtalar joint in a manner similar to the Broden view and can sometimes be helpful when the possibility of subtalar instability must be considered (Fig. 2).

## Nonsurgical Treatment

Nonsurgical treatment of chronic lateral ankle instability focuses on bracing and physical therapy. Mechanical instability of the ankle cannot be corrected through nonsurgical means, but symptoms of ankle instability often can be treated nonsurgically and improved with therapy.

Bracing for ankle instability is most effective when a well-defined activity, such as participation in a sport, is associated with the problem. A variety of functional ankle braces are available, usually in the form of a lace-up ankle sleeve with supplemental wraps that restrict inversion by connecting the lateral side of the calcaneus to the anterior aspect of the ankle. Taping techniques are equally effective. Braces and taping have both been shown to be effective in reducing the incidence of recurrent ankle sprains in athletes.

These therapeutic approaches are limited mechanically because the protective benefits they provide are easily overpowered by forces generated during major unexpected inversion episodes. Some studies show that the mechanical benefit of taping may be lost after as little as 10 minutes of heavy athletic participation. Braces and taping presumably enhance ankle proprioception by stimulating mechanoreceptors in the skin, which may be more important than the mechanical benefit they provide. The peroneal reaction time to sudden unexpected inversion can be reduced as much as 20% by taping the ankle.

Quantitatively, the action of the peroneal tendons is clearly more important than external support. Maximal peroneal contraction has been shown to be up to five times more powerful at resisting inversion forces than external braces alone. The effectiveness of the peroneal muscles is limited primarily by timing. It takes approximately 120 ms for the reflex arc to generate significant mechanical force in a resting peroneal muscle after an unexpected inversion displacement.

It is also clear that the peroneal musculature is not entirely at rest during vigorous activities. Running, jumping, and cutting motions all result in preactivation of the peroneal musculature before impact of the foot with the ground. There is also evidence that the peroneal musculature exerts a secondary, passive role in preventing displacement of the talus, even when it is not actively contracting. Therefore, peroneal musculature strengthening can play a role in conservative therapy for lateral ankle ligament laxity.

Physical therapy in the rehabilitation of chronic lateral ankle laxity includes postural and proprioceptive training. In particular, the use of wobble boards or disks has been advocated to assess and improve balance and stability. Limited studies have found impaired performance in single-leg balance and proprioceptive activities by patients with lateral ankle instability. This may represent a preexisting condition that predisposes patients to injury or may result from the injury.

## Surgical Treatment

Surgical intervention is eventually required in a subset of patients. Appropriate indications for surgery include demonstrable mechanical instability and the presence of functional instability of the ankle. Occasionally, patients wish to know what risks they incur by not undergoing a reconstructive procedure. Although there is no clear understanding of the long-term outcomes of ankle instability that is not surgically treated, the results gleaned from CT and MRI have led to a growing appreciation of the traumatic origin of most osteochondral lesions of the talus, and it is likely that continued exposure to major sprain episodes increases the risk of their development. Anecdotal evidence suggests that marginal osteophytes and early arthrosis are associated with recurrent cutting activities seen in some sports such as soccer (leading to "footballer's ankle") and that recurrent minor subluxation of the ankle is likely a causative factor. Although there is no consensus that mechanical instability alone is problematic, continued functional instability likely constitutes risk.

### Direct Anatomic Repair

Historically, the lateral ankle ligaments were believed to be irreparable once injured, and several reconstructive techniques were advocated. Broström, extending his experimentation with the surgical repair of acute ankle sprains to chronic conditions, performed simple suture repairs of the ATFL and the CFL based on the work of Stener and others in successful late repairs of the metacarpophalangeal ligaments in the hand. Broström's results remain the standard for direct anatomic repair. Patient satisfaction and mechanical stability are achieved in approximately 85% of cases.

Direct anatomic repair is technically straightforward. Tendons are not used as a graft. The anatomic origins and insertions of the ligaments themselves are not altered, and subtalar motion typically is not limited.

The Broström procedure can be accomplished through an oblique incision just off the anterior border of the distal fibula or through a vertical incision. The oblique incision advocated by Broström results in minimal scarring when made in Langer's lines. Care must be taken to avoid the superficial peroneal and sural nerves, which are typically found at the dorsal and plantar apices of the incision, respectively. A vertical incision, which results in a much more noticeable scar, provides a useful approach when pathology of the peroneal sheath must be explored or when a patient's tissues may be damaged and the possibility exists for converting to a tendon-weave reconstruction.

Multiple methods for repair of the lateral ankle ligaments have been described, including suture to the stump of the ligament and insertion of the margin of the ATFL into a fibular bone trough using sutures passed through bone. The latter remains the most popular technique. Re-

**TABLE 1 | Beighton Scoring Table for General Ligamentous Laxity**

| Criteria | Left | Right |
|---|---|---|
| 1. Little finger dorsiflexion > 90° | 0 or 1 | 0 or 1 |
| 2. Thumb apposition to flexor forearm | 0 or 1 | 0 or 1 |
| 3. Elbow hyperextension > 10° | 0 or 1 | 0 or 1 |
| 4. Knee hyperextension > 10° | 0 or 1 | 0 or 1 |
| 5. Trunk flexion, palms touching floor | 0 or 1 | |
| Total | 0 to 9 | |

*(Reproduced with permission from Beighton P, Solomon L, Soskolne CL: Articular mobility in an African population. Ann Rheum Dis 1973;32:413-418.)*

cent reports have indicated that small suture anchors in the fibula can provide good clinical results.

Most authors advocate a period of 2 to 3 weeks of initial immobilization after direct repair. Active range-of-motion exercises are then initiated, and a removable cast boot is used to protect the repair as the patient regains mobility. Strengthening exercises are begun after 4 to 6 weeks.

The main limitation of the Broström procedure lies in patient factors. The quality of the residual ankle ligaments plays a critical role in achieving a successful outcome. Three genetic conditions have been clearly associated with excessive ligamentous laxity: classic Ehlers-Danlos syndrome, Marfan syndrome, and osteogenesis imperfecta. In addition to these usually obvious conditions, the explosive growth of genetic testing in the last 30 years has led to a greater understanding of the spectrum of normal and abnormal ligamentous laxity. Benign joint hypermobility syndrome (BJHS) is now widely recognized and believed to represent a variety of undetermined genetic deficiencies in the protein constituents of ligament. Most authorities now recognize BJHS as synonymous with the type III variant of Ehlers-Danlos syndrome. In addition, global ligamentous laxity can be acquired through the physiologic effect of various disorders, including rheumatic fever, chronic alcoholism, and hyperparathyroidism. Systematic training of a joint can also result in chronic laxity, as may occur with professional dancers. In general, the diagnosis of generalized ligamentous laxity can be based on physical examination criteria. The Beighton instability scoring system, resulting in a Beighton score, is often used to evaluate BJHS (Table 1). There is no known correlation between a patient's Beighton score and the success or failure of the Broström procedure, but the physical test results of the Beighton instability scoring system should be included in the evaluation of patients with lateral ankle ligament laxity. In addition, these patients should be alerted to the fact that even in uninjured joints, the degree of passive and active motion is excessive and, for them, normal.

### Modifications to Direct Anatomic Repair

Several modifications of direct anatomic repair have been advocated to increase the initial strength of the construct or address specific problems. In the widely used modification of the Broström suture technique described by Karlsson and associates, the ATFL margin is inserted into a bone trough using bone sutures. Another modification by Gould, which is commonly referred to as the modified Broström, involves mobilizing the superior margin of the inferior extensor retinaculum after a standard direct repair and suturing it to the repaired margin of the ATFL (Fig. 3). The retinaculum originates from the lateral surface of the calcaneus anterior to the insertion of the CFL. With the incorporation of the inferior extensor retinaculum, this procedure is not strictly anatomic and mildly limits subtalar motion. However, the procedure improves resistance to direct inversion stress.

In another variation, the repair is done in standard fashion and then distally based periosteal flaps are elevated off the fibula and turned down over the suture line to provide reinforcement. The technique provides reinforcement of the primary repair without violating any native anatomic course of the ligament and has been shown to produce good clinical results.

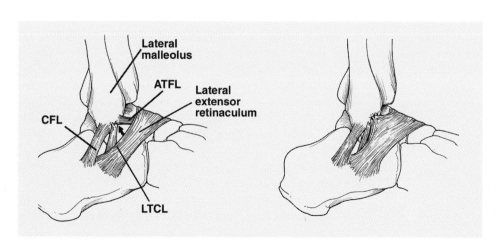

**Figure 3** Gould modification of Broström direct repair. CFL = calcaneofibular ligament. ATFL = anterior talofibular ligament. LTCL = lateral talocalcaneal ligament. *(Reproduced from Colville MR: Surgical treatment of the unstable ankle. J Am Acad Orthop Surg 1998; 6:368-377.)*

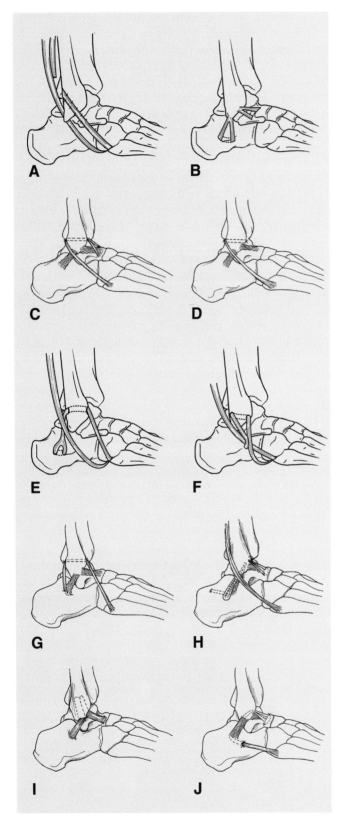

**Figure 4** Illustrations of various tenodesis/augmentation methods. **A**, Nilsonne (1932). **B**, Elmslie (1934). **C**, Watson-Jones (1940). **D**, Evans (1953). **E**, Windfield (1953). **F**, Pouzet (1954). **G**, Chrisman and Snook (1969). **H**, Anderson (1985). **I**, Sjølin (1991). **J**, Colville and Grondel (1995). *(C, D, G, H, I, and J reproduced from Colville MR: Surgical treatment of the unstable ankle. J Am Acad Orthop Surg 1998;6:368-377.)*

## Reconstruction Using Grafts

Indications for augmented reconstruction include a history of a failed Broström procedure, excessively attenuated soft tissues, or a genetic hypermobility disorder. Lateral ankle ligament reconstruction using tendon grafts predates that of direct anatomic repair. The most popular procedures have focused on tenodesis of the peroneus longus or peroneus brevis tendon (Fig. 4).

Nilsonne described simple tenodesis of the peroneus brevis to the fibula in the 1930s, but the procedure is most associated with Evans, who popularized it in the 1950s. The peroneus brevis was originally sutured to the lateral periosteum of the fibula, but in later and more common versions of the procedure, it was divided, routed through an oblique hole drilled in the fibula, and resutured to itself proximally. The Evans procedure has been universally associated with dramatic loss of subtalar motion. It eliminates inversion instability of the ankle, but it does not restrict anterior translation of the talus on the tibia. For these reasons, the Evans procedure alone is seldom used.

In an effort to improve control of the anterior subluxation of the talus, Watson-Jones proposed routing the peroneus brevis tendon through a posterior-to-anterior hole drilled in the fibula and then through a tunnel in the talar neck before returning it to the fibular malleolus, where it is sutured to itself. This technique provides a near anatomic reconstruction of the ATFL and retains nearly the same course of the tendon from the fibula to the fifth metatarsal as in the Evans procedure. Thus, the Watson-Jones procedure is also associated with dramatic loss of subtalar motion, although it represents a dramatic improvement in control of the tibiotalar joint. Other authors later recommended using only half of the peroneus brevis tendon for Watson-Jones procedures to preserve more peroneal tendon function. This modification was also widely adopted for other tenodesis procedures.

Elmslie proposed the first procedure to reconstruct both the ATFL and the CFL in 1934. His reconstruction used a free fascia lata graft routed through tunnels in the calcaneus, fibula, and anterolateral talar neck. Fascia lata grafts proved ineffective, and Chrisman and Snook developed a modification in 1969 in which they routed the anterior half of the peroneus brevis tendon through a tunnel in the anterolateral neck of the talus, posteriorly through the fibula, and then inferiorly to the calcaneus. In the Chrisman-Snook procedure, the ATFL and CFL are more nearly approximated than in the Watson-Jones procedure. Using an ad hoc rating system, the original authors reported 45 of 48 ankles to have good or excellent results at the time of long-term follow-up. However, like other nonanatomic reconstructions, the Chrisman-Snook procedure has been shown to significantly restrict subtalar motion.

The Chrisman-Snook procedure was further modified by Colville and Grondel in 1995 by changing the orientation of the fibular tunnel back to an oblique course and routing the split peroneus brevis tendon first through a calcaneal tunnel, then through the fibula, and finally through a talar tunnel. This technique attempts to reconstruct the ligaments in the most nearly anatomic fashion. The reported clinical results indicate a resolution of the functional ankle instability, with much less restriction of subtalar motion than with the other procedures.

### Other Graft Materials

The split peroneus brevis tendon has been the most extensively used graft material for ankle tenodesis. Concern over the preservation of peroneal function remains an issue. Small series have reported the use of Achilles tendon allografts with no apparent problems at short-term follow-up. The use of hamstring autografts also has been reported in a small series. Both possibilities will likely see further investigation in the near future.

### Associated Hindfoot Varus

Recognition of associated hindfoot varus is critical to the success of lateral ankle ligament reconstruction. Hindfoot varus can develop slowly as part of a neuromuscular cavovarus foot or can be a normal anatomic variant. Any degree of hindfoot varus is potentially pathologic with functional ankle instability. A review of hindfoot alignment that was analyzed using CT found an increased incidence of hindfoot varus in a group of 12 patients with functional ankle instability when compared with controls.

Distinguishing the cause of hindfoot varus is critical. Some deformities are purely dynamic and result from weak peroneal musculature. Others result as an accommodation to a fixed forefoot valgus deformity or plantar flexed first ray. The Coleman lateral standing block test can be used to determine whether hindfoot varus is fixed or flexible. If the condition is fixed, a closing wedge Dwyer calcaneal osteotomy with a lateral translation of the tuberosity fragment should be added to an ankle reconstruction. The osteotomy can be done through a relatively small incision and heals reliably. Partial weight bearing can often be instituted as early as 1 month after surgery. If the hindfoot varus is a result of the tripod effect from a plantar flexed first ray, dorsiflexion osteotomy of the first metatarsal may be indicated in addition to ankle ligament repair. Sometimes both osteotomies are needed.

### Arthroscopy as an Adjunct to Surgical Treatment

Some investigators advocate routine arthroscopy at the time of ankle reconstruction because of the high incidence of associated intra-articular injuries with chronic ankle instability. Chondral and osteochondral injuries are consistently reported in 15% to 25% of patients. Although care must be taken to avoid excessive fluid ex-

travasation when arthroscopy is done immediately before an open reconstruction, the procedure adds minimal morbidity and allows adequate inspection of the entire joint. There is no arthroscopic technique for stabilizing the ATFL that offers advantages over direct open repair. Thermal capsular shrinkage entails considerable risk in the repair of ankle instability because of the proximity of the superficial and deep peroneal nerves and the limited capacity of the often thin soft tissues to dissipate heat.

## Summary

The treatment of lateral ankle instability continues to involve the subtle "art of medicine" at every stage: diagnosis, therapy, and surgical management. Two clear themes have emerged with time. First, respecting the native anatomy of the ankle ligaments when undertaking any surgical repair is critical to a successful outcome. Second, efforts to objectify the indications for surgery have failed both because of subtle differences in patient biology and, equally important, differences in patient goals. Treating lateral ankle instability is therefore likely to remain challenging for even the most experienced practitioner for many years to come.

## Annotated Bibliography

### Pathomechanics

Fernandes N, Allison GT, Hopper D: Peroneal latency in normal and injured ankles at varying angles of pertubation. *Clin Orthop* 2000;375:193-200.

In 34 soccer and rugby players with self-reported functional ankle instability, surface electromyograms were recorded over the peroneal muscles following activation of a trap-door mechanism to suddenly and unexpectedly invert the ankle. No statistical difference in the electrical peroneal latency was noted between the patients' injured and uninjured sides, but a slightly decreased latency of 6 ms for the dominant leg was noted.

Scranton PE Jr, McDermott JE, Rogers JV: The relationship between chronic ankle instability and variations in mortise anatomy and impingement spurs. *Foot Ankle Int* 2000;21:657-664.

In a study of 35 patients undergoing a Broström procedure for ankle instability and 100 adult volunteers, the incidence of asymmetric but asymptomatic ankle laxity was 11% in the control group. Those undergoing ankle surgery had a 3.37 times increased incidence of spurs and loose bodies. The fibula was found to have a 38° range of position relative to the axis of the talus and the medial malleolus.

Van Bergeyk AB, Younger A, Carson B: CT analysis of hindfoot alignment in chronic lateral ankle instability. *Foot Ankle Int* 2002;23:37-42.

A prospective case control study comparing axial and coronal CT scans of 14 ankles with chronic lateral instability to 12 controls found a significant difference in the angle between the calcaneus and the vertical plane between the two groups; 6.4°

varus from vertical in those with instability was found compared with 2.7° in those with no instability. This method suggested an anatomic correlation with recurrent ankle instability and suggested that calcaneal osteotomy to correct extreme hindfoot valgus may have a role in the surgical treatment of chronic ankle instability.

## Diagnosis

Bonnin M, Tavernier T, Bouysset M: Split lesions of the peroneus brevis tendon in chronic ankle laxity. *Am J Sports Med* 1997;25:699-703.

In 18 patients with split lesions of the peroneal brevis tendon, symptoms developed in three phases: ankle sprain, chronic instability, and posterolateral pain. The split lesion of the peroneus brevis tendon may have resulted from chronic ankle laxity. The authors suggest that the peroneal tendons should be checked at the time of surgery for ankle instability. In addition to the procedure done to stabilize the ankle, a specific surgical treatment may be needed to repair the lesion.

DiGiovanni BF, Fraga CJ, Cohen BE, Shereff MJ: Associated injuries found in chronic lateral ankle instability. *Foot Ankle Int* 2000;21:809-815.

In 61 patients with primary lateral ligament reconstruction for chronic instability, none had isolated lateral ligament injuries; 77% had peroneal tenosynovitis, 67% had anterolateral impingement lesions, 54% had attenuation of the peroneal retinaculum, and 49% had ankle synovitis. Other less common but significant injuries included intra-articular loose bodies, peroneus brevis tears, osteochondral talar lesions, and medial ankle tendon tenosynovitis.

Frost SC, Amendola A: Is stress radiography necessary in the diagnosis of acute or chronic ankle instability? *Clin J Sport Med* 1999;9:40-45.

From an analysis of the literature, the authors concluded that talar tilt and anterior drawer stress radiographs have no clinical relevance in acute ankle injuries. The large variability in talar tilt and anterior drawer values in both injured and uninjured ankles precludes their routine use for evaluation of chronic injuries.

Hintermann B, Boss A, Schafer D: Arthroscopic findings in patients with chronic ankle instability. *Am J Sports Med* 2002;30:402-409.

Preoperative ankle arthroscopy of 148 ankles with chronic instability found rupture or elongation of the ATFL in 86%, of the CFL in 64%, and of the deltoid ligament in 40%. Cartilage damage was noted in 66% of ankles with lateral ligament injuries; 98% of those with deltoid ligament injuries had cartilage damage.

Karlsson J, Brandsson S, Kalebo P, Eriksson BI: Surgical treatment of concomitant chronic ankle instability and longitudinal rupture of the peroneus brevis tendon. *Scand J Med Sci Sports* 1998;8:42-49.

In this report on surgical treatment of 19 ankles with combined instability of the lateral ankle ligaments and longitudinal rupture of the peroneus brevis tendon, the authors stress that peroneus brevis tendon rupture should be suspected in patients with lateral ligamentous instability and retromalleolar pain and that tendon rupture should be repaired or reconstructed at the time of ligament surgery.

Komenda GA, Ferkel RD: Arthroscopic findings associated with the unstable ankle. *Foot Ankle Int* 1999;20:708-713.

Before lateral ankle stabilization, arthroscopic examination of 55 ankles with chronic lateral instability identified intra-articular abnormalities in 93%. These included loose bodies, synovitis, osteochondral lesions of the talus, ossicles, osteophytes, adhesions, and chondromalacia. There was a 25% frequency of chondral injuries; there was no correlation between the presence of osteochondral lesions or amount of talar tilt and results.

## Surgical Treatment

Becker HP, Ebner S, Ebner D, et al: 12-year outcome after modified Watson-Jones tenodesis for ankle instability. *Clin Orthop* 1999;358:194-204.

At 12-year follow-up after a modified Watson-Jones tenodesis procedure, 18 of 25 patients (72%) had excellent to good clinical results. The authors concluded that this procedure effectively corrected lateral ankle instability with no clinical deterioration with time and no influence on gait.

Girard P, Anderson RB, Davis WH, Isear JA, Kiebzak GM: Clinical evaluation of the modified Broström-Evans procedure to restore ankle stability. *Foot Ankle Int* 1999;20:246-252.

At an average 30-month follow-up of 21 lateral ankle reconstructions using the modified Broström procedure with augmentation with a portion of the peroneus brevis tendon, the only significant difference from the uninjured ankle was a loss of inversion and eversion. The authors concluded that the procedure is technically simple and provides a greater static restraint for inversion stress without evidence of dramatic over tightening or loss of peroneal strength.

Kaikkonen A, Lehtonen H, Kannus P, Jarvinen M: Long-term functional outcome after surgery of chronic ankle instability: A 5-year follow-up study of the modified Evans procedure. *Scand J Med Sci Sports* 1999;9:239-244.

On long-term (mean, 4.6 years) follow-up of 38 Evans tenodesis procedures, 25 patients (52%) considered the operated ankle much better than before surgery; however, objective evaluation found excellent or good results in only 17 patients (35%). Functional impairment was most evident in a patient's ability to walk down a staircase and to balance on a square beam.

Kitaoka HB, Lee MD, Morrey BF, Cass JR: Acute repair and delayed reconstruction for lateral ankle instability: Twenty-year follow-up study. *J Orthop Trauma* 1997;11: 530-535.

A comparison of 53 primary ligament repairs and 31 delayed reconstruction procedures showed that clinical and radiographic results were similar in the two groups. It was concluded that most severe (grade III) ankle sprains can be treated nonsurgically; if residual instability occurs, satisfactory results can be achieved with late reconstruction.

Krips R, van Dijk CN, Halasi PT, et al: Long-term outcome of anatomical reconstruction versus tenodesis for the treatment of chronic anterolateral instability of the ankle joint: A multicenter study. *Foot Ankle Int* 2001;22: 415-421.

This retrospective, multicenter study included 25 patients with anatomic reconstructions and 29 patients with tenodesis for chronic anterolateral ankle instability. At follow-up of more than 12 years, 15 of the 25 patients (60%) with anatomic reconstructions had excellent results compared with only 8 of 29 patients (25%) with tenodesis procedures. The authors concluded that a tenodesis procedure does not restore the normal anatomy of the lateral ankle ligament and has results inferior to those occurring after anatomic reconstruction.

Messer TM, Cummins CA, Ahn J, Kelikian AS: Outcome of the modified Broström procedure for chronic lateral ankle instability using suture anchors. *Foot Ankle Int* 2000;21:996-1003.

At a mean follow-up of almost 3 years, 20 of 22 patients (91%) had good or excellent functional results after modified Broström procedures using suture anchors. The authors concluded that the use of suture anchors is a simple and effective adaptation of the modified Broström procedure, which results in good or excellent outcomes with few complications in most patients.

Thermann H, Zwipp H, Tscherne H: Treatment algorithm of chronic ankle and subtalar instability. *Foot Ankle Int* 1997;18:163-169.

In a follow-up study of 131 reconstructive procedures, 113 Evans tenodesis procedures, and 42 Chrisman-Snook procedures, no patient had clinically important ankle instability. Of those patients with reconstruction or tenodesis procedures, 90% had good or excellent results. Patients who had an Evans tenodesis procedure had 3.3° less talar tilt than did patients with a reconstructive procedure. The Chrisman-Snook procedure resulted in a mean supination deficit of 7.2° in 20 patients.

## Classic Bibliography

Broström L: Sprained ankles VI: Surgical treatment of "chronic" ligament ruptures. *Acta Chir Scand* 1966;132: 551-565.

Chrisman OD, Snook GA: Reconstruction of lateral ligament tears of the ankle: An experimental study and clinical evaluation of seven patients treated by a new modification of the Elmslie procedure. *J Bone Joint Surg Am* 1969;51:904-912.

Colville MR, Grondel RJ: Anatomic reconstruction of the lateral ankle ligaments using a split peroneus brevis tendon graft. *Am J Sports Med* 1995;23:210-213.

Evans DL: Recurrent instability of the ankle: A method of surgical treatment. *Proc R Soc Med* 1953;46:343-344.

Gould N: Repair of lateral ligament of ankle. *Foot Ankle* 1987;8:55-58.

Inman VT: *The Joints of the Ankle*. Baltimore, MD, Williams & Wilkins, 1976.

Isman RE, Inman VT: Anthropometric studies of the human foot and ankle. *Bull Prosthet Res* 1969;10:97-129.

Konradsen L, Ravn JB: Prolonged peroneal reaction time in ankle instability. *Int J Sports Med* 1991;12:290-292.

Nilsonne H: Making a new ligament in ankle sprain. *J Bone Joint Surg* 1932;14:380-381.

Snook GA, Chrisman OD, Wilson TC: Long-term results of the Chrisman-Snook operation for reconstruction of the lateral ligaments of the ankle. *J Bone Joint Surg Am* 1985;67:1-7.

Watson-Jones R: *Fractures and Other Bone and Joint Injuries*. Edinburgh, Scotland, E & S Livingstone, 1940.

# Chapter 11

# Heel Pain

Christopher L. Tisdel, MD

## Introduction

Pain at the plantar surface of the heel is the most common complaint of patients treated in orthopaedic foot and ankle clinics throughout the United States. It is estimated that more than 2 million Americans will seek treatment for plantar heel pain each year. Multiple etiologies for plantar heel pain have been described in the literature, along with an often confusing array of treatment options. When a proper history is obtained and a thorough physical examination is done to confirm the diagnosis of plantar fasciitis, then an appropriate conservative treatment protocol that is safe and inexpensive can usually alleviate the source of plantar heel pain. Proximal plantar fasciitis is believed to be the most common cause of heel pain, accounting for about 80% of patients with symptoms. Nonsurgical treatment of proximal plantar fasciitis has a reported success rate of 85% to 95%, but it may require 6 to 12 months for all pain to resolve. Nonetheless, educating patients and physicians about the causes, natural history, and safe treatment options for plantar heel pain can help reduce patient and physician concerns regarding the duration of treatment and associated costs.

## Anatomy

The anatomy of the plantar heel illustrates its role as a supportive shock absorber during ambulation (Fig. 1). A healthy individual absorbs 110% of body weight at the heel with each heel-strike while walking and 200% of body weight while running. From heel-strike to the toe-off phase of the gait cycle, the plantar fascia is the major support of the longitudinal arch. During toe-off, the plantar fascia is passively tensioned by the windlass mechanism, which elevates the longitudinal arch and locks the transverse tarsal joints to accommodate forward propulsion. Therefore, a tension stress is applied to the origin of the plantar fascia on the calcaneus throughout the weight-bearing phase of gait.

The plantar fascia is a tough, fibrous layer composed of both collagen and elastin fibers. It has a subcutaneous origin from the os calcis and inserts into the five plantar flexor tendon sheaths and bases of the proximal phalan-

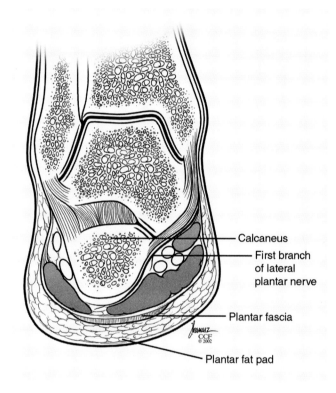

Figure 1 Coronal cross section of the hindfoot. *(Reproduced with permission from the Cleveland Clinic Foundation, Cleveland, OH.)*

ges. The plantar fascia is divided into three areas: central, medial, and lateral. The central component is the major functional and anatomic portion of the plantar fascia, with the lateral and medial components primarily investing fascial layers (Fig. 2).

The heel pad and plantar fascia are important supportive structures that protect the underlying bones, muscles, vessels, and nerves of the hindfoot. In particular, the distal branches of the posterior tibial nerve course through the subcalcaneal region. The calcaneal nerve branches arise directly from the posterior tibial nerve and are sensory nerves to the medial and plantar heel dermis. The medial and lateral plantar nerve branches then proceed into the plantar foot through their respective fora-

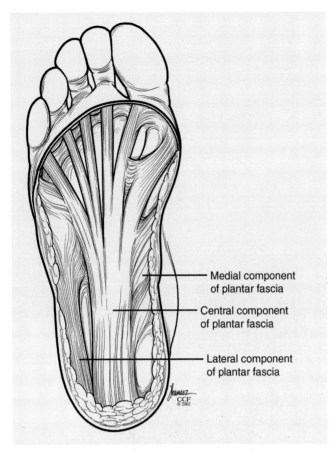

**Figure 2** Anatomic components of the plantar fasciitis. *(Reproduced with permission from the Cleveland Clinic Foundation, Cleveland, OH.)*

men within the origin of the abductor hallucis muscle, thus comprising the distal tarsal tunnel. The first branch of the lateral plantar nerve, the nerve to the abductor dig-

iti minimi muscle, passes deep to the abductor hallucis muscle fascia and plantar fascia. It provides motor and sensory nerve fibers to the plantar calcaneus and intrinsic hindfoot muscles (Fig. 3).

## History and Physical Examination

A complete history and physical examination are essential in the proper diagnosis and treatment of plantar heel pain. Patients usually describe a gradual onset of deep, aching pain in the plantar heel that is not associated with significant trauma. The pain is well localized to the plantar medial aspect of the heel without signs of inflammation or neuropathic symptoms. With further questioning, subtle increases in ambulatory activities often are reported to have preceded the reported onset of pain. In addition, patients often report that pain is aggravated by weight-bearing activities and relieved by rest and that pain is most severe during the initial steps taken after a period of rest, such as arising from bed in the morning or standing up from a chair or car seat. This described start-up pain improves with walking or stretching of the plantar fascia, but it may be exacerbated again by prolonged standing activities. With time, symptoms may worsen to result in pain with every step and an antalgic gait pattern as well as visible swelling in the tender area compared with the asymptomatic and less involved heel if symptoms are bilateral. Patients may learn to walk with their foot in an equinovarus position to avoid bearing weight on the painful plantar medial heel, which can result in lateral metatarsalgia, muscular aches in the leg, and knee and back pain.

Most etiologies of plantar heel pain can be ruled in or out by a complete history (Table 1). Pain radiating distal or proximal with associated numbness or paresthesias is

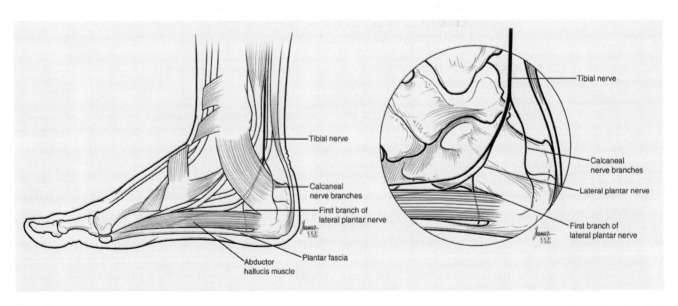

**Figure 3** **A,** Medial anatomy of the plantar fascia and tibial nerve branches. **B,** Close-up view of medial hindfoot. *(Reproduced with permission from the Cleveland Clinic Foundation, Cleveland, OH.)*

**TABLE 1 | Differential Diagnosis for Plantar Heel Pain**

Plantar fasciitis

Calcaneal stress fracture

Fat pad atrophy (central heel pain)

Compressive or metabolic neuropathies

Inflammatory arthropathies
  Rheumatoid arthritis
  Seronegative spondyloarthropathies
  Systemic lupus erythematosus
  Crystalline arthropathies
  Psoriatic arthritis

Ischemia

Infection

Neoplasm

Acute trauma/fracture

likely neuropathic in origin, whereas pain associated with hindfoot warmth and swelling is likely either the result of a stress fracture or infection. Significant associated weight loss or night pain may be indicative of a hindfoot neoplasm. Tenderness on the medial and lateral sides of the posterior tuberosity of the calcaneus is often indicative of a stress fracture in osteopenic patients.

The most common cause of plantar heel pain in both the athletic and nonathletic populations is proximal plantar fasciitis. It usually presents as a unilateral condition in a middle-aged, overweight patient who remains active by walking and performing standing activities. A tight Achilles tendon or a pes planus or pes cavus deformity can increase the loading of the plantar fascia during normal standing activities and may be associated with plantar fasciitis. During rest (for example, at night while the patient sleeps), the foot relaxes into a plantar flexed position, allowing the inflamed fascia to shorten and tighten. With the initiation of weight bearing on the affected foot, the contracted fascia is stretched and produces start-up pain.

Specimens of the inflamed fascia obtained during surgery often reveal collagen necrosis, angiofibroblastic hyperplasia, chondroid metaplasia, and matrix calcification. These changes are consistent with a reparative inflammatory response secondary to an overuse phenomenon.

In elderly patients, atrophy of the plantar fat pad can produce central heel pain syndrome. Fat pad atrophy may also occur in patients with connective tissue disorders or those with a history of multiple plantar foot corticosteroid injections. These patients describe pain with any weight bearing, especially when wearing hard-soled shoes and standing or walking on hard floor surfaces. There is no radiation of pain to the plantar fascia and no improvement after a period of walking (unlike the start-up pain associated with plantar fasciitis).

Entrapment of the first branch of the lateral plantar nerve is an often overlooked cause of plantar medial heel pain. Entrapment occurs as the nerve changes course

from a vertical to a horizontal direction around the medial plantar heel, where it is compressed between the deep fascia of the abductor hallucis muscle and the medial head of the quadratus plantae muscle. Isolated compression of this nerve is rare; it usually occurs in running athletes, ballet dancers, and figure skaters and is often associated with abductor hallucis muscle hypertrophy. Another site of potential first branch nerve entrapment is just distal to the medial calcaneal tuberosity, and nerve entrapment here occurs in association with inflammatory changes of the proximal plantar fascia. This association of plantar fasciitis and compression of the first branch of the lateral plantar nerve suggests that the diagnosis and treatment of these two conditions can overlap.

During physical examination, the lower extremity should be exposed and observed during stance and gait, and any deviations from a normal foot type and gait pattern should be noted. Examination of the foot should rule out neurovascular disorders. Swelling and warmth of the hindfoot accompanied by painful medial-lateral compression of the calcaneus indicates a stress fracture. Plantar fasciitis is usually associated with localized pain to the origin of the fascia on the medial tuberosity of the calcaneus. Stretching the fascia by passive dorsiflexion of the ankle and metatarsophalangeal joints and firm palpation of the plantar medial heel may be necessary to locate tenderness. The absence of a point of tenderness may place the diagnosis in doubt. Pain identified more medial over the origin of the abductor hallucis muscle is also commonly noted and may indicate compression of the first branch of the lateral plantar nerve. Distinguishing pain associated with compression of the first branch of the lateral plantar nerve from pain associated with plantar fasciitis can be difficult during physical examination (Fig. 4). Pain located over the central plantar heel, with appreciable atrophy of the heel pad, may be found in elderly patients. This central heel pain syndrome is distinct from plantar fasciitis and requires different treatment. A complete examination should include evaluation for Achilles tendon contracture, painless range of motion of the ankle and subtalar complex, and pain-free percussion of the tarsal tunnel. Any deviations from local pain isolated to the plantar heel should raise the possibility of other diagnoses. A plantar heel pain syndrome usually is accompanied by unilateral symptoms. Bilateral heel pain, multiple sites of enthesopathy, or joint pain suggest the possible presence of a systemic rheumatologic condition.

Although plantar heel pain syndromes are primarily defined by a detailed history and thorough physical examination, ancillary tests may be appropriate to help confirm the diagnosis. Weight-bearing radiographs of the foot should be negative in patients with plantar fasciitis except on the lateral view where a plantar calcaneal traction osteophyte is found in approximately 50% of all patients with plantar fasciitis. However, because radiographs demonstrate the presence of plantar heel spurs in many

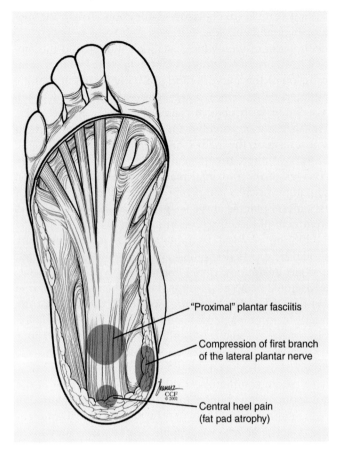

"Proximal" plantar fasciitis

Compression of first branch of the lateral plantar nerve

Central heel pain (fat pad atrophy)

**Figure 4** Common sites of plantar heel pain. *(Reproduced with permission from the Cleveland Clinic Foundation, Cleveland, OH.)*

asymptomatic patients, the radiographic presence of a heel spur adds little to the clinical diagnosis or management.

Although technetium bone scans can demonstrate increased uptake at the origin of the fascia in patients with plantar fasciitis and increased uptake throughout the entire calcaneus in patients with calcaneal stress fractures, it is rarely indicated to confirm the diagnosis. Nonetheless, bone scanning can be a valuable tool for ruling out musculoskeletal sources of pain and can be diagnostically helpful for patients with vague or recalcitrant symptoms. MRI of the foot is also rarely indicated, but it is helpful in defining soft-tissue or bone lesions of the hindfoot. MRI findings in patients with plantar fasciitis include edema, thickening of the fascia, and marrow edema within the plantar calcaneus. These findings are consistent with chronic inflammation and offer little diagnostic information that cannot be otherwise determined by physical examination.

Ultrasound examination of the plantar heel can identify a thickened plantar fascia, but ultrasound results are highly dependent on the expertise of the ultrasound technician. Its use in diagnosing plantar fasciitis is more common in investigational studies of injections or extracorporeal shock wave therapy (ESWT).

## Nonsurgical Treatment

Nonsurgical treatment of plantar fasciitis is successful in more than 90% of patients. However, complete pain relief may require many months to more than a year of compliance with a treatment protocol. Treatment protocol compliance can be greatly improved by educating patients about plantar heel pain and enlisting them as active participants in their own treatment.

Several studies have concluded that Achilles tendon and plantar fascia stretching effectively treats plantar heel pain. In these studies, patients were instructed to stretch three to four times a day and were given handouts illustrating proper stretching techniques. Because stretching can irritate the fascia and posterior leg muscles for 2 to 4 weeks before pain improvement begins, warning patients about this adverse effect helped prevent noncompliance. In addition, use of over-the-counter cushioned heel cups or pads and supportive shock-absorbing shoes helped lessen daily discomfort. One multicenter, prospective, randomized study compared the use of custom-made orthotics and over-the-counter shoe inserts in the early treatment of plantar fasciitis and reported that over-the-counter shoe inserts were more effective. Results from this same study also helped verify the efficacy of Achilles tendon and plantar fascia stretching in the treatment of plantar fasciitis.

Because plantar fasciitis is an overuse inflammatory condition, activity modification is an essential component of any treatment protocol. Avoiding high-impact foot activities and maintaining aerobic fitness by swimming, biking, or use of an elliptical walker is encouraged. Use of nonsteroidal anti-inflammatory medications (if not contraindicated) or applying ice can help reduce inflammatory pain, especially in the early treatment stages.

Patients should return for follow-up examination if their pain is not improved in 2 months. A night splint can then be used. Night splints have been shown to help alleviate morning start-up pain by maintaining fascia stretching during sleep. A corticosteroid injection can also be administered to help alleviate pain. To avoid infiltration of the plantar fat pad and prevent its subsequent atrophy, a medial approach with the needle directed deeply toward the origin of the plantar fascia is recommended. Corticosteroid injections have been successful in the short-term relief of heel pain. Multiple corticosteroid injections, however, can cause a plantar fascia rupture and have not been associated with any long-term benefits. If the plantar fascia ruptures or lengthens by attenuation, some patients will experience lateral midfoot pain, suggesting column overload. These symptoms may be disabling for many months but usually resolve.

Recalcitrant plantar heel pain has been shown to be relieved by use of a short leg walking cast. In one retrospective study, patients selected casting as the most effective pain-relieving treatment modality. Another study, however, documented a cure rate of only 42% when casting was used for an average of 6 weeks. Nevertheless, a 3- to 6-week course of casting is generally an effective way to relieve pain in many patients. This should be followed by another course of stretching, use of shoe inserts, and shoe and activity modification until a complete resolution of pain results.

When patients fail to respond to nonsurgical treatment, additional medical workup should be considered. Because rheumatoid arthritis or other seronegative spondyloarthropathies can be associated with chronic heel pain, laboratory studies should include a complete blood cell count, and differential white blood cell count, and assessment of erythrocyte sedimentation rate, rheumatoid factor, antinuclear antibodies, HLA B27, and uric acid levels. Prolonged medical management emphasizing the use of anti-inflammatory modalities is the treatment of choice for patients with inflammatory enthesopathies. Young patients with bilateral heel pain that is unresponsive to conventional treatment are particularly at risk for one of the seronegative spondyloarthropathies (eg, Reiter's syndrome, ankylosing spondylitis, and psoriatic arthritis).

Patients with central heel pain secondary to fat pad atrophy are also treated nonsurgically. For these patients, shock-absorbing footwear, plastic heel cups, custom-made orthoses, and activity modifications are generally effective in relieving central heel pain.

## Surgical Treatment

The American Orthopaedic Foot and Ankle Society (AOFAS) has developed a position statement on the use of endoscopic and open heel surgery to treat plantar heel pain (http:www.aofas.org). The treatment guidelines contained in this position statement are still widely accepted and intended to protect patients with heel pain from inappropriate invasive procedures. Noting that more than 90% of patients respond favorably to safe and inexpensive forms of nonsurgical treatment within 6 to 10 months, the AOFAS recommends nonsurgical treatment for a minimum of 6 months and preferably 12 months before considering surgery. After a complete medical evaluation, the AOFAS recommends that surgery should be considered for the remaining patients only after an in-depth discussion of procedure options and risks. The AOFAS discourages the use of endoscopic plantar fasciotomy in patients with coexistent nerve compression as a probable source of pain.

Appropriate surgical treatment for plantar heel pain has resulted in pain relief success rates ranging from 50% to 100%. Recent long-term surgical outcome studies emphasize prolonged postoperative recovery from pain (6 to 8 months) and report complete satisfaction with surgical outcomes in only approximately 50% of patients. Despite these data, 80% to 90% of patients can expect only mild pain or no pain with minimal activity restrictions as a final outcome after surgery.

### Isolated Plantar Fasciotomy

When pain is isolated to only the origin of the central plantar fascia band, an isolated plantar fasciotomy may be considered. With the patient supine and commonly under ankle block anesthesia, a 2- to 3-cm incision is made obliquely in the plantar medial hindfoot. After the plantar fascia is bluntly exposed, 50% of the medial fascia is released. Biomechanical studies warn against complete release of the fascia, with severe drop of the medial and lateral columns of the foot as a probable outcome. In clinical practice, patients with a previous rupture or complete plantar fascia release have some degree of flatfoot deformity, walk with less energy and force on the affected side, and commonly report lateral midfoot discomfort. Releasing only the medial 50% of the plantar fascia treats the site of inflammation and lessens the severity of mechanical adverse effects.

The use of endoscopic plantar fascia release has gained popularity. When done correctly in patients with isolated plantar fasciitis, this approach results in less morbidity and a more rapid return to function postoperatively. However, during this technically challenging procedure, the surgeon's ability to see surrounding structures may be impaired, and the lateral plantar nerve may be at risk for injury. An endoscopic release is not appropriate for patients with suspected compression of the first branch of the lateral plantar nerve.

### Partial Plantar Fasciotomy With Distal Tarsal Tunnel Release

When surgery is indicated, patients with pain near the origin of the abductor hallucis muscle should undergo decompression of the first branch of the lateral plantar nerve in addition to the previously described open partial plantar fasciotomy. Plantar medial heel pain, especially when chronic, can be related to multiple causes. Distinguishing isolated plantar fasciitis from compression of the first branch of the lateral plantar nerve can be difficult during preoperative examination. Releasing the nerve and fascia in all instances contributes little morbidity and is gaining popularity because it treats both causes of plantar medial heel pain. The technique also releases the deep fascia of the abductor hallucis muscle, freeing the first branch of the lateral plantar nerve as it courses around the medial band of the quadratus plantae.

A plantar heel spur excision is not routinely done as part of plantar heel pain surgery. On rare occasions, an osteophyte may be large enough to compress the first branch of the lateral plantar nerve, or it may be directed plantarly and warrant removal. Careful dissection of the flexor digitorum brevis muscle origin is necessary to remove the spur, and care should be taken to avoid injury to surrounding vessels and nerves. Postoperative pain, swelling, and ecchymosis are usually greater and prolong the recovery after heel spur excision.

## Extracorporeal Shock Wave Therapy

Studies demonstrating the effectiveness of ESWT, a new noninvasive treatment for chronic plantar fasciitis, have led to the recent approval of this technique by the US Food and Drug Administration. Use of externally applied energy to alleviate musculoskeletal pain has been explored internationally for years. Treatment of plantar heel pain with ESWT has been popular in Europe since published reports of its successful use first appeared in the 1990s.

The specific biologic effects of ESWT on musculoskeletal tissues are not fully understood. Animal studies have revealed that ESWT may create a zone of microdisruption that stimulates new bone and tissue formation. Other theories suggest that ESWT damages nociceptor cell membranes, thereby disrupting the transmission of pain signals. ESWT usually uses a fluid medium, typically water, to propagate the shock waves that are then transmitted into tissues via a coupling gel. Three techniques for generating shock waves have been studied for use in treating heel pain: electrohydraulic, electromagnetic, and piezoelectric. The US Food and Drug Administration has recently approved electrohydraulic (high-power) and electromagnetic (low-power) devices for the treatment of chronic plantar heel pain.

Several placebo-controlled trials of ESWT for plantar fasciitis have reported pain relief benefits. One such study showed that 56% more of the patients treated with high-power ESWT had a successful result compared with the placebo group. However, a more recent controlled trial of low-power ESWT for plantar fasciitis revealed no significant differences in reports of heel pain relief between active treatment and placebo groups at 6 and 12 weeks. Because it is less expensive and results in fewer complications than open surgery, ESWT is a promising treatment option for chronic plantar heel pain. However, additional well-constructed outcome studies are needed to determine whether low-power or high-power ESWT is more effective in the treatment of plantar heel pain.

## Summary

Plantar heel pain is a common foot disorder, usually caused by proximal plantar fasciitis. Nonsurgical treatment is effective in most patients with plantar fasciitis, but pain resolution may require up to 1 year. If surgery is required, no more than half of the fascia should be released to avoid functional deficits. Decompression of the lateral plantar nerve is added in patients with pain near the origin of the abductor hallucis muscle and is becoming a routine part of plantar fascia release procedures. Occasionally, plantar heel spur excision is needed, but this adds to the morbidity of the procedure and prolongs re-

covery time.

## Annotated Bibliography

### History and Physical Examination

Pfeffer GB: Plantar heel pain. *Instr Course Lect* 2001;50: 521-531.

This chapter discusses the etiology, clinical presentation, and treatment options for patients with plantar heel pain.

### Nonsurgical Treatment

Crawford F, Atkins D, Young P, Edwards J: Steroid injection for heel pain: Evidence of short-term effectiveness: A randomized controlled trial. *Rheumatology (Oxford)* 1999;38:974-977.

This double-blind, randomized controlled trial compared the effects of a steroid injection and a local anesthetic injection in the treatment of plantar heel pain. A statistically significant reduction of pain in favor of the steroid group was noted at 1 month, and no differences were detected between the two groups at 3 and 6 months.

Geppert MJ, Mizel MS: Management of heel pain in the inflammatory arthritides. *Clin Orthop* 1998;349:93-99.

Systemic conditions associated with heel pain are reviewed, and a conservative treatment protocol is presented, with emphasis on obtaining the correct diagnosis.

Pfeffer G, Bacchetti P, Deland J, et al: Comparison of custom and prefabricated orthoses in the initial treatment of proximal plantar fasciitis. *Foot Ankle Int* 1999;20:214-221.

This multicenter, prospective randomized trial compared several nonsurgical treatments for proximal plantar fasciitis. Five different treatment groups (a total of 236 patients) were evaluated 8 weeks after treatment began. The percentage of patients reporting improvement was 95% for the group that used stretching combined with silicone inserts, 88% for the group that used rubber inserts, 81% for the group that used felt inserts, 72% for the group that used stretching alone, and 68% for the group that used custom-made orthotics.

### Surgical Treatment

Davies MS, Weiss GA, Saxby TS: Plantar fasciitis: How successful is surgical intervention? *Foot Ankle Int* 1999; 20:803-807.

In this longitudinal outcome study, 43 patients (47 heels) underwent plantar fasciotomy and decompression of the nerve to the abductor digiti minimi. At a mean follow-up of 31.4 months, 76% of heels were pain free or minimally painful, but only 49% of patients were completely satisfied with the outcome.

Murphy GA, Pneumaticos SG, Kamaric E, Noble PC, Trevino SG, Baxter DE: Biomechanical consequences of sequential plantar fascia release. *Foot Ankle Int* 1998;19: 149-152.

This cadaver study describes the mechanical consequences of a complete versus partial release of the plantar fascia.

*Extracorporeal Shock Wave Therapy*

Buchbinder R, Ptasznik R, Gordon J, Buchanan J, Prabaharan V, Forbes A: Ultrasound-guided extracorporeal shock wave therapy for plantar fasciitis: A randomized controlled trial. *JAMA* 2002;288:1364-1372.

In this well-designed, double-blind, randomized, placebo-controlled trial of low-power ESWT for the treatment of heel pain, no significant differences were noted between active treatment and placebo groups.

Haupt G: Use of extracorporeal shock waves in the treatment of pseudarthrosis, tendinopathy and other orthopedic diseases. *J Urol* 1997;158:4-11.

This review article summarizes the uses of shock waves in the treatment of various orthopaedic conditions and describes the physiology and theories regarding the modes of action of ESWT.

Ogden JA, Alvarez R, Levitt R, Cross GL, Marlow M: Shock wave therapy for chronic proximal plantar fasciitis. *Clin Orthop* 2001;387:47-59.

This randomized placebo-controlled, double-blinded study was conducted to determine the safety and effectiveness of high-power ESWT in the treatment of plantar fasciitis. Three hundred two patients enrolled in the study, and 56% more of the patients in the treatment group had a successful result when evaluated at 3 months.

## Classic Bibliography

Amis J, Jennings L, Graham D, Graham CE: Painful heel syndrome: Radiographic and treatment assessment. *Foot Ankle* 1988;9:91-95.

Anderson RB, Foster MD: Operative treatment of subcalcaneal pain. *Foot Ankle* 1989;9:317-323.

Baxter DE, Pfeffer GB: Treatment of chronic heel pain by surgical release of the first branch of the lateral plantar nerve. *Clin Orthop* 1992;279:229-236.

Bordelon RL: Subcalcaneal pain: A method of evaluation and plan for treatment. *Clin Orthop* 1983;177:49-53.

Daly PJ, Kitaoka HB, Chao EY: Plantar fasciotomy for intractable plantar fasciitis: Clinical results and biomechanical evaluation. *Foot Ankle* 1992;13:188-195.

Davis PF, Severud E, Baxter DE: Painful heel syndrome: Results of nonoperative treatment. *Foot Ankle Int* 1994;15:531-535.

Furey JG: Plantar fasciitis: The painful heel syndrome. *J Bone Joint Surg Am* 1975;57:672-673.

Gill LH, Kiebzak GM: Outcome of nonsurgical treatment for plantar fasciitis. *Foot Ankle Int* 1996;17:527-532.

Hicks JH: The mechanics of the foot: The plantar aponeurosis and the arch. *J Anat* 1954;88:25-31.

Jahss MH, Kummer F, Michelson JD: Investigations into the fat pads of the sole of the foot: Heel pressure studies. *Foot Ankle* 1992;13:227-232.

Lapidus PW, Guidotti FP: Painful heel: Report of 323 patients with 364 painful heels. *Clin Orthop* 1965;39:178-186.

Sammarco GJ, Helfrey RB: Surgical treatment of recalcitrant plantar fasciitis. *Foot Ankle Int* 1996;17:520-526.

Sarrafian SK: Functional characteristics of the foot and plantar aponeurosis under tibiotalar loading. *Foot Ankle* 1987;8:4-18.

Schon LC, Glennon TP, Baxter DE: Heel pain syndrome: Electrodiagnostic support for nerve entrapment. *Foot Ankle* 1993;14:129-135.

Tisdel CL, Harper MC: Chronic plantar heel pain: Treatment with short leg walking cast. *Foot Ankle Int* 1996;17:41-42.

Wapner KL, Sharkey PF: The use of night splints for treatment of recalcitrant plantar fasciitis. *Foot Ankle* 1991;12:135-137.

# Section 4

# Neurologic Disorders and Injuries

Section Editor:
G. Andrew Murphy, MD

# Chapter 12

# The Diabetic Foot

Gregory C. Berlet, MD

Naomi N. Shields, MD

## Introduction

Diabetes mellitus has a strong economic impact on the US health care system and on the quality of life of patients and their families and caregivers. It is estimated that approximately 17 million Americans—6.2% of the US population—have diabetes mellitus, with almost 1 million new cases diagnosed each year in people age 20 years or older. Approximately one fifth of the US population older than 65 years (7 million people) have diabetes. These numbers are expected to rise along with the increase in the average age of the population. The economic impact of diabetes in the United States is formidable. An estimated $98 billion in direct and indirect medical costs was spent on diabetes in 1997 in the United States.

Diabetes is a multisystem disease; its effects on the cardiovascular, renal, retinal, nervous, and immune systems all contribute to diabetic foot complications. Lower extremity infections (primarily of the foot) are the primary reason for hospital admission of diabetic patients. Up to 20% of diabetic patients have at least one serious foot infection during their lifetime. Foot ulcers contribute to lower extremity amputations, with as many as two thirds of nontraumatic amputations occurring as the result of diabetes mellitus. Eighty-five percent of diabetes-related lower extremity amputations are preceded by a foot ulcer. Early treatment of ulceration and infection, combined with patient education, can contribute to reducing the incidence of amputation and enhancing the quality of life for diabetic patients.

## Basic Science and Pathophysiology of Diabetes Mellitus

### Neurologic Disease

Diabetic neuropathy has been defined as a demonstrable disorder, either clinically evident or subclinical, that occurs in the setting of diabetes mellitus without other causes for peripheral neuropathy. It includes manifestations in the somatic and/or autonomic parts of the peripheral nervous system. Ten percent of all diabetic patients have some form of sensory, motor, or autonomic dysfunction at the time diabetes mellitus is diagnosed. Fifty percent develop neuropathy within 25 years of diagnosis. No single etiologic pathway has been confirmed for all diabetic neuropathy. It is likely that a combination of metabolic factors (for example, glycosylation of proteins, decreased availability of nerve growth factors, and immunologic factors) and microvascular insufficiency results in the final common pathway of neuropathic changes.

Sensory neuropathy is the most prevalent and obvious nerve dysfunction in diabetic patients. Sensory nerve dysfunction affects as many as 70% of diabetic patients and is a major factor precipitating foot ulceration. In one study, the critical triad of neuropathy, repetitive trauma, and foot deformity was present in 63% of patients with ulceration. Twenty-five percent to 33% of neuropathies are associated with pain. Pain can be superficial (burning, tingling, or allodynia), shooting/electric-like, or cramping/aching. Sensory disturbances show a length-related pattern with stocking and glove distribution resulting from a dying-back distal axonopathy (starting at the periphery and proceeding axially).

Motor neuropathy is clinically most evident by the presence of claw toes caused by intrinsic muscle weakness and an equinus position of the ankle resulting from Achilles tendon contracture. The combination of these factors transfers stress to the forefoot, leading to focal high pressures and resultant skin breakdown. Claw toes occur because of loss of flexor function of the intrinsic muscles, resulting in hyperextension of the metatarsophalangeal joints and flexion of the proximal interphalangeal joints by the unopposed flexor and external extrinsic muscles. Pressure is placed on the dorsal surface of the clawed toes as they come in contact with the toe box of the shoe, and increased pressure occurs underneath the metatarsal heads. Achilles tendon contracture leads to excessive pressure to the distal metatarsals, resulting in an increased risk of ulceration. This scenario has been confirmed by several studies showing that treatment of forefoot ulceration with Achilles tendon lengthening reduces healing time and decreases reulceration rates.

Autonomic dysfunction is the most commonly overlooked manifestation of peripheral neuropathy. Autonomic neuropathy occurs when the autonomic nervous system is unable to control the blood vessel tone and sweat and lubricating glands (eccrine and apocrine glands) in the foot. The skin dries and cracks, allowing the ingress of microbes. In addition, standing foot pressure can be as high as 400 kPa in given areas, which necessitates fine regulation of blood vessels to ensure adequate oxygenation of tissues and avoidance of local anoxia, which can lead to cell death and ulceration. In patients with autonomic neuropathy, repetitive (even mild) trauma can result in preulcerative and ulcerative lesions over areas receiving shear and axial stress.

### Vascular Disease

Vascular disease resulting from diabetes mellitus may be the underlying etiology of most diabetes-related complications. The leading cause of death among diabetic patients is heart disease; approximately 73% of patients with diabetes mellitus also have concurrent hypertension. The risk of a cerebrovascular accident is two to four times higher among patients with diabetes.

Atherosclerosis is more common in diabetic patients and affects them at a younger age. Atherosclerotic plaques in nondiabetic patients are found in the intimal layer of the blood vessel and are patchy rather than circumferential, whereas these plaques in diabetic patients are found in the media layer of the blood vessel and are more diffuse and circumferential. Vasculopathy in diabetic patients is often bilateral and tends to progress more rapidly. The iliac and femoral vessels are often affected. Atherosclerotic disease typically occurs at or distal to the popliteal trifurcation and involves the anterior tibialis, posterior tibialis, and peroneal arteries. Surgical treatment (for example, endarterectomies and bypass procedures) can improve distal ischemia and contribute to healing of foot lesions.

## Physical Examination

The identification of peripheral neuropathy is necessary to lower the risk of subsequent infection and ulceration. Current clinical recommendations call for a comprehensive foot examination at least once a year for all patients with diabetes to identify high-risk foot conditions. Patients with high-risk foot conditions may require more frequent evaluation. Patients with neuropathy should have a visual inspection of their feet during every visit with their health care provider.

A comprehensive examination of the foot includes the assessment of skin, hair, nails, musculoskeletal structures, vascular status, and protective sensation. Footwear should be inspected for blood or other discharges, abnormal wear pattern, foreign objects, proper fit, appropriate material, and foot protection. The patient should be provided with information on self-examination of the feet and the importance of blood glucose monitoring.

Patients are assigned a risk category based on the history of ulceration, deformity, previous amputation, absence of pedal pulses, and loss of sensation. The risk categories are graded from 0 to 3 based on the likelihood of foot complications (Table 1). A patient with feet of normal appearance and normal sensation with or without minor deformity (risk category 0) should have a basic knowledge of foot care, a yearly examination, and regular footwear. On the other end of the spectrum are patients with an insensate foot with deformity and a history of ulceration (risk category 3). Patients in risk category 3 should perform daily foot self-examination; undergo patient-risk education; wear custom-fabricated, pressure-dissipating accommodative foot orthoses and inlay-depth, soft-leather, adjustable-lacing shoes; have follow-up monitoring every 2 months and immediate clinical evaluation of any new skin or nail problems; and should be evaluated by an orthopaedic foot and ankle surgeon.

Sensory neuropathy can be assessed using Semmes-Weinstein monofilaments. Protective sensation is indicated by the patient's ability to perceive a 5.07 monofilament applied perpendicular to the skin.

Vascular perfusion is assessed by the presence (or absence) of dorsalis pedis and posterior tibial pulses. Skin that is thin, fragile, shiny, and hairless is an indication of decreased vascular supply. In addition, all corns, calluses, preulcerative lesions (eg, intradermal hemorrhage and blisters), or open ulcerations should be documented. Toenails should also be examined to determine whether they are ingrown, deformed, or fungal. Thick toenails may indicate vascular or fungal disease.

## Diagnostic Studies

### Vascular Evaluation

All patients with nonhealing wounds or evidence of ischemia should undergo a vascular evaluation. Doppler ultrasonography is effective in assessing the adequacy of circulation. Data are reported as both absolute pressure and the ratio of foot and ankle pressure to brachial Doppler arterial pressure. Pneumatic tourniquets at least one and one half times the circumference of the limb are used, and readings are taken using Doppler probes. Current guidelines indicate that toe pressures should be greater than 40 mm Hg and the ankle brachial index should be greater than 45 mm Hg to be considered favorable for healing. Waveforms should be taken because calcification in a lower extremity can result in a false elevated reading. In the presence of such a reading, a monophasic waveform indicates the presence of a calcified vessel and a triphasic waveform confirms the presence of a vessel with normal elasticity.

Transcutaneous oxygen measurement does not produce false readings when calcified vessels are present. A value of greater than 30 mm Hg is predictive of circulation adequate for healing. Toe pressures of at least 40 mm Hg are better predictors for healing than the ankle-brachial index.

| TABLE 1 | Risk Categories for Foot Complications* | |
| --- | --- | --- |
| Category | Risk Factors | Treatment Recommendations |
| 0 | No history of ulceration<br>No deformity<br>No previous amputation<br>Pedal pulses present<br>No sensory loss | Instruct in basic foot care<br>Yearly foot examination<br>Regular footwear |
| 1 | No history of ulceration<br>No deformity<br>No previous amputation<br>Pedal pulses present<br>Sensory loss | Daily foot self-examination<br>Diabetic foot patient education<br>Depth shoes or running shoes<br>Nonmolded soft inlays<br>Possible total contact orthoses<br>Foot examination by physician every 6 months |
| 2 | No history of ulceration<br>Moderate (prelesion) deformity (ie, hallux rigidus, metatarsal head prominence, claw or hammer toes, callus, plantar bony prominence, hallux valgus, or dorsal exostosis)<br>Pedal pulses present<br>Single lesser ray amputation<br>Sensory loss | Daily foot self-examination<br>Diabetic foot patient education<br>Depth shoes or running shoes<br>Custom-molded foot orthoses<br>Adjuncts: silicon toe sleeves, lambs wool, foam toe separators, hammer toe crests, or metatarsal pad<br>External shoe modifications: metatarsal bar, rocker sole, extended steel shank, or medial or lateral wedges<br>Foot examination by physician every 4 months |
| 3 | History of ulceration<br>Presence of deformity (ie, Charcot deformity, hallux rigidus, metatarsal head prominence, claw or hammer toes, callus, plantar bony prominence, hallux valgus, or dorsal exostosis)<br>Previous amputation (multiple ray, first ray, transmetatarsal, or Chopart)<br>Pedal pulses present or absent<br>Sensory loss | Daily foot self-examination<br>Patient-at-risk diabetic foot education<br>Custom-fabricated, pressure-dissipating accommodative foot orthoses<br>Inlay-depth, soft-leather, adjustable-lacing shoes<br>External shoe modifications: rocker soles, extended steel shanks, solid ankle cushion heels, well filled with low-density materials<br>Unweighting orthoses (patella tendon bearing brace, ankle-foot orthosis)<br>Foot examinations by physician every 2 months<br>Immediate clinical evaluation of any new skin or nail problem<br>Consider evaluation by orthopaedic foot and ankle surgeon |

*Patients are assigned a risk category (0 to 3) based on the likelihood of foot complications. Factors considered in each category include history of ulceration, presence or absence of deformity, previous amputation (partial or full) of either foot, presence or absence of pedal pulses, and degree of sensory loss (neuropathy).

### Arteriography

If noninvasive vascular studies reveal ischemia, arteriography is useful in specifically assessing the occluded vessels. However, arteriography is expensive and may lead to complications that include allergic reaction to the dye, pseudoaneurysm, and acute renal failure in patients with compromised renal function or dehydration. As an alternative, magnetic resonance arteriography can be done, but this test is more useful in evaluating large vessels.

### Radiographic Studies

Clinical findings are still the mainstay for diagnosing musculoskeletal infections, especially osteomyelitis. No single complementary imaging technique has 100% specificity and sensitivity for every case of musculoskeletal infection. When osteomyelitis is suspected, plain radiography should be the first step of the diagnostic-imaging workup, followed by three-phase bone scintigraphy and then the use of infection-specific radiopharmaceutical agents. Studies using technetium Tc 99m with MRI and bone marrow studies are recommended for difficult cases to improve sensitivity and specificity, particularly when trying to differentiate osteomyelitis from Charcot arthropathy.

## Outpatient Management of Common Benign Conditions and Preventive Care

### Skin and Nail Care

Skin and nail care is important in the management and prevention of diabetic foot problems. Educational material is available from many sources to inform patients with diabetes about routine foot care, precautions to take to avoid foot injury, and the use of appropriate shoes. Diabetic patients should be instructed to daily inspect the skin on their feet, to avoid soaking their feet in hot water and trimming their own calluses, to apply lotion or emollient to their feet regularly after bathing for maintenance of skin moisture, and to wear appropriately fitting footwear. These patients frequently have hyperkeratotic skin changes and are more susceptible to fissuring and less resistant to trauma with loss of normal moisture in the foot from neuropathy. Therefore, it is important to recognize that calluses and corns develop secondary to pressure and to treat these aggressively with appropriate shoe wear and possibly orthotic devices. At times, surgical realignment or decompression of underlying bony pressure points may be necessary. Fungal infections of the skin should be diagnosed by evaluating scrapings using potassium hydroxide. When fungal infections are present, dermatologic consultation is appropriate.

Diabetic patients, their families, and caregivers must be involved in the care of the diabetic foot. Common concerns include routine toenail care, ingrown toenails, and onychomycotic nail infection. Toenail care guidelines include trimming toenails straight across and leaving the medial and lateral corners distal to the nail folds intact to minimize risk of ingrown toenails or to seek professional assistance with toenail care. Sanding with a high-speed burr by a health care provider may be used to treat thick, deformed toenails. All infections secondary to ingrown toenails should be treated by taking appropriate cultures and prescribing culture-guided antibiotics, decompressing periungual abscesses, and if infections frequently recur, partial or complete matricectomy should be done for permanent nail ablation. Footwear and orthotics should be examined for proper fit. Onychomycosis may need aggressive treatment in a diabetic patient to decrease the risk of secondary infection, fungal systemic infection, and complications from abnormal toenail growth. Laboratory confirmation of onychomycosis is recommended before beginning treatment. Currently, antifungal medications are applied topically (miconazole, griseofulvin, or the newer amolforine, a topical lacquer painted on the nail for 6 months) or taken orally (griseofulvin [for 12 to 18 months], itraconazole [for 3 months] or terbinafine hydrochloride [for 3 months]). Topically applied antifungal medications have a lower cure rate than oral antifungal medications; however, patients taking oral medications must be monitored for liver toxicity or congestive heart failure.

### Brace and Orthotic Management
Braces and orthoses are important in the long-term management of diabetic patients. These devices provide stability, limit motion, accommodate deformities, unload pressure, and distribute forces evenly throughout the foot, which promotes the healing of ulcerations or preulcerative lesions as well as providing prophylactic treatment.

Improper or poorly fitting footwear is a significant cause of diabetic foot ulcerations. Low-risk patients without deformity, loss of protective sensation, prior amputa-

tion, or previous foot ulcers who have an intact vascular supply should be advised regarding appropriate footwear and have their feet examined regularly. Patients in high-risk categories should be considered for special footwear (eg, extra-depth, therapeutic or custom-molded shoes) combined with custom-molded inserts as appropriate. The Medicare therapeutic shoe bill provides some coverage for at-risk Medicare-eligible patients.

To minimize diabetic foot ulcerations, shoes should have an appropriate width and shape for the patient's foot, a deep toe box to accommodate deformities, and as few seams as possible. The orthosis should also be accommodative and can be made from a variety of polyethylene blown foams combined with rubber or soft leather. The shoe sole should be supportive and cushioning and of sufficient thickness to limit foot penetration by sharp objects. Rigid orthoses should be avoided, especially in patients with neuropathy and those with rigid deformities. Orthoses and shoes may be modified with posting, wedges, rocker soles, bars, and amputation fillers. They may also be used in conjunction with a variety of ankle-foot orthoses (AFOs).

## Ulceration
### Epidemiology
Fifteen percent of diabetic patients develop foot ulcers. Ulcers occur in diabetic patients as a result of peripheral neuropathy, peripheral arterial disease, or a combination of both. With chronic open wounds, the risk of osteomyelitis and amputation increases. Wounds fail to heal from a combination of local wound factors, including infection (soft-tissue cellulitis or abscess or bony osteomyelitis), recurring trauma to a wound combined with a patient's limited ability to sense pressure applied to it, continued pressure from a bony prominence, ischemia, foreign body, or treatment with a wound-inhibiting agent. Systemic factors include white blood cell ineffectiveness caused by poor glucose control; malnutrition; the use of immunosuppressive drugs, steroids, or tobacco; peripheral vascular disease; venous insufficiency; and extremity swelling resulting from venous insufficiency or congestive heart failure.

### Microbiology
Diabetic foot infections are often polymicrobial, with both aerobic and anaerobic gram-positive and gram-negative bacteria present. Therefore, adequate "deep-tissue" cultures and bacterial colony counts must often be obtained for diagnosis. Consultation with an infectious disease specialist is recommended when a diabetic foot infection is identified because the resistance patterns for many bacteria as well as the spectrum of available antibiotics have changed radically. Diabetic foot infections that do not threaten the limb can be treated with either oral or parenteral antibiotics. Limb-threatening and life-

**TABLE 2 | Wagner Ulcer Classification System**

| Grade | Description |
|-------|-------------|
| 0 | Skin intact |
| 1 | Superficial |
| 2 | Deeper, full-thickness extension |
| 3 | Deep abscess formation or osteomyelitis |
| 4 | Partial gangrene of the forefoot |
| 5 | Extensive gangrene |

Reproduced from Wagner F: A classification and treatment program for diabetic neuropathic and dysvascular foot problems. Instr Course Lect 1979;25-143-165.

threatening infections, however, are treated with parenteral antibiotics. Antibiotics used to treat osteomyelitis may be taken for 4 to 6 weeks, depending on the bacterial agent and the extent of bony débridement. Adequate bony débridement mechanically eradicates the foci of infection (particularly infected bone). The bony fragment(s) should not only be cultured but also studied histologically to confirm a diagnosis of osteomyelitis, which may otherwise require many weeks of intravenous antibiotics.

## Vascular Management

Evaluation of the vascular status of a diabetic patient with a foot infection should include a patient history to identify previous vascular compromise, surgery, claudication, or dependent rubor. In addition, physical examination should include assessment of pulses, hair on the toes and affected foot, skin shine, and bleeding at ulceration edges. Tests that aid in the evaluation of vascular status include ankle-brachial index tests (which may identify artificially high ankle-brachial indices as a result of vascular calcification and incompressibility), Doppler ultrasonography with assessment of digital arterial pressures, transcutaneous toe oxygen measurement, and arteriography.

Peripheral arterial disease in diabetic patients occurs at a much younger age and with more rapid involvement than in nondiabetic patients. It is often multisegmental and bilateral and involves the small branches of the tibial and peroneal arteries. It should be noted that the pedal vessels are usually spared. If ischemia is present, vascular surgery should be considered. Arterial bypass to the dorsalis pedis and posterior tibial artery can help salvage an ischemic foot or allow a more distal amputation, thereby preserving limb length.

## Evaluation and Staging

When evaluating a diabetic patient with a foot ulcer, the history includes the date of ulcer onset, length of time present, inciting factors, level of glucose control (ideally hemoglobin $A^{1c} < 7.0\%$), systemic signs (such as fever or malaise), vascular status, tobacco usage, prior treatments and results, previous wounds, medical comorbidities (cardiac, visual, and renal), and immunosuppressive status. Evaluation of the ulcer includes noting the location, size, margins (callus, hyperkeratotic edges, eschars, granulation tissue, etc), depth (probing to bone correlates highly with presence of osteomyelitis), drainage, odor, presence of lymphangitis, presence and extent of cellulitis, and associated swelling and erythema. Physical examination also includes assessment of pulses, sensory status including monofilament evaluation, general skin condition, limb swelling, bony architecture for stability and deformity, skin dryness, Achilles tendon tightness, joint motion limitations, and gait and balance, as well as evaluation of the contralateral limb for any significant deformities, calluses, or preulcerative lesions.

Radiologic evaluation includes three-view plain radiographs of the foot or ankle as appropriate. Nuclear studies using technetium Tc 99m, gallium 67, or indium 111 can be used to evaluate soft-tissue infection or osteomyelitis, Charcot arthropathy, or a combination of infection and arthropathy. MRI has proved highly sensitive and specific for localizing the extent and planes of infection, but it may not distinguish Charcot arthropathy from infections with high specificity.

Laboratory studies include white blood cell count with differential, erythrocyte sedimentation rate, C-reactive protein level, albumin and prealbumin serum levels, and wound cultures (deep and postdébridement, if possible).

Diabetic foot wound classification systems include those of Wagner (Table 2) and Brodsky (Table 3). Brodsky's classification differentiates neuropathic ulcers and ischemic ulcers and offers treatment recommendations for each grade of ulceration.

## Nonsurgical Treatment

### Débridement Principles

Débridement is the keystone of management of diabetic foot ulcerations. Sharp débridement can often be done as an outpatient procedure. Extensive débridement of all necrotic tissue (eschar, slough, and hyperkeratotic callus) to a clean wound base and margins often converts a nonhealing wound into a healing wound. Care should be taken to remove all overhanging edges to allow epithelial contact with the granulation base. Conversion of a circular wound to an elliptical wound also assists with wound healing. Once initial débridement is completed, sharp débridement done weekly or biweekly can increase the healing rate and speed. Once wound healing is complete, appropriate protective footwear and orthoses should be ordered and the patient educated regarding the risk of recurrence.

### Wound Care

Wound care principles emphasize the use of dressings that maintain a moist environment, which helps prevent tissue dehydration and cell death and accelerates wound healing. In addition to providing a moist environment,

| TABLE 3 | Brodsky's Depth/Ischemia Classification of Diabetic Foot Lesions | |
| --- | --- | --- |
| Grade | Definition | Treatment |
| **Depth Classification** | | |
| 0 | The at-risk foot. Previous ulcer or neuropathy with deformity that may cause new ulceration | Patient education, regular examination, appropriate footwear and insoles |
| 1 | Superficial ulceration, not infected | External pressure relief using total contact cast, walking brace, or special footwear |
| 2 | Deep ulceration exposing tendon or joint (with or without superficial infection) | Surgical débridement<br>Wound care<br>Pressure relief if closed and converts to grade 1<br>Antibiotics as needed |
| 3 | Extensive ulceration with exposed bone and/or deep infection (ie, osteomyelitis or abscess) | Surgical débridement<br>Ray or partial foot amputations<br>Intravenous antibiotics<br>Pressure relief if wound converts to grade 1 |
| **Ischemic Classification** | | |
| A | Not ischemic | Adequate vascularity for healing |
| B | Ischemia without gangrene | Vascular evaluation (Doppler ultrasonography with assessment of digital arterial pressures, transcutaneous toe oxygen measurement, and arteriography)<br>Vascular reconstruction as needed |
| C | Partial (forefoot) gangrene of foot | Vascular evaluation<br>Vascular reconstruction (proximal and/or distal bypass or angioplasty)<br>Partial foot amputation |
| D | Complete foot gangrene | Vascular evaluation<br>Major extremity amputation (below-knee or above-knee) with possible proximal vascular reconstruction) |

Reproduced with permission from Brodsky JW: The diabetic foot, in Mann RA, Coughlin MJ (eds): Surgery of the Foot and Ankle, ed 7. St Louis, MO, Mosby-Year Book, 1999.

the ideal dressing absorbs exudation from the wound, does not cause wound desiccation, acts as a barrier to further contamination, and is easily removable. Because wounds have varying amounts of exudate, dressings should be selected on their absorption ability. Basic classifications of wound care agents are shown in Table 4.

Treatment should include frequent wound débridements combined with pressure off-loading and appropriate wound dressings. Antibiotic therapy may be particularly helpful when cellulitis or inadequate arterial flow is present, but it should not be used on a long-term basis. If vascular evaluation suggests an ischemic component, an additional evaluation by a vascular specialist is warranted and vascular reconstruction considered.

In general, an attempt should be made to convert a chronic wound to an acute wound and initiate wound neovascularity and the healing process. The healing process has three stages: inflammation, which lasts from injury to 2 to 5 days; proliferation (tissue formation), which lasts from 2 days to 3 weeks; and tissue remodeling and maturation, which lasts from 3 weeks to 2 years.

### Total Contact Casting and Mechanical Relief

Total contact casting represents the gold standard for off-loading plantar ulcerations. Off-loading decreases me-

chanical stress and trauma to the wound and helps optimize the wound-healing environment. Total contact cast application requires technical skill and frequent changes to accommodate changes in extremity size and allow for wound assessment and débridement. Because complications can result from total contact cast application, it is contraindicated in patients with deeply infected wounds or ischemic ulcerations.

Although other off-loading options are available, including prefabricated walking boots, healing sandals, assistive devices (crutches, walkers, and wheelchairs), and bed rest, total contact casting is still the preferred method of nonsurgical treatment. In a recent randomized, controlled trial comparing the effectiveness of total contact casts, removable pneumatic walking braces, and diabetic healing sandals, it was concluded that the rate of healing in patients using total contact casts was five times faster than in a combined group of patients who did not have casts.

### Surgical Treatment
#### Soft-Tissue Management
Drainage of abscesses is vital to limit further tissue necrosis and spread of infection (especially along tendon sheaths). Multiple débridements to viable bleeding tissues

**TABLE 4 | Basic Classifications of Wound Care Agents**

**Topical wound agents**
Saline
Hydrogels
Antiseptic agents (Dakin's solution, acetic acid)
Antibiotic ointments (silver sulfadiazine, bacitracin-polymyxin-neomycin)
Betadine
Growth factor
**Wound dressings**
Transparent films
Hydrocolloids
Foams
Alginates
Absorptive wound fillers
Antimicrobial dressings
Hydrogels
Gauze
**Hyperbaric oxygen**
**Débridement**
**Off-loading**
Crutches/walker
Bed rest
Total contact cast
Removable walking boots
Wheelchair
Healing sandals
**Wound closure**
Secondary healing
Primary closure
Skin graft
Local skin flaps
Muscle, myocutaneous, fascial, or fasciocutaneous flaps
Free flaps
Vacuum-assisted closure
Skin substitutes-bioengineered skin
**Systemic factors**
Nutritional
Diabetes control
Tobacco cessation

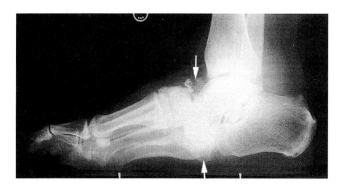

**Figure 1** Uniplant (sagittal) disruption of the naviculocuneiform articulation. Note site of collapse deformity (top arrow) and position of cuboid (bottom arrow); this planar position of the cuboid is the usual site of ulceration after subluxation and collapse.

## Charcot Arthropathy

### Epidemiology

Charcot arthropathy, also known as neuropathic arthropathy, is a progressive deterioration of weight-bearing joints, most commonly in the foot and ankle (Fig. 1). The pathogenesis of the Charcot foot has been explained by two major theories, neurotraumatic and neurovascular. The neurotraumatic theory attributes bony destruction to the loss of pain sensation and proprioception combined with repetitive mechanical trauma to the foot. The neurovascular theory suggests that joint destruction is secondary to an autonomic dysfunction with loss of normal vasomotor control, particularly at entheses. Hyperemia and periarticular osteopenia result. Repetitive minor trauma (walking), in turn, causes joint instability and bone fragmentation. The hypertrophic osteoarthropathy is explained by the healing of the fracture-dislocations in patients who have not had adequate immobilization because of their lack of protective sensation. The radiographs of these patients resemble hypertrophic nonunions with the resultant deformity as a result of the mechanical consequences of weight bearing. It has been estimated that approximately 25% to 50% of patients with Charcot arthropathy remember a minor traumatic event; however, multiple cases of spontaneous Charcot joint changes occurring in diabetic patients at rest and cases associated with foot infections support hyperemia as a potential cause. It is likely that a combination of neurotraumatic and neurovascular dysfunction is responsible for Charcot changes in most patients with Charcot arthropathy.

Charcot arthropathy was once thought to be an unusual complication of diabetic peripheral neuropathy. With the incidence of neuropathy starting at 10% at the time of diagnosis of diabetes mellitus and increasing up to 50% after 25 years of diabetes mellitus, neuropathic arthropathy is quite prevalent among diabetic patients. The incidence of Charcot arthropathy in the diabetic population ranges up to 7.5%, with 9% to 35% of patients

may be necessary. Articular surfaces should be removed and preservation of tendon peritenon, when possible, is advised to preserve healthy tendon. The wound should remain moist to limit tissue desiccation; consultation for timely wound coverage is encouraged.

### Management of Deformity

Ostectomy to remove underlying bony prominences will allow many ulcerations to heal. Achilles tendon lengthening to unload forefoot and midfoot ulcerations assists both healing and maintenance of ulcer healing. Prophylactic correction of deformities such as hammer toes and claw toes should be considered to limit ulcer occurrence or recurrence.

having bilateral involvement. The development of Charcot arthropathy requires a well-perfused foot, which precludes ischemic peripheral vascular disease at the time of initial onset of this condition. The goal of treatment for patients with Charcot arthropathy is to maintain functional ambulation. A plantigrade foot that is able to fit into an accommodative shoe and remain free of ulceration best serves this goal.

### Classification and Staging

The classic Eichenholtz classification system is used to stage Charcot arthropathy. Stage I, the developmental or fragmentation stage (acute Charcot), is characterized by periarticular fracture and joint subluxation with risk of instability and deformity. Stage II, the coalescence stage (subacute Charcot), is characterized by resorption of bone debris and soft-tissue homeostasis. Stage III, the consolidation or reparative stage (chronic Charcot), is characterized by restabilization of the foot with fibrous or bony arthrodesis of the involved joints. The Eichenholtz classification system did not originally include a pre-fragmentation stage (clinical stage), the point at which early diagnosis and intervention are critical to prevent long-term sequelae. Therefore, stage 0, the acute inflammatory phase, has been added, which represents the pre-fragmentation clinical setting.

Early presentation (stage 0) of Charcot arthropathy is characterized by a swollen, erythematous, warm, hyperemic foot. Open wounds are rare at this stage. Most patients will have some discomfort from pain despite a dense sensory neuropathy. Radiographs reveal periarticular soft-tissue swelling and varying degrees of osteopenia.

Stages 0 and I Charcot arthropathy are often confused with infection despite a patient's lack of a significantly elevated white blood cell count or fever. Patients with diabetes usually show a fluctuation in blood glucose levels when a significant infection is present, and maintenance of normal blood glucose levels should discount infection in the differential diagnosis. Imaging with bone scanning can be misleading. MRI is the best imaging modality to differentiate an abscess from soft-tissue swelling. The most accurate combination of radiologic procedures to differentiate a Charcot arthropathy from osteomyelitis is not clear. However, there is evidence that a combination of radionuclide scanning and MRI is as accurate in this differentiation as any single or combined study currently available.

### Management

The challenges to treatment of Charcot arthropathy include (1) when to allow weight bearing in the acute phase of the disease process, (2) whether prefabricated devices are as successful as a total contact cast in the acute phase, (3) the use of early surgical stabilization versus accommodation if and when deformity develops, and (4) the decision to proceed with late reconstruction versus accommodation or amputation in the late stages marked by deformity.

Most patients with acute Charcot arthropathy can be treated effectively by relieving pressure with total contact casting, which permits an even distribution of plantar foot pressures across the plantar surface. The literature on this controversial subject varies regarding treatment recommendations. However, most authors agree that total contact casting with guarded ambulation yields a successful healing rate of 75%, with minimal risk of a Charcot process being produced in the contralateral limb. Successful healing is difficult to define; however, in general, it implies consolidation of the disease process and results in a foot in a plantigrade position with no or minimal deformity. More commonly, it implies that minor degrees of deformity are successfully accommodated by shoe orthoses or brace management or are rendered treatable by these means after minor surgery, such as removal of bony prominences in weight-bearing areas. Casts are changed every 2 to 4 weeks until warmth, erythema, and edema have resolved in the affected limb (that is, soft-tissue homeostasis has returned) and radiographs show evidence of stabilization. Weight-bearing radiographs should be obtained every 4 to 6 weeks until stability is ensured or sooner if there is an acute change. Total contact casting usually continues for up to 4 months; when the active disease phase is complete, the patient can be fitted with an AFO, followed by custom-made shoes and accommodative orthoses. The continued use of an AFO, such as a double upright brace with limited motion or locked-ankle rocker sole and appropriate T strap, may be required in some patients to prevent recurrent plantar ulceration.

Patients with Wagner grade 3, 4, or 5 ulcers should undergo incision, drainage, and antibiotic therapy and exhibit evidence of wound improvement before total contact cast application. Ulcers should be evaluated and débridement done at the time of cast changes.

An alternative to total contact casting for the treatment of neuropathic plantar ulceration is a prefabricated pneumatic walking brace, which has been found to decrease forefoot and midfoot plantar pressure in a manner comparable to that of a total contact cast. Benefits include more frequent wound surveillance, ability to apply several types of dressings, and ease of application. Limitations include severe foot deformity and patient noncompliance, both of which can make the use of a prefabricated pneumatic brace less effective.

Early stabilization of Charcot joints has been advocated as a way to prevent late deformity, which can be very challenging to accommodate with footwear and difficult to surgically reconstruct. Surgery done in the inflammatory phase of Charcot arthropathy has a high rate of nonunion, metal fatigue, and wound complications, including superficial and deep infection and late deformity, the prevention of which was the initial impetus for open

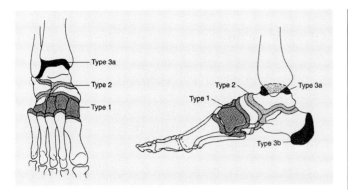

**Figure 2** Anatomic classification system for Charcot arthropathy of the foot. Type 1 involves tarsometatarsal and naviculocuneiform joints. Type 2 involves subtalar, talonavicular, or calcaneocuboid joints. Type 3a involves the tibiotalar joint; type 3b involves pathologic fracture of the tubercle of the calcaneus. *(Reproduced with permission from Brodsky JW: The diabetic foot, in Mann RA, Coughlin MJ (eds): Surgery of the Foot and Ankle, ed 7. St Louis, MO, Mosby- Year Book, 1999, p 949.)*

reduction and internal fixation. Complex spatial frames with minimal skin incisions may decrease these risks and allow earlier surgical intervention.

When deformity develops, the orthopaedic surgeon must decide whether the deformity is manageable with a combination of nonsurgical treatments such as inlay-depth shoes, accommodative foot orthoses, and AFOs. If a plantigrade weight-bearing surface cannot be achieved, surgical stabilization or reconstruction requires rigid stabilization in a compromised biomechanical environment using internal fixation, which, as a whole, is not designed for structures as small as the foot nor is it designed to maintain bony stability for the prolonged periods needed to achieve bony stabilization. Reconstruction of the deformed neuropathic foot is best done in Eichenholtz stage III when soft-tissue stability and some degree of bony stability have been achieved.

Surgical treatment of Charcot deformities can lead to a number of complications. Consequently, patients with a chronic, stable Charcot foot and a residual exostosis beneath a recurrent or nonhealing ulcer can be treated with an exostectomy, which carries less risk of serious complications. A joint stabilization procedure may be necessary in patients with subluxation that produces a markedly unstable extremity.

### Anatomic-Based Management of the Charcot Foot

Anatomic classification based on location can help simplify treatment recommendations. Residual deformity is specific to the joints affected. One Charcot anatomic classification system is shown in Figure 2.

### *Type 1 (Tarsometatarsal)*

Type 1 Charcot arthropathy affects the tarsometatarsal and naviculocuneiform joints. This anatomic location represents the area in which approximately 60% of all Charcot arthropathy of the foot occurs. The most common problems associated with type 1 involvement are bony prominences

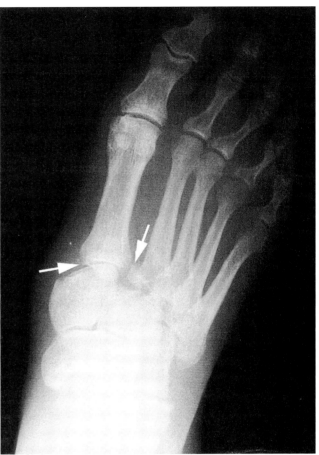

**Figure 3** Multiplane disruption of the metatarsal-tarsal area in a middle-aged female patient. This is the most common type of Charcot arthropathy in diabetic patients.

placing the foot at risk for ulceration (Fig. 3).

The treatment of acute type 1 Charcot arthropathy is total contact casting with protected weight bearing followed by an AFO when soft-tissue homeostasis is present. In acute dislocation with minimal fragmentation but imminent skin compromise, surgical reduction and stabilization may be indicated. The selection of an open or closed procedure depends on the ability of the surgeon to achieve a plantigrade foot with continued casting and guarded weight bearing. Surgical approaches vary, but the trend is to minimize skin incisions rather than rely on the ability to achieve solid joint fusion and expect long periods until consolidation has been achieved.

When type 1 Charcot arthropathy results in chronic ulceration from plantar or medial pressure, an ostectomy usually promotes healing, even of chronic ulcers. One potential complication from ostectomy is iatrogenic midfoot instability, which can usually be avoided by confirming midfoot stability preoperatively.

### *Type 2 (Transverse Tarsal)*

The transverse tarsal and subtalar joints are involved in approximately 35% of patients with Charcot changes in the foot. The most common problem with type 2 involvement is persistent hindfoot instability and ulceration, particularly medially over the dislocated talar head.

Treatment of acute type 2 Charcot arthropathy includes total contact casting with protected weight bearing followed by an AFO with the goal of avoiding complete dislocation, with the talar head plantar-medial and the hindfoot in marked valgus. For patients with this multiplane (frontal, sagittal, and axial plane) deformity, an ulcer-free foot is difficult to maintain using braces and appropriate footwear. In these patients, closed reduction, temporary fixation, casting, and prolonged avoidance of weight bearing is a reasonable treatment option. Weight bearing in a total contact cast may be unwise for Chopart dislocations with multiplane deformity because medial pressure from the talar head secondary to peritalar subluxation is difficult to accommodate orthotically and can result in ulceration.

Chronic type 2 Charcot arthropathy with recalcitrant or recurrent ulceration may require a reconstructive triple arthrodesis and Achilles tendon lengthening. If unbraceable ankle valgus has evolved from the chronic severe planovalgus hindfoot/midfoot deformity, then a pantalar fusion may be required. This is a formidable procedure in an insensate foot and ankle and is a common precursor to major limb amputation.

### Type 3 (Ankle)

Type 3 Charcot arthropathy affects the ankle in approximately 5% of patients with Charcot changes in the foot. The goal of treatment for patients with type 3 Charcot arthropathy is to keep the foot in anatomic alignment with the weight-bearing axis of the leg. Initial care includes total contact casting and no weight bearing until complete bony consolidation has occurred, followed by an AFO. With chronic, unbraceable deformity and/or ulceration, ankle or tibiotalocalcaneal arthrodesis may be necessary. The goal of surgical treatment is achievement of a stable limb with good weight-bearing alignment. Nonunions are common with type 3 Charcot arthropathy, and the choice of internal fixation should be carefully considered.

## Amputation

Diabetic patients have a 15% to 20% higher risk for lower extremity amputations than the general population and account for more than 50% of all extremity amputations. Eighty thousand diabetic-related amputations per year are performed in the United States, 50% of which may be preventable. After the initial amputation, an amputee has a 30% risk of requiring a contralateral amputation within 3 years, and 60% of diabetic patients die within 5 years of the first amputation. Costs to patients and society are high. It is therefore vital to prevent as many amputations as possible by reducing risk factors through ap-

propriate foot care, patient education, aggressive early treatment of ulcers and infections, and optimal glucose level control. Many major amputations are the result of antibiotic-resistant osteomyelitis (for example, methicillin–resistant *Staphylococcus aureus*) that can develop adjacent to a chronic wound.

When a patient is a candidate for amputation, selection of the amputation level is critical and should be based on careful consideration of wound-healing factors, such as nutritional status (prealbumin level), absolute lymphocyte count, peripheral vascular status, tissue oxygenation/perfusion, and tobacco usage. Patient functional status should be considered with a goal of creating a stable, plantigrade, shoeable, braceable foot and providing maximal function with no additional soft-tissue breakdown. Options include partial-digital, digital, ray-resection (digital and metatarsal), transmetatarsal, Chopart (midtarsal), Syme (tibiotalar disarticulation), and below-knee and above-knee amputations. With midfoot amputations, tendon transfer to balance residual foot function and Achilles tendon lengthening are often helpful to prevent recurrent soft-tissue breakdown in the distal stump. After amputation, appropriate footwear and bracing must be provided.

The soft-tissue envelope and intact skin should be maintained as needed for primary closure when amputation is performed. This often means that asymmetric, nonstandard flaps must be created, particularly in the presence of plantar ulcerations or infection. If possible, the use of split-thickness skin grafts should be avoided on the distal aspect or weight-bearing surface of the stump. With digital dry gangrene, observation with autoamputation is reasonable. In general, maximizing foot length while avoiding the use of split-thickness skin grafts is preferred. In a patient with ischemia, vascular evaluation and, if possible, improvement of arterial flow often allows the salvage of a longer limb. If urgent amputation is needed, vascular reconstruction can be done between initial débridement and secondary treatment to maximize limb salvage potential. Initial débridement should remove all infected and nonviable necrotic tissue. Later débridements usually allow secondary closure. Primary closure can be done when all tissue is well vascularized, no apparently infected tissue remains, and closure can be done without skin tension. Once healing has occurred, it is necessary to provide appropriate bracing, accommodative shoe insoles and footwear, patient education, and rehabilitation guidelines.

## Summary

The most important aspect of treatment of diabetic foot disorders is prevention or early treatment of ulceration and infection to decrease the likelihood of amputation. Appropriate footwear, braces, and accommodative shoe insoles help prevent ulcers and promote healing of small, well-vascularized, superficial ulcers. Débridement(s) and careful wound care are essential in the management of diabetic foot ulcers. Total contact casting can provide mechanical off-loading by pressure distribution to optimize the wound-healing environment. The development of severe Charcot arthropathy may require surgical stabilization or reconstruction, but these procedures are difficult in diabetic patients and postoperative complications are frequent and can be catastrophic. The combination of late removal of bony prominences after healing has occurred and continued accommodative orthotic management is a safer, more predictable mode of treatment for this difficult to treat clinical entity in the diabetic patient.

## Annotated Bibliography

### General

American Diabetes Association: The impact of diabetes. Available at: http://www.diabetes.org/info/facts/impact/default.jsp. Accessed October 10, 2003.

This Web site provides useful epidemiologic and economic data that emphasize the significant socioeconomic cost of diabetes.

### Basic Science and Pathophysiology of Diabetes Mellitus

Armstrong DG, Stacpoole-Shea S, Nguyen H, Harkless LB: Lengthening of the Achilles tendon in diabetic patients who are at high risk for ulceration of the foot. *J Bone Joint Surg Am* 1999;81:535-538.

Ten patients with diabetes and a history of neuropathic plantar ulceration of the forefoot participated in a laboratory gait trial. The authors conclude that peak pressures on the plantar aspect of the forefoot are significantly reduced following percutaneous lengthening of the Achilles tendon in patients with diabetes who are at high risk for foot ulceration.

### Physical Examination/Diagnostic Evaluation

Armstrong DG, Lavery LA, Harkless LB: Validation of a diabetic wound classification system: The contribution of depth, infection, and ischemia to risk of amputation. *Diabetes Care* 1998;21:855-859.

In this prospective study, the medical records of 360 patients who were treated for foot wounds were reviewed. The authors report an increased prevalence of amputation as wound depth increased and found that patients were 11 times more likely to receive amputation if the wound probed to bone. They conclude that outcomes deteriorated with increasing grade and stage of wounds.

### Outpatient Management of Common Benign Conditions and Preventive Care

American Diabetes Association: Consensus Development Conference on Diabetic Foot Wound Care: 7-8 April 1999, Boston, Massachusetts. *Diabetes Care* 1999; 22:1354-1360.

A summary of a multidisciplinary, eight-member panel after input from 25 experts and the audience on treatment issues concerning diabetic foot wounds is presented.

Pinzur MS, Slovenkai MP, Trepman E: Guidelines for diabetic foot care: The Diabetes Committee of the American Orthopaedic Foot and Ankle Society. *Foot Ankle Int* 1999;20:695-702.

This article provides guidelines for diabetic foot care, including diabetic foot screening, patient education, basic treatment, and referrals to a specialist.

### Ulceration

Armstrong DG, Nguyen HC, Lavery LA, van Schie CH, Boulton AJ, Harkless LB: Off-loading the diabetic foot wound: A randomized clinical trial. *Diabetes Care* 2001; 24:1019-1022.

In this prospective clinical trial, 63 diabetic patients with diabetic foot ulcers were randomized to be treated with either a total contact cast, half-shoe, or removable cast walker. The authors report that diabetic ulcers healed in 89.5% of the total contact cast group, 65% of the half-shoe group, and 58.3% of the removable cast walker group. Time to healing was also statistically shorter for patients treated with a total contact cast.

Caravaggi C, Faglia E, De Giglio R, et al: Effectiveness and safety of a nonremovable fiberglass off-bearing cast versus a therapeutic shoe in the treatment of neuropathic foot ulcers: A randomized study. *Diabetes Care* 2000;23: 1746-1751.

In this randomized controlled study, 50 diabetic patients with neuropathic plantar ulcers were treated with either a cloth shoe with a rigid sole and unloading alkaform insole (shoe group) or a nonremovable off-bearing fiberglass cast (cast group). Patients had weekly follow-ups. The authors report that the reduction in ulcer area occurred more rapidly in the cast group. The ulcers of 50% of patients in the cast group healed after 30 days versus 20.8% in the shoe group.

Ledermann HP, Morrison WB, Schweitzer ME: MR image analysis of pedal osteomyelitis: Distribution, patterns of spread, and frequency of associated ulceration and septic arthritis. *Radiology* 2002;223:747-755.

This study evaluates the anatomic distribution of osteomyelitis and septic arthritis in 161 patients with advanced pedal infection and compares ulcer location with the distribution of osteomyelitis and septic arthritis. Contrast-enhanced MRI findings were analyzed. The authors discuss patterns of spread from contiguous infections.

Mueller MJ, Sinacone DR, Hastings MK, Strube MJ, Johnson JE: Effect of Achilles tendon lengthening on neuropathic plantar ulcers. *J Bone Joint Surg Am* 2003; 85:1436-1445.

This study compared outcomes of 64 patients with diabetes mellitus and a neuropathic plantar ulcer treated with total contact casting with and without an Achilles tendon lengthening.

There were 33 patients in the group that underwent total contact casting alone and 31 patients in the group that underwent total contact casting with Achilles tendon lengthening. At 7 months follow-up, the risk for ulcer recurrence in the Achilles tendon lengthening group was 75% less at 7 months and 52% less at 2 years than that in the total contact casting group.

Nishimoto GS, Attinger CE, Cooper PS: Lengthening the Achilles tendon for the treatment of diabetic plantar forefoot ulceration. *Surg Clin North Am* 2003;83:707-726.

This review reports that gastrocnemius recession is safer than percutaneous Achilles tendon lengthening but has a 16% incidence of late recurrence of plantar forefoot ulceration.

### Charcot Arthropathy

Pinzur MS, Shields N, Trepman E, Dawson P, Evans A: Current practice patterns in the treatment of Charcot foot. *Foot Ankle Int* 2000;21:916-920.

This article reports the results of a two-part survey of patients and surgeons regarding treatment patterns for and current footwear use of patients with Charcot osteoarthropathy of the foot and ankle.

### Amputation

Peters EJ, Childs MR, Wunderlich RP, Harkless LB, Armstrong DG, Lavery LA: Functional status of persons with diabetes-related lower-extremity amputations. *Diabetes Care* 2001;24:1799-1804.

This article studies the effect that diabetes-related lower-extremity amputations have on quality of life as measured with the Sickness Impact Profile. One hundred twenty-four patients with diabetes were evaluated (35 with an amputation and 89 control subjects who had not undergone amputation). The patients who had undergone transtibial amputation had a significantly higher total impairment score than patients who had not undergone amputation. This is in contrast to patients with toe or midfoot amputations, for whom total impairment scores were not significantly higher than those for the control subjects.

## Classic Bibliography

Eichenholtz SN (ed): *Charcot Joints*. Springfield, IL, CC Thomas, 1966.

Grayson ML, Gibbons GW, Balogh K, Levin E, Karchmer AW: Probing to bone in infected pedal ulcers: A clinical sign of underlying osteomyelitis in diabetic patients. *JAMA* 1995;273:721-723.

Lin SS, Lee TH, Wapner KL: Plantar forefoot ulceration with equinus deformity of the ankle in diabetic patients: The effect of tendo-Achilles lengthening and total contact casting. *Orthopedics* 1996;19:465-475.

Myerson MS, Henderson MR, Saxby T, Short KW: Management of midfoot diabetic neuropathy. *Foot Ankle Int* 1994;15:233-241.

Myerson M, Papa J, Eaton K, Wilson K: The total-contact cast for management of neuropathic plantar ulceration of the foot. *J Bone Joint Surg Am* 1992;74:261-269.

Pecoraro RE, Reiber GE, Burgess EM: Pathways to diabetic limb amputation: Basis for prevention. *Diabetes Care* 1990;13:513-521.

Pinzur MS, Gold J, Schwartz D, Gross N: Energy demands for walking in dysvascular amputees as related to the level of amputation. *Orthopedics* 1992;15:1033-1036.

Steed DL, Donohoe D, Webster MW, Lindsley L: Effect of extensive debridement and treatment on the healing of diabetic foot ulcers: Diabetic Ulcer Study Group. *J Am Coll Surg* 1996;183:61-64.

Wagner FW Jr: The dysvascular foot: A system for diagnosis and treatment. *Foot Ankle* 1981;2:64-122.

# Chapter 13

# Charcot-Marie-Tooth Disease and the Cavovarus Foot

John S. Kirchner, MD

## Introduction

Charcot-Marie-Tooth disease represents a wide spectrum of distinct, inherited, peripheral motor-sensory neuropathies. It affects 1 in 2,500 people annually, making it the most commonly occurring inherited neuropathy in the United States. Charcot-Marie-Tooth disease was first described by Charcot and Marie in France in 1886 and simultaneously by Tooth in England. Primarily affecting motor function in a distal to proximal fashion, Charcot-Marie-Tooth disease is a progressive peripheral neuropathy that is thought to result from an abnormality of myelination. It falls within a subgroup of disorders known as the hereditary motor and sensory neuropathies, of which it is the most common.

Charcot-Marie-Tooth disease was further delineated by Dyck and associates using electrodiagnostic criteria. Type 1, also known as hypertrophic Charcot-Marie-Tooth disease, is an autosomal dominant disorder characterized by thickened nerves with abnormally fatty myelin that spontaneously breaks down, resulting in demyelination and uniform slowing of nerve conduction velocities. Type 1 is the most common form, occurring in approximately 50% of patients with Charcot-Marie-Tooth disease. Further subclassification of type 1 depends on the precise genetic mutation. Type 2, also known as neuronal or atrophic Charcot-Marie-Tooth disease, is an autosomal dominant disorder with incomplete penetration. It is characterized by near-normal nerve conduction velocities and the deterioration of the axons. Type 2 occurs in approximately 20% of patients with Charcot-Marie-Tooth disease. Type 3, also known as Dejerine-Sottas disease, is inherited as an autosomal dominant trait and is histologically characterized by marked segmental demyelination with thinning of the myelin around the nerves. Type 4 is a rare autosomal recessive form of the disease. Another type, CMT-X, is the X-chromosome–linked form of Charcot-Marie-Tooth disease; males are primarily affected, and females are either unaffected or minimally affected. This type occurs in approximately 10% to 20% of patients with Charcot-Marie-Tooth disease.

## Pathophysiology

The classic symptom of Charcot-Marie-Tooth disease is a cavovarus foot deformity that is caused by selective muscle weakness that leads to imbalance between agonist and antagonist muscles (Table 1 and Fig. 1). One study noted atrophy and weakness in the anterior compartment, peroneus brevis muscle, and small intrinsic muscles of the foot, suggesting that the anterior muscle compartment weakens, while the posterior muscles retain near-normal strength. Late in the disease course, the peroneus brevis muscle is selectively affected, while the peroneus longus muscle remains minimally involved. The subsequent deformities result from this muscle imbalance (Fig. 2). The peroneus longus muscle, which is opposed by a weak anterior tibial muscle, causes plantar flexion of the first ray. This plantar flexion causes a compensatory varus hindfoot alignment because the foot functions in weight bearing as a tripodal system from heel strike to midstance. As the plantar flexed first ray strikes the ground before the fifth ray, the foot, to compensate, supinates, bringing the midfoot and hindfoot into a varus position to achieve foot flat (Fig. 3).

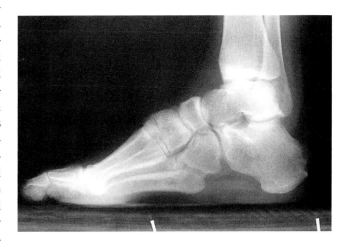

**Figure 1** Lateral radiograph of a typical cavovarus foot deformity in a patient with Charcot-Marie-Tooth disease.

**TABLE 1 | Foot Deformities in Charcot-Marie-Tooth Disease**

| Deformity | Weak Agonist Muscle(s) | Intact Antagonist Muscle(s) | Action |
|---|---|---|---|
| Equinus | Tibialis anterior | Gastrocnemius-soleus and peroneus longus | Pulls the foot in a plantar direction |
| Hindfoot varus | Peroneus brevis | Tibialis posterior | Inverts the subtalar joint |
| Forefoot valgus | Tibialis anterior | Peroneus longus | Pulls the first ray in a plantar direction |
| Pes cavus | Foot intrinsics | Foot extrinsics | Raises the longitudinal arch |
| Toe deformities | Foot intrinsics | Foot extrinsics, especially if the extensor hallucis longus/extensor digitorum longus is used for ankle dorsiflexion with a weak tibialis anterior | Claw toes, long extensors can accentuate metatarsophalangeal hyperextension if intact |

*(Reproduced with permission from Guyton GP, Mann RA: The pathogenesis and surgical management of foot deformity in Charcot-Marie-Tooth disease. Foot Ankle Clin 2000;5:317-326.)*

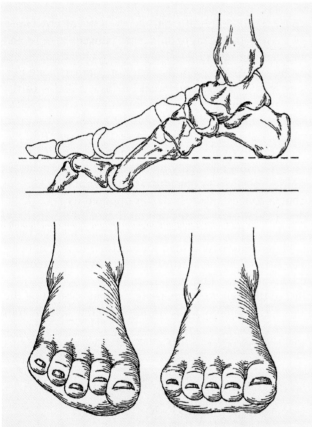

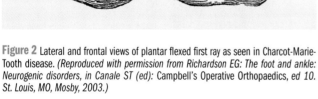

**Figure 2** Lateral and frontal views of plantar flexed first ray as seen in Charcot-Marie-Tooth disease. *(Reproduced with permission from Richardson EG: The foot and ankle: Neurogenic disorders, in Canale ST (ed): Campbell's Operative Orthopaedics, ed 10. St. Louis, MO, Mosby, 2003.)*

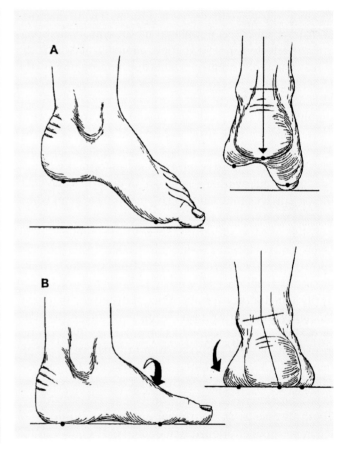

**Figure 3** When the plantar flexed first ray strikes the ground (**A**), the heel is forced into varus (**B**). *(Reproduced with permission from Richardson EG: The foot and ankle: Neurogenic disorders, in Canale ST (ed): Campbell's Operative Orthopaedics, ed 10. St. Louis, MO, Mosby, 2003.)*

As the peroneus brevis muscle becomes weaker, foot and ankle eversion is compromised, allowing the posterior tibial musculotendinous unit to chronically maintain a varus position of the foot. In time, equinus deformities of the ankle and hindfoot contribute to the varus position. This occurs because weakness of the anterior tibial muscle results in an unopposed or weakly opposed gastrocnemius-soleus complex and because the posterior tibial muscle is an accessory ankle plantar flexor. The varus moment at the hindfoot and ankle is further compounded by the complex, approximately 90° rotation of the gastrocnemius-soleus complex as it inserts onto the calcaneus, bringing the soleus muscle to the medial side of the Achilles tendon insertion. The intrinsic muscles of the foot weaken early in the ascending demyelination process, allowing the extrinsic flexors and extensors to create the typical claw toe deformity.

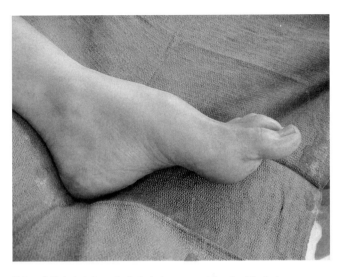

Figure 4 Clinical photograph of a typical cavovarus deformity of the foot.

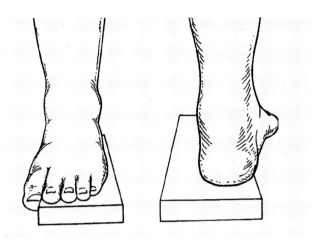

Figure 5 Coleman lateral standing block test. The plantar flexed first metatarsal is allowed to hang free from the block; supple hind part of the foot then corrects. *(Reproduced with permission from Richardson EG: The foot and ankle: Neurogenic disorders, in Canale ST (ed): Campbell's Operative Orthopaedics, ed 10. St. Louis, MO, Mosby, 2003.)*

| TABLE 2 |Surgical Procedures for Foot Deformities in Patients With Charcot-Marie-Tooth Disease |
|---|---|
| **Soft-Tissue Procedures** | |
| Plantar fascia release | Plantar fascia becomes secondarily tight and contributes to the cavus deformity |
| Achilles tendon lengthening | Equinus contracture may be caused by the relative overpull of the gastrocnemius-soleus complex |
| Extensor tendon recession or lengthening to more proximal insertion | May eliminate long extensor contribution to claw toe deformity as well as improve extensor digitorum longus power as an ankle dorsiflexor |
| Extensor hallucis longus transfer to first metatarsophalangeal neck (Jones procedure) | Improves extensor hallucis longus function as ankle dorsiflexor and eliminates extensor hallucis longus as deforming force in extension deformity of the hallux metatarsophalangeal joint |
| Peroneus longus to brevis transfer | Eliminates first ray plantar flexing force and strengthens eversion, which typically is weak |
| Transfer of posterior tibial tendon to dorsum of foot | Converts relatively strong posterior tibial tendon from a cavus-producing vector to an ankle dorsiflexor |
| Claw toe procedures | Include flexor-to-extensor transfer (Girdlestone), plantar dermotomy, flexor tenotomy, and extensor recession |
| **Bony Procedures** | |
| Interphalangeal joint fusion | Part of treatment of rigid claw toe deformity |
| Metatarsal osteotomies | Dorsiflexing, closing wedge osteotomy of the first metatarsal or all metatarsals |
| Midfoot osteotomies | Variety of closing wedge and translational osteotomies between the midtarsal and tarsal-metatarsal joints; normal muscle balance considered prerequisite |
| Calcaneal osteotomies | For rigid hindfoot varus; variety of configurations has been described, including lateral closing wedge osteotomy and crescentic osteotomy |
| Triple arthrodesis | Usually salvage procedure for severe, rigid cavovarus deformity |

In addition, the extrinsic extensors (extensor hallucis longus and extensor digitorum longus) weaken, allowing the long toe flexors to increase the claw toe deformity.

Because this disease process is progressive, the foot of a patient with Charcot-Marie-Tooth disease initially is supple and correctable. However, the deformities gradually become fixed. It is important to understand that Charcot-Marie-Tooth disease involves a dynamic disease process that affects treatment recommendations. Whether the multiple foot and ankle deformities are supple or fixed is of marked importance, and the end result of progressive involvement is often fixed deformity.

## History and Physical Examination

Because Charcot-Marie-Tooth disease is an inherited, demyelinating, distal-to-proximal peripheral neuropathy in which the feet are affected first and most severely, it is important to obtain a complete family history. Early loss of intrinsic muscle strength of the foot followed by selective extrinsic lower leg muscle weakness produces progressive deformities. Most patients in the first or second decade of life express concerns about high-arched feet, painful plantar callosities, and possibly mild gait disturbances. However, as the disease progresses, recurrent lateral ankle sprains can occur as a result of both the varus deformity and a weak peroneus brevis muscle. The varus deformity and peroneus brevis muscle weakness usually are more or less symmetric.

Physical examination is an extremely important component of the evaluation of patients with Charcot-Marie-Tooth disease and begins with observation of the barefoot gait. This allows the evaluating physician to observe the subtle dynamic overpowering of the anterior compartment and the peroneus brevis muscle. Standing evaluations should be performed with the patient facing the evaluating physician and then turned away; hindfoot, midfoot, and forefoot weight-bearing positions should be documented during each evaluation. The most common findings are claw toes, wasting of the midfoot, elevation of the arch, and dorsal talar bossing (Fig. 4). In addition, atrophy of the anterior muscles below the knee usually is visible. Fixed hindfoot varus is evaluated using the Coleman lateral standing block test, during which the patient stands on a wooden block and allows the first ray to hang off the block (Fig. 5). If the hindfoot corrects to a neutral or valgus alignment, the diagnosis of a flexible hindfoot (subtalar joint) and at least a partially fixed plantar flexed first metatarsal is made.

Ankle jerk reflexes usually are absent, and sensory examination using electromyography may be normal or highly abnormal; however, abnormal motor findings usually are greater than abnormal sensory findings. Semmes-Weinstein monofilament testing is an effective screening tool for peripheral sensory neuropathy. Any equinus contracture must be documented, particularly if plantar forefoot sensation is diminished. Proprioception and vibratory sensation usually are lost first, and muscle-strength testing must be detailed and the results well documented for comparison with future examination results. Routine radiographs include weight-bearing AP and lateral views of both feet.

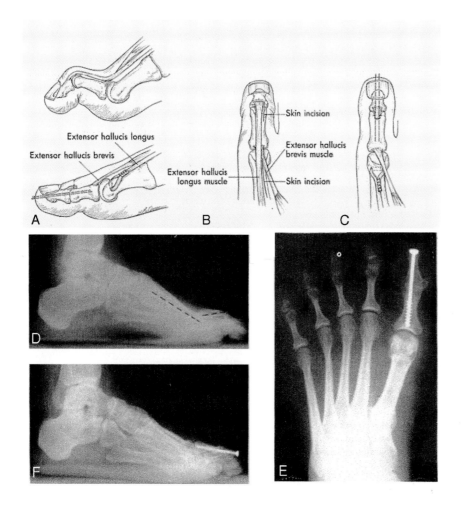

**Figure 6** Schematic representation (**A** through **C**) and radiographic illustration (**D** through **F**) of the Jones procedure. *(Reproduced with permission from Paulos L, Coleman SS, Samuelson KM: Pes cavovarus: Review of a surgical approach using selective soft-tissue procedures. J Bone Joint Surg Am 1980;62:942-953.)*

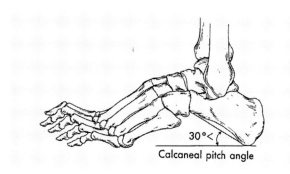

**Figure 7** Calcaneal pitch angle measures the degree of calcaneal deformity. *(Reproduced with permission from Richardson EG: The foot and ankle: Neurogenic disorders, in Canale ST (ed): Campbell's Operative Orthopaedics, ed 10. St. Louis, MO, Mosby, 2003.)*

## Surgical Treatment

When surgery is indicated in patients with Charcot-Marie-Tooth disease, it is essential to determine whether the deformity is fixed or flexible. Each component of the foot deformity should be evaluated individually before a complete surgical plan is established (Table 2). Assessment of each anatomic region of the foot (forefoot, midfoot, hindfoot, and ankle) is recommended.

### Forefoot (Claw Toes)

In the forefoot, the most common deformity, claw toes, is evident when the ankle and heel are brought to neutral position, resulting in a plantar flexed first metatarsal and forefoot valgus (eversion or pronation).

For fixed lesser toe deformities, metatarsophalangeal joint capsulotomy and proximal interphalangeal joint resection with or without arthrodesis are recommended. This is combined with tendon rebalancing, including extensor tendon lengthening, as well as flexor to extensor transfers. For flexible deformities, the flexor to extensor tendon transfer is commonly used, bringing the two limbs of the flexor tendon around the waist of the proximal phalanx of the lesser toe and suturing them dorsally. The clawed hallux is treated with interphalangeal joint arthrodesis and transfer of the extensor hallucis tendon to the neck of the first metatarsal (Jones procedure) (Fig. 6).

### Midfoot (Cavus)

Anterior cavus deformity occurs when the calcaneus is not in the correct position (ie, calcaneal pitch angle is > 30°) (Fig. 7). This is caused by a plantar flexed first ray resulting from muscle imbalance (ie, weak anterior tibialis and strong peroneus longus muscles) and secondary shortening and contracture of the plantar fascia. In patients with a flexible foot who have no degenerative arthritic changes in the midfoot, release of the plantar fascia, dorsal closing wedge osteotomy of the first metatarsal, and transfer of the peroneus longus muscle to the peroneus brevis muscle at the ankle are indicated. In middle-aged patients with fixed cavus deformity, closing wedge osteotomies of multiple metatarsals (Fig. 8) with plantar fascial release or midtarsal arthrodesis are recommended. Options for midtarsal arthrodesis include tarsometatarsal arthrodesis (Fig. 9), Cole dorsal tarsal closing wedge osteotomy (Fig. 10), and Japas V-osteotomy (Fig. 11).

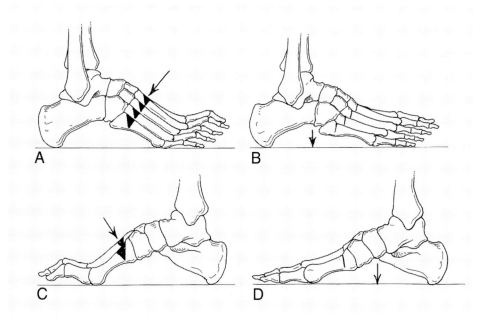

**Figure 8** Multiple metatarsal dorsal closing wedge osteotomies illustrating the degree of arch correction that is possible distal to the apex of the arch. **A** and **B**, Lateral views of the foot emphasizing the second, third, fourth, and fifth metatarsals. **A** shows the location of the wedges and the amount of bone removed (arrow); **B** shows the amount of arch correction provided by this procedure (arrow). **C** and **D**, Medial views of the foot. **C** shows the location of the wedges and the amount of bone removed (arrow); **D** shows the amount of arch correction provided by this procedure (arrow).

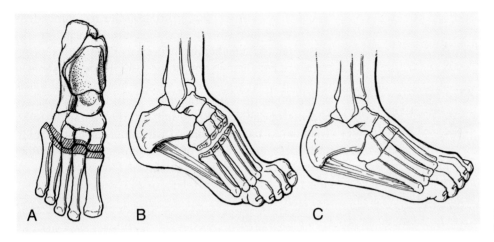

**Figure 9** Plantar (**A**) and lateral (**B** and **C**) views of tarsometatarsal arthrodeses.

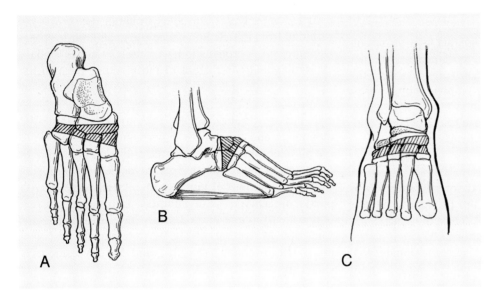

**Figure 10** Plantar (**A**), lateral (**B**), and dorsal (**C**) views of Cole dorsal tarsal closing wedge osteotomy.

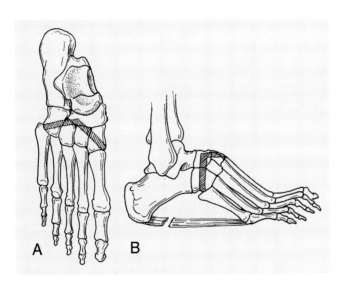

**Figure 11** Plantar (**A**) and lateral (**B**) views of Japas V-osteotomy of tarsus.

## Hindfoot (Varus)

Varus hindfoot deformity also is caused by the distal to proximal weakening of intrinsic and selective extrinsic muscles. If the Coleman lateral standing block test (Fig. 5) demonstrates a flexible, correctable heel varus, a calcaneal lateral closing wedge osteotomy and lateral translation of the tuberosity fragment when needed should correct the hindfoot varus. However, this procedure must be combined with correction of the initial deformity (ie, correction of a plantar flexed first metatarsal and release of the plantar fascia). Good results have been reported in almost 90% of patients after combined sliding calcaneal and closing wedge metatarsal osteotomies (Fig. 12) with plantar fascia release as needed. Cited as advantages of this procedure are correction of all components of the cavovarus deformity; production of a more stable, functional ankle; improvement in gait; avoidance of postoperative bracing; and preservation of the joints of the hindfoot and midfoot.

To maintain correction, a tendon balancing procedure also is required. Transfer of the peroneus longus tendon

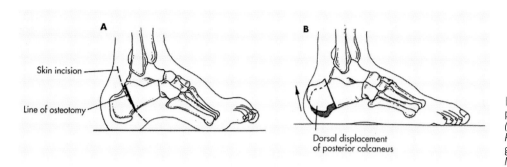

Figure 12 **A**, Cavovarus deformity. **B**, Status post-osteotomy with dorsal displacement. *(Reproduced with permission from Mann RA: Pes cavus, in Coughlin MJ, Mann RA (eds): Surgery of the Foot and Ankle, ed 7. St. Louis, MO, Mosby, 1999, p 780.)*

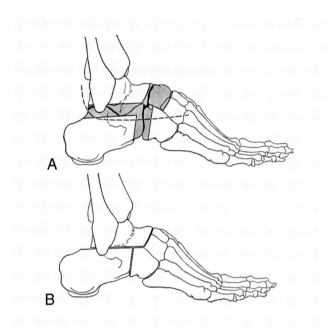

Figure 13 Arthrodesis. **A**, Bony resections. **B**, Apposition of bony fragments. *(Reproduced with permission from Richardson EG: The foot and ankle: Neurogenic disorders, in Canale ST (ed): Campbell's Operative Orthopaedics, ed 10. St. Louis, MO, Mosby, 2003, p 2813.)*

to the peroneus brevis musculotendinous unit and the posterior tibial musculotendinous unit to the dorsum of the foot are recommended. If the patient is willing to wear an ankle-foot orthosis at least part of the time postoperatively, transfer of only the peroneus longus to the peroneus brevis is a viable option.

In older patients with fixed deformity and/or degenerative arthritic changes in the subtalar and/or midtarsal joints, triple arthrodesis is recommended (Fig. 13). Combined with transfer of the posterior tibial musculotendinous unit through the interosseous membrane to the dorsum of the midfoot as a single or staged procedure, triple arthrodesis will correct and maintain the correction of a marked deformity. Radiographically, progressive degenerative changes at the ankle joint can be expected but often do not correlate with clinical symptoms. An Achilles tendon lengthening also may be required for equinocavovarus deformity secondary to Charcot-Marie-Tooth disease.

## Nonsurgical Treatment

If the patient is in the second or third decade of life and has muscle weakness and an awkward gait, then correction of forefoot, midfoot, and/or hindfoot deformities without arthrodesis (using, for example, tendon transfer, soft-tissue release, and osteotomy) is recommended because it can help prevent fixed deformity, which, is difficult to treat with a brace in this age group. In some of these patients, however, correction of flexible deformities may still require bracing. In addition, a young patient with muscle weakness and an awkward gait (toe-heel or foot flat-heel) may not have a normal heel-toe gait after surgery. It is important to keep in mind that although surgery can correct painless deformities that cause problems with gait and shoe wear, the development of periarticular pain can compromise an otherwise successful procedure. Therefore, goals of surgical and nonsurgical treatment, complications, and recovery should be thoroughly discussed with the patient and family. Because pain can adversely affect function just as much as muscle weakness, deformity, and an awkward gait, caution should be key when considering surgical treatment for patients with a progressive peripheral neuropathy.

Molded (custom-made) or manufactured ankle-foot orthoses that fit inside shoes, a double upright brace with a locked or limited motion ankle and an outside T strap (varus-correcting T strap), shoes with a rocker sole, and modified footwear with molded insoles posted laterally all may improve gait, reduce symptoms of ankle instability, and improve function.

Physical therapy may aid in strengthening uninvolved muscles, which weaken with no antagonist muscle counterbalance. Proprioceptive conditioning may also help improve balance and reduce the proclivity to ankle sprain. However, both strengthening and proprioception have limited effect if the neuropathy is severe and progresses rapidly.

## Summary

Charcot-Marie-Tooth disease encompasses several distinct, inherited, peripheral neuropathies that affect motor function. One of the most common deformities caused by the muscle imbalance associated with Charcot-Marie

Tooth disease is cavovarus foot deformity. Nonsurgical treatment with braces and orthoses may improve gait and function in patients with flexible deformities. Surgical treatment requires correction of all components of the deformity in the hindfoot, midfoot, and forefoot. Combinations of calcaneal and metatarsal osteotomies, tendon transfers, and soft-tissue releases may be necessary to obtain a stable, plantigrade foot. Triple arthrodesis generally is indicated for older patients with severe, fixed deformities.

## Annotated Bibliography

Cooper PS: Application of external fixators for management of Charcot deformities of the foot and ankle. *Foot Ankle Clin* 2002;7:207-254.

According to the author, external fixation has advantages over other fixation methods in the areas of treatment of osteoporosis and osteomyelitis, wound healing, and compliance issues.

Guyton GP, Mann RA: The pathogenesis and surgical management of foot deformity in Charcot-Marie-Tooth disease. *Foot Ankle Clin* 2000;5:317-326.

Various deformities of the foot caused by Charcot-Marie-Tooth disease are described and treatment recommendations are discussed.

Hildebrandt G, Holler E, Woenkhaus M, et al: Acute deterioration of Charcot-Marie-Tooth disease IA (CMT IA) following 2 mg of vincristine chemotherapy. *Ann Oncol* 2000;11:743-747.

Severe to life-threatening neuropathy has been reported in patients with hereditary neuropathies who receive vincristine. The authors report such an occurrence in a patient undergoing treatment with vincristine for non-Hodgkin's lymphoma. No neurologic problems were present before treatment, but during treatment, the patient gradually developed dysphagia, dysarthria, muscular weakness of all extremities, areflexia, paraesthesia of the fingertips, and bilateral sensory impairment of her feet and legs. Symptoms resolved over 6 months after vincristine therapy was discontinued.

Pakarinen TK, Laine HJ, Honokonen SE, Peltonen J, Oksala H, Lahtela J: Charcot arthropathy of the diabetic foot: Current concepts and review of 36 cases. *Scand J Surg* 2002;91:195-201.

In a review of 36 patients with Charcot-Marie-Tooth disease foot deformities, the delay in diagnosis averaged 29 weeks. Fourteen surgical procedures were done in 10 patients. The authors cite as prerequisites for successful reconstructive surgery correct timing, adequate fixation, and a long postoperative non–weight-bearing period.

Pinzur MS: Charcot's foot. *Foot Ankle Clin* 2000;5:897-912.

This review of Charcot-Marie-Tooth disease describes evaluation, disease progression, and treatment.

Sammarco GJ, Taylor RL: Cavovarus foot treated with combined calcaneus and metatarsal osteotomies. *Foot Ankle Int* 2001;22:19-30.

Lateral sliding elevating calcaneal osteotomies combined with dorsolateral closing wedge osteotomies of one or more metatarsal bases were used to successfully treat severe symptomatic cavovarus foot deformity in 89% of patients. The authors report that this procedure provides a pain-free, plantigrade foot with a lower longitudinal arch and a stable ankle without sacrificing motion.

## Classic Bibliography

Bentzon PGK: Pes cavus and the M. peroneus longus. *Acta Orthop Scand* 1932;4:50-52.

Charcot JM, Marie P: Sur une forme particulaiere d'atrophie musculaire progressive, souvent familiale de'butatant par les pieds et les jambes et atteignant plus tard les mains. *Rev Med* 1886;6:97-138.

Dyck PJ, Lambert EG: Lower motor and primary sensory neuron diseases with peroneal muscular atrophy, I: Neurologic, genetic, and electrophysiologic findings in hereditary polyneuropathies. *Arch Neurol* 1968;18:603-618.

Dyck PJ, Ott J, Moore SB, Swanson CJ, Lambert EH: Linkage evidence for genetic heterogeneity among kinships with hereditary motor and sensory neuropathy, type I. *Mayo Clin Proc* 1983;58:430-435.

Holmes JR, Hansen ST Jr: Foot and ankle manifestations of Charcot-Marie-Tooth disease. *Foot Ankle* 1993;14:476-486.

Jones R: An operation for paralytic calcaneocavus. *Am J Orthop Surg* 1908;5:371.

Paulos L, Coleman SS, Samuelson KM: Pes cavovarus: Review of a surgical approach using selective soft-tissue procedures. *J Bone Joint Surg Am* 1980;62:942-953.

Sabir M, Lyttle D: Pathogenesis of Charcot-Marie-Tooth disease: Gait analysis and electrophysiologic, genetic, histopathologic, and enzyme studies in a kinship. *Clin Orthop* 1984;184:223-235.

Santavirta S, Turunen V, Ylinen P, Konttinen YT, Tallroth K: Foot and ankle fusions in Charcot-Marie-Tooth disease. *Arch Orthop Trauma Surg* 1993;112:175-179.

Skre H: Genetic and clinical aspects of Charcot-Marie-Tooth's disease. *Clin Genet* 1974;6:98-118.

Thometz JG, Gould JS: Cavus deformity, in *The Child's Foot and Ankle*, ed 1. New York, NY, Raven Press, 1992, pp 343-353.

Tooth HH: *The Peroneal Type of Progressive Muscular Atrophy*. London, England, HK, 1886.

# Chapter 14

# Interdigital Neuroma and Tarsal Tunnel Syndrome

Wen Chao, MD

## Introduction

Interdigital neuroma and tarsal tunnel syndrome are static nerve disorders that can occur in the foot and ankle. This chapter reviews the pathophysiology, clinical presentation, diagnostic studies, treatment, and complications of these two disease entities.

## Interdigital Neuroma

Interdigital neuroma (IDN) is a disease process that affects the interdigital nerve as it courses under the transverse metatarsal ligament. With dorsiflexion of the toes, as occurs when walking or running, the interdigital nerve compresses against the distal end of the transverse metatarsal ligament. With chronic irritation, fusiform swelling and pathologic changes of the nerve can occur (Fig. 1). The most common histologic findings associated with IDN are perineural fibrosis, degeneration of the nerve fibers, and thickening and hyalinization of the endoneural blood vessels. The mechanism of injury and histologic appearance of the nerve help confirm that this is a form of entrapment neuropathy and repetitive injury of the interdigital nerve rather than a neuroma. Nonetheless, the term "neuroma" is commonly used to describe this disease process.

The incidence of IDN is much greater in females than males, implicating shoes with high heels and narrow toe boxes as a major cause of this disease process. The incidence of second and third web-space involvement is comparable in both clinical and cadaveric studies. As many as 90% of IDNs reportedly occur in the third web space, whereas IDNs almost never occur in the first or fourth web space. Other anatomic factors such as deviation of the toe, inflammation of the intermetatarsal bursa, or thickening of the transverse metatarsal ligament can also cause symptoms of IDN. In addition, trauma to the forefoot may contribute to the development of IDN.

### History and Physical Examination

Patients with IDNs commonly report pain on the plantar aspect of the foot that may be located between or just distal to the metatarsal heads. The pain is usually neuritic and accompanied by a burning sensation, radiating distally into the involved toes. Patients may describe the feeling of something moving around or a wrinkle in the sock in the plantar aspect of the foot. The symptoms are typically aggravated by activity, such as walking or running, or by certain footwear, especially shoes with high heels or narrow toe boxes. Symptoms are often relieved by stopping the aggravating activity, removing the shoe, and rubbing the forefoot.

Physical examination should start by observing both feet with the patient standing. Any deviation or subluxation of the toes or swelling of the involved foot is noted. The metatarsophalangeal (MTP) joints are examined, and areas of periarticular tenderness and range of motion are identified. Because the second MTP joint, where synovitis often occurs, is adjacent to the web space in which an IDN may be located, the meticulous palpation of specific anatomic features will help differentiate synovitis from IDN, particularly in the second web space. Instability of the second MTP joint should be recorded, if present. Next, the involved web space is palpated from a proximal to distal direction. This may reproduce the neuritic pain. Another helpful test is to squeeze the foot in a medial to lateral direction while palpating the web space, which may result in a click or grinding feeling (Mulder's sign). If this test reproduces the patient's pain, it is diagnostic of an IDN. A painless Mulder's sign can be a normal finding. Sensory examination of the toes is usually normal.

### Diagnostic Studies

Although the diagnosis of an IDN is best made by thorough history and careful physical examination, weight-bearing radiographs of the involved foot may be helpful to rule out a bone-related problem, such as a stress fracture of the metatarsal neck. The efficacy of other imaging modalities in the diagnosis of IDN is still controversial. Nonetheless, published studies have reported the successful use of ultrasonography and MRI in the diagnosis of IDN.

One recent study showed that ultrasonography findings, when compared with histologic and surgical findings, correctly identified an IDN in 85% of patients and that

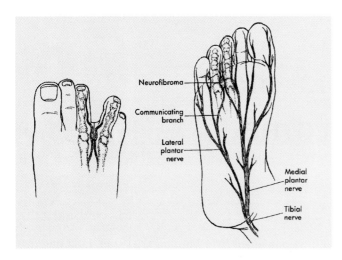

**Figure 1** The most common anatomic location of interdigital neuroma; plantar and dorsal views. *(Adapted with permission from McElvenny RY: J Bone Joint Surg 1943; 25:675.)*

identification of the interdigital nerve in continuity with a mass increases diagnostic confidence. This study also reported that a mass more than 20 mm long in the web space suggests the presence of an abnormality other than a neuroma. Another study reported the successful use of ultrasonography in confirming the recurrence of a neuroma at an average of 19.2 months after resection. Ultrasonography detected the presence of a recurrent neuroma in 13 of 20 patients, 11 of whom underwent repeated neuroma excision. Histologic findings confirmed recurrent neuroma in 10 of the 11 patients.

The value of MRI in diagnosing IDN is less clear. A review of the recent literature reveals that the optimal sequence for MRI evaluation of IDN continues to be a source of debate. One recent study showed that T1-weighted axial and coronal images with an axial fast-spin echo T2-weighted sequence detected IDNs more consistently than an enhanced T1 fat-suppressed sequence.

Another helpful diagnostic procedure involves the injection of anesthetic solution into the web space. If the symptoms temporarily resolve, even with the patient trying to reproduce the pain, then the diagnosis of IDN is more likely. This test is helpful in detecting concomitant problems as well. By temporarily eliminating the neuritic pain, the patient may be able to better localize other sources of pain, if present. Concomitant problems that may be present or may be the cause of pain include fat pad atrophy; problems related to the MTP joint, such as synovitis, instability, subluxation, dislocation, and arthritis; osteonecrosis of the metatarsal head; stress fracture of the metatarsal neck; soft-tissue tumors, such as synovial cyst or ganglion cyst; bursitis; and other diseases of the nerve.

### Nonsurgical Treatment

The nonsurgical treatment of IDN is often successful. Neuroma symptoms may be relieved by wearing shoes with wider toe boxes, stiffer soles, and lower heels. In addition, a metatarsal pad can help alleviate excessive pressure under the metatarsal heads. Several studies have shown that corticosteroid injections can also effectively treat IDNs. One such study showed that pain was relieved in 80% of patients after one injection. Forty-six percent of the patients reported pain relief lasting longer than 3 months. Another study reported that multiple corticosteroid injections (average 3.8) resulted in complete resolution of pain after 2 years in 60% of patients with IDNs. The results of a three-stage treatment protocol were as follows: the first stage consisted of patient education, footwear modifications, and metatarsal head relief; the second stage consisted of corticosteroid and local anesthetic injections into the involved web space; and the third stage consisted of surgical excision for patients in whom the first two stages of treatment failed. Overall, 85% of the patients reported improvement with the treatment program. Twenty-one percent of the patients required surgical excision of the nerve, of which 96% reported satisfactory results.

### Surgical Treatment

Surgical treatment is indicated when nonsurgical treatment fails. Several surgical techniques have been described, including nerve resection, release of the intermetatarsal ligament with or without neurolysis, and transposition of the nerve into the intermuscular space. The most common surgical treatment for IDN is excision of the neuroma. The goal of the surgical excision is to resect the nerve as proximal to the weight-bearing area of the metatarsal heads as possible. This helps to avoid the development of a painful stump neuroma.

### Clinical Outcomes

A recent long-term follow-up study of IDN resection using a dorsal approach revealed an overall satisfaction rate of excellent or good in 85% of the patients after more than 5 years. Multiple clinical studies have demonstrated that releasing the intermetatarsal ligament alone or combined with neurolysis can also be effective in relieving pain associated with IDN. One such study compared the treatment of IDN by resection with a technique in which the interdigital nerve was transposed into the intermuscular space between the adductor hallucis and the interosseous muscles after division of the digital nerves distal to the IDN. For the first 6 months after surgery, the resection group reported a slightly lower level of pain. However, at 12-month follow-up and again at 36- to 48-month follow-up, the resection group reported a higher average pain level than the transposition group.

The surgical approach for excision can be either dorsal or plantar. The dorsal approach is most frequently used and recommended. However, some surgeons recommend the plantar approach. One report examined the use of 172 plantar incisions in 137 patients for various problems of the forefoot, including resection of IDNs and stump neuromas. The satisfaction rate was 96%. These results are similar to those reported for resection of a single IDN. In this group of patients, the authors noted dense sensory loss of the plantar aspect of the third metatarsal head to the tip of the third toe and no disability. They suggested that dense sensory loss to the third toe can be avoided by resecting the larger of the two IDNs, releasing the intermetatarsal ligament, and performing neurolysis of the smaller IDN.

### Complications

Because the success rate for resection of a symptomatic IDN is in the range of 85%, approximately 15% of patients have residual pain. This may be explained by inaccurate diagnosis, incorrect web space selection, or a painful stump neuroma, which always develops when a nerve is transected. The difference between a symptomatic and an asymptomatic stump neuroma is its location. Therefore, during surgical resection, the nerve must be resected as proximal to the metatarsal heads as possible so that the stump neuroma is not near the weight-bearing surface. The relationship between the interdigital nerve and the metatarsal heads can vary. An accessory nerve branch may travel obliquely under the metatarsal head to join the interdigital nerve. After resection of the interdigital nerve, the accessory branch may retract under the weight-bearing surface of the metatarsal head and cause a painful stump neuroma; this complication can be prevented by suturing the accessory nerve branch proximal to the weight-bearing surface of the foot.

Despite meticulous surgical technique, pain can recur. Recurrent pain may be comparable to the initial pain or localized and electric-like. The physical examination of the involved foot should be as comprehensive as that for a primary IDN to help rule out other causes of pain. In addition, the differential diagnoses for the primary IDN must be reconsidered for the recurrent IDN. The initial treatment of recurrent IDN symptoms is nonsurgical and includes wearing shoes with wider toe boxes and stiffer soles, the use of a metatarsal pad, and corticosteroid injections. Surgical intervention is indicated when nonsurgical options fail. Because the results of both approaches are similar, the surgical approach for recurrent IDN can be either dorsal or plantar. However, patients with recurrent IDN should be informed that the success rate for re-excision (about 60% to 70%) is less than that for primary excision of an IDN, regardless of the surgical approach.

## Tarsal Tunnel Syndrome

Entrapment neuropathy of the posterior tibial nerve or one of its branches is called tarsal tunnel syndrome. Although many reports have compared this entity to carpal tunnel syndrome, tarsal tunnel syndrome is a different clinical entity in many respects, including anatomy, etiol-

ogy, pathophysiology, clinical presentation, diagnostic study results, and patient response to nonsurgical and surgical treatments.

The tarsal tunnel is bordered anteriorly by the medial malleolus and laterally by the posterior process of the talus, sustentaculum tali, and medial calcaneus. The laciniate ligament (flexor retinaculum) courses over the contents of the tarsal tunnel, which include the posterior tibial tendon; flexor digitorum longus; flexor hallucis longus; and posterior tibial nerve, artery, and vein. The laciniate ligament is continuous with the superficial and deep aponeurosis of the leg posteriorly and proximally and with the fascia of the abductor hallucis distally. Each tendinous structure within the tarsal tunnel travels in its own synovial sheath and is contained within a separate fibro-osseous compartment covered by fibrous projections from the laciniate ligament to the calcaneal periosteum. The posterior tibial nerve and artery are commonly attached to these projections by a layer of dense fatty tissue. A recent study of the vascular supply of the nerves in the tarsal tunnel revealed that the blood supply to the posterior tibial nerve and its branches comes directly from the corresponding artery and that there are many interconnections both proximally and distally along the primary longitudinal vessels. These findings indicate that the posterior tibial, medial, and lateral plantar nerves receive an abundant vascular supply from their accompanying arteries.

The posterior tibial nerve has three branches: medial calcaneal, medial, and lateral plantar. In one large cadaveric study, the posterior tibial nerve divided into medial and lateral plantar branches within the tarsal tunnel in 93% to 96% of the specimens and proximal to it in the remaining 4% to 7%. In addition, the medial calcaneal nerve branched from the posterior tibial nerve in 69% to 90% and from the lateral plantar nerve in 10% to 31%. This branching can occur proximal to, within, or distal to the tarsal tunnel. Distal to the tarsal tunnel, the medial and lateral plantar nerve each travels in its own fibrous tunnel. The lateral plantar nerve courses through a fibrous arch formed by the fascia of the abductor hallucis muscle medially and the fascia of flexor digitorum longus and quadratus plantae laterally, emerging between the flexor digitorum brevis and the calcaneus as it courses to the abductor digiti minimi.

There are many causes of tarsal tunnel syndrome, including trauma, space-occupying lesions, and deformities of the foot. Often, no exact etiology can be found in patients with symptoms of tarsal tunnel syndrome, but in patients in whom an etiology is obvious, trauma is the most common cause. Displaced fractures of the bony structures around the tarsal tunnel, sprains of the deltoid ligament, and injuries to the tendinous structures within the tarsal tunnel often decrease the cross-sectional area of the tarsal tunnel, causing compression of the posterior tibial nerve. Scarring of the posterior tibial nerve from hemorrhage in the tarsal tunnel can occur after trauma and has been associated with the failure of tarsal tunnel release.

Space-occupying lesions compressing the posterior tibial nerve can occur inside or outside of the tarsal tunnel and include ganglia, lipoma, and neurilemoma. Nerve compression can also be caused by bony exostosis, a medial talocalcaneal bar, a hypertrophic flexor retinaculum, a hypertrophic or accessory abductor hallucis muscle, an accessory flexor digitorum longus muscle, rapid weight gain, fluid retention, and chronic thrombophlebitis. Proliferative synovitis and tenosynovitis, especially when associated with inflammatory arthropathies, can cause an inflammatory mass to form in the tarsal tunnel. A recent study of 30 feet with tarsal tunnel syndrome caused by ganglia found that 63% of the patients reported numbness or pain in the toes and sole of the foot and paresthesias in the distribution of the medial plantar nerve. Most ganglia originated from the talocalcaneal joint, and five were associated with talocalcaneal coalitions. Another study examined seven patients with tarsal tunnel syndrome caused by talocalcaneal coalition and a ganglion. All of the patients had pain, sensory disturbance in the sole of the foot, and a positive Tinel's sign.

Both varus and valgus heel deformities can be associated with tarsal tunnel syndrome. With a varus heel deformity, the forefoot compensates by pronation. It has been suggested that in a pronated forefoot, the shortening of the abductor hallucis muscle decreases the cross-sectional area of the tarsal tunnel. In addition, the pronation of the forefoot places an increased stretch on the posterior tibial nerve. Many reports have shown that the valgus heel and abducted forefoot in a pes planus deformity also cause increasing tension on the posterior tibial nerve. A recent cadaveric study demonstrated that tension on the posterior tibial nerve was significantly increased in a surgically created pes planus foot during dorsiflexion, eversion, and combined dorsiflexion-eversion. A subsequent study demonstrated that after tarsal tunnel release in a surgically created pes planus, the tension on the posterior tibial nerve was further increased during eversion and combined dorsiflexion-eversion without significant effect during dorsiflexion. Triple arthrodesis in anatomic position and distraction calcaneocuboid arthrodesis were effective in decreasing the tension on the posterior tibial nerve. Another cadaveric study reported an increase in the tarsal tunnel compartment pressure when the foot and ankle were positioned into full eversion and full inversion.

### History and Physical Examination

The clinical symptoms of tarsal tunnel syndrome can be diffuse and poorly localized. Patients may report pain or paresthesias. The pain can be described as burning, tingling, or numbing; intermittent or constant; or localized or global and can radiate distally or proximally. History

of a concomitant proximal nerve entrapment helps diagnose a double crush syndrome. The symptoms of tarsal tunnel syndrome are usually aggravated by walking, standing, or running and are relieved by rest. Patients sometimes have pain at night.

On physical examination, any varus or valgus deformity of the foot should be noted. Tinel's sign along the posterior tibial nerve may or may not be present. The results of sensory examination along the distribution of the posterior tibial nerve branches are usually normal. The earliest sign of sensory disturbance is a decrease in two-point discrimination on the plantar surface of the foot. Motor deficit, which is difficult to assess, is uncommon. A recent study described a new diagnostic test in which the affected ankle is placed into full eversion and dorsiflexion, while all of the MTP joints are maximally dorsiflexed and held for 5 to 10 seconds. Because this maneuver may intensify or induce some symptoms of tarsal tunnel syndrome, it can facilitate diagnosis.

### Diagnostic Studies

Although there is no single test that can definitively make the diagnosis of tarsal tunnel syndrome, electrodiagnostic studies (eg, electromyography) are accurate up to 90% of the time. Because early signs of tarsal tunnel syndrome are primarily sensory, sensory nerve conduction studies are more sensitive than motor nerve conduction studies. The diagnosis of tarsal tunnel syndrome is strengthened when all three of the following exist: pain and paresthesias in the foot, positive Tinel's sign, and positive electrodiagnostic study results. Electrodiagnostic studies also help to rule out double crush syndrome and other neurologic problems, such as peripheral neuropathy. Radiologic studies aid in the diagnosis of tarsal tunnel syndrome by evaluating the anatomy within the tarsal tunnel. Weight-bearing radiographs of the foot and ankle can help identify bony abnormality around the tarsal tunnel and the presence of any biomechanical deformity of the foot. MRI is effective in assessing specific structures within the tarsal tunnel and identifying any space-occupying lesion, which may be compressing the posterior tibial nerve. MRI is also useful in preoperative planning because it can localize a lesion and identify its relationship to the posterior tibial nerve. In one study, MRI scans were abnormal in 88% of patients with tarsal tunnel syndrome.

### Nonsurgical Treatment

The initial treatment of tarsal tunnel syndrome is nonsurgical, the goal of which is to decrease tension and compression around the posterior tibial nerve. Nonsteroidal anti-inflammatory drugs, local corticosteroid injections, and immobilization may decrease inflammation in the tendinous structures around the nerve, particularly if tenosynovitis is present. After a corticosteroid injection, a period of immobilization and protected weight bearing is recommended to prevent rupture of the tendinous

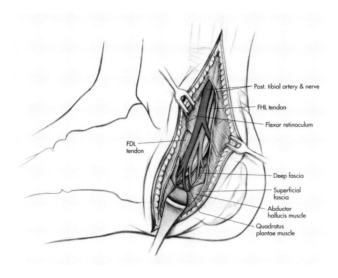

**Figure 2** Surgical treatment of tarsal tunnel syndrome. FHL = flexor hallucis longus, FDL = flexor digitorum longus. *(Reproduced with permission from Lutter LD (ed): Atlas of Adult Foot and Ankle Surgery. St. Louis, MO, Mosby-Year Books, 1997, p 209.)*

Labels on figure: Post. tibial artery & nerve; FHL tendon; Flexor retinaculum; FDL tendon; Deep fascia; Superficial fascia; Abductor hallucis muscle; Quadratus plantae muscle

structures within the tarsal tunnel, especially the posterior tibial nerve. The tension on the posterior tibial nerve can be diminished by immobilization or the use of a foot orthosis. Methods of immobilization include off-the-shelf or custom-molded, rigid ankle-foot orthoses or a short leg cast. Various types of foot orthoses may be effective for flexible deformities. For a flexible valgus heel deformity, medial longitudinal arch supports and medial heel wedges can be effective. However, for more severe deformities, either University of California Biomechanics Laboratory (UCBL) orthoses or custom-molded ankle-foot orthoses are required.

### Surgical Treatment

Surgical treatment of tarsal tunnel syndrome is indicated when nonsurgical treatment fails. The surgery involves decompressing the entire tarsal tunnel 3 to 5 cm proximal to the flexor retinaculum and distally to include release of the deep fascia of the abductor hallucis (Fig. 2). As part of the distal release, the medial and lateral plantar nerves are identified and decompressed. If a more distal involvement of either the medial or lateral plantar nerve is identified, further plantar release of either nerve may be required. Care must be taken to protect the smaller medial calcaneal nerve, which readily blends with the deep subcutaneous and superficial fascial layers. If a space-occupying lesion is present, distal release of either the medial or lateral plantar nerve may not be necessary. The success of surgical treatment of tarsal tunnel syndrome is most predictable when a space-occupying lesion is removed.

### Clinical Outcomes

Successful outcomes of surgical treatment for tarsal tunnel syndrome have been reported in up to 91% of patients in one series, with patients reporting being so improved by the surgery that they would have it again or reporting an absence of symptoms. However, another retrospective study demonstrated that only 44% of 30 patients (14 of 32 feet) had good or excellent results after a mean 31-month follow-up. Many of the patients in this study underwent previous surgeries on the foot, and three of five who reported complete satisfaction had another lesion that was surgically treated at the same time as the tarsal tunnel syndrome. In light of these results, the authors cautioned against decompression of the posterior tibial nerve unless there is an associated lesion near or within the tarsal tunnel. Another study examined the outcome of surgery after long-standing tarsal tunnel syndrome. In this study, 18 patients with long-standing tarsal tunnel syndrome (median, 60 months) underwent surgery. Sixty-one percent of the patients had complete relief of symptoms after surgery at a median 18-month follow-up. The authors concluded that surgical decompression was beneficial in most patients with long-standing tarsal tunnel syndrome. A study that reviewed the diagnosis, surgical technique, and functional outcome in patients with tarsal tunnel syndrome reported that the most common clinical presentation of this disease process included pain, paresthesias, and numbness. The authors also reported that electrodiagnostic study results were abnormal in 81% of patients and 72% were satisfied with the surgical outcome. In addition, in most of the patients with idiopathic tarsal tunnel syndrome impingement at the abductor hallucis fascia was discovered during surgery.

### Complications

Complications after tarsal tunnel release include infection, delay in wound healing, hypertrophic scar, or persistent pain. The persistence of symptoms after surgery may be related to inadequate release, chronic disease with motor involvement, epineural scarring of the posterior tibial nerve, or double crush syndrome, or may be idiopathic. In one study, older age was associated with an increased failure rate of tarsal tunnel release. Unfortunately, after ruling out double crush syndrome, inadequate release with or without epineural scarring is the only cause of persistent symptoms that can be treated with additional surgery.

For patients with recurrent or persistent pain after tarsal tunnel release, a complete history and thorough physical examination are the most reliable tools for identifying the problem. For example, an inadequate release can be distinguished from scarring of the posterior tibial nerve by noting the length and location of the previous incision and the history of the patient's symptoms. If the patient has a history of initial relief of symptoms and then later reports recurrent symptoms, epineural scarring may be the cause. If the patient has a history of persistent pain, paresthesias, and numbness along the medial and/or lateral plantar nerves, then inadequate release may be the source of the recurrent symptoms because the area of inadequate release is usually distal. The initial treatment for the recurrent symptoms after failure of tarsal tunnel release is similar to that for preoperative symptoms.

The clinical result after revision tarsal tunnel release depends on the etiology of the recurrent symptoms. One study examined 13 revision tarsal tunnel releases that were divided into three groups. The first group had extensive scarring around the nerve with an adequate release. The second group had extensive scarring around the nerve with inadequate release. The third group did not have significant scarring around the nerve but had inadequate release. The outcomes of revision tarsal tunnel release were the best for the third group and the poorest for the first group. The second group had overall improvement of symptoms, but results were not as good as those of the third group. The authors advised against revision posterior tibial nerve epineurolysis if the initial release was adequate. For patients with epineural scarring, other treatment options include peripheral nerve stimulation, vein wrapping around the nerve after epineurolysis, or radial forearm free flap. However, the outcome of these treatment methods is still under investigation.

## Summary

The diagnosis and treatment of interdigital neuroma and tarsal tunnel syndrome require thorough clinical evaluation and workup and meticulous surgical skills. For these two static nerve disorders, the treatment of surgical complications are complex and can be challenging.

## Annotated Bibliography

### Interdigital Neuroma

Colgrove RC, Huang EY, Barth AH, Greene MA: Interdigital neuroma: Intermuscular neuroma transposition compared with resection. *Foot Ankle Int* 2000;21:206-211.

The result of resection of the interdigital nerve was compared with transposition of the interdigital nerve into an intermuscular position between the adductor hallucis and the interossei muscle. Transposition of the interdigital nerve produced better long-term results than resection of the nerve.

Coughlin MJ, Pinsonneault T: Operative treatment of interdigital neuroma: A long-term follow-up study. *J Bone Joint Surg Am* 2001;83:1321-1328.

This long-term follow-up study of IDN resection using a dorsal approach revealed an overall satisfaction rate of excellent or good in 85% of patients after more than 5 years.

Levine SE, Myerson MS, Shapiro PP, Shapiro SL: Ultrasonographic diagnosis of recurrence after excision of an interdigital neuroma. *Foot Ankle Int* 1998;19:79-84.

Ultrasonography detected the presence of a recurrent neuroma in 13 of 20 patients in this study.

Miller SD: Technique tip: Forefoot pain: Diagnosing metatarsophalangeal joint synovitis from interdigital neuroma. *Foot Ankle Int* 2001;22:914-915.

The techniques of diagnosing MTP joint synovitis from IDN are outlined in this report.

Quinn TJ, Jacobson JA, Craig JG, van Holsbeeck MT: Sonography of Morton's neuromas. *AJR Am J Roentgenol* 2000;174:1723-1728.

Ultrasonography correctly identified an IDN in 85% of patients in this study.

Williams JW, Meaney J, Whitehouse GH, Klenerman L, Hussein Z: MRI in the investigation of Morton's neuroma: Which sequences? *Clin Radiol* 1997;52:46-49.

T1-weighted axial and coronal images with an axial fast-spin echo T2-weighted sequence detected IDN more consistently than an enhanced T1 fat-suppressed sequence.

### Tarsal Tunnel Syndrome

Bailie DS, Kelikian AS: Tarsal tunnel syndrome: Diagnosis, surgical technique, and functional outcome. *Foot Ankle Int* 1998;19:65-72.

This review of the diagnosis, surgical technique, and functional outcome in patients with tarsal tunnel syndrome showed that the most common clinical presentation of this disease process included pain, paresthesias, and numbness. The electrodiagnostic study results were abnormal in 81% of patients and 72% were satisfied with the surgical outcome.

Daniels TR, Lau JT, Hearn TC: The effects of foot position and load on tibial nerve tension. *Foot Ankle Int* 1998;19:73-78.

In this cadaveric study, the tension on the posterior tibial nerve was significantly increased in a surgically created pes planus foot during dorsiflexion, eversion, and combined dorsiflexion-eversion.

Flanigan DC, Cassell M, Saltzman CL: Vascular supply of nerves in the tarsal tunnel. *Foot Ankle Int* 1997;18:288-292.

This study showed that the blood supply to the posterior tibial nerve and its branches comes directly from the corresponding artery.

Kinoshita M, Okuda R, Morikawa J, Jotoku T, Abe M: The dorsiflexion-eversion test for diagnosis of tarsal tunnel syndrome. *J Bone Joint Surg Am* 2001;83:1835-1839.

This study described the dorsiflexion-eversion test in which the affected ankle is placed into full eversion and dorsiflexion as all of the MTP joints are maximally dorsiflexed and held for 5 to 10 seconds to facilitate the diagnosis of tarsal tunnel syndrome.

Lau JT, Daniels TR: Tarsal tunnel syndrome: A review of the literature. *Foot Ankle Int* 1999;20:201-209.

This recent review article describes the anatomy, pathophysiology, clinical presentation, diagnosis, and treatment results of tarsal tunnel syndrome.

Lau JT, Daniels TR: Effects of tarsal tunnel release and stabilization procedures on tibial nerve tension in a surgically created pes planus foot. *Foot Ankle Int* 1998;19: 770-777.

In this cadaveric study, after tarsal tunnel release in a surgically created pes planus, the tension on the posterior tibial nerve was further increased during eversion and combined dorsiflexion-eversion without significant effect during dorsiflexion. Triple arthrodesis and distraction calcaneocuboid arthrodesis were effective in decreasing the tension on the posterior tibial nerve.

Nagaoka M, Satou K: Tarsal tunnel syndrome caused by ganglia. *J Bone Joint Surg Br* 1999;81:607-610.

Of 30 feet with tarsal tunnel syndrome caused by ganglia, 63% of patients had numbness or pain in the toes and sole of the foot and paresthesias in the distribution of the medial plantar nerve.

Takakura Y, Kumai T, Takaoka T, Tamai S: Tarsal tunnel syndrome caused by coalition associated with a ganglion. *J Bone Joint Surg Br* 1998;80:130-133.

In a study of seven patients with tarsal tunnel syndrome caused by talocalcaneal coalition and a ganglion, pain, sensory disturbance in the sole of the foot, and a positive Tinel's sign were reported.

Trepman E, Kadel NJ, Chisholm K, Razzano L: Effect of foot and ankle position on tarsal tunnel compartment pressure. *Foot Ankle Int* 1999;20:721-726.

This cadaveric study showed an increase in tarsal tunnel compartment pressure when the foot and ankle were positioned into full eversion and full inversion.

Turan I, Rivero-Melian C, Guntner P, Rolf C: Tarsal tunnel syndrome: Outcome of surgery in longstanding cases. *Clin Orthop* 1997;343:151-156.

Sixty-one percent of the patients with long-standing tarsal tunnel syndrome (median, 60 months) had complete relief of symptoms after surgery at a median 18-month follow-up.

## Classic Bibliography

Benedetti RS, Baxter DE, Davis PF: Clinical results of simultaneous adjacent interdigital neurectomy in the foot. *Foot Ankle Int* 1996;17:264-268.

Bennett GL, Graham CE, Mauldin DM: Morton's interdigital neuroma: A comprehensive treatment protocol. *Foot Ankle Int* 1995;16:760-763.

Cimino WR: Tarsal tunnel syndrome: Review of the literature. *Foot Ankle* 1990;11:47-52.

Davis TJ, Schon LC: Branches of the tibial nerve: Anatomic variations. *Foot Ankle Int* 1995;16:21-29.

Greenfield J, Rea J Jr, Ilfeld FW: Morton's interdigital neuroma: Indications for treatment by local injections versus surgery. *Clin Orthop* 1984;185:142-144.

Levitsky KA, Alman BA, Jevsevar DS, Morehead J: Digital nerves of the foot: Anatomic variations and implications regarding the pathogenesis of interdigital neuroma. *Foot Ankle* 1993;14:208-214.

Mann RA, Reynolds JC: Interdigital neuroma: A critical clinical analysis. *Foot Ankle* 1983;3:238-243.

Pfeiffer WH, Cracchiolo A III: Clinical results after tarsal tunnel decompression. *J Bone Joint Surg Am* 1994;76: 1222-1230.

Rasmussen MR, Kitaoka HB, Patzer GL: Nonoperative treatment of plantar interdigital neuroma with a single corticosteroid injection. *Clin Orthop* 1996;326:188-193.

Richardson EG, Brotzman SB, Graves SC: The plantar incision for procedures involving the forefoot: An evaluation of one hundred and fifty incisions in one hundred and fifteen patients. *J Bone Joint Surg Am* 1993;75:726-731.

Shapiro PP, Shapiro SL: Sonographic evaluation of interdigital neuromas. *Foot Ankle Int* 1995;16:604-606.

Skalley TC, Schon LC, Hinton RY, Myerson MS: Clinical results following revision tibial nerve release. *Foot Ankle Int* 1994;15:360-367.

Takakura Y, Kitada C, Sugimoto K, Tanaka Y, Tamai S: Tarsal tunnel syndrome: Causes and results of operative treatment. *J Bone Joint Surg Br* 1991;73:125-128.

Weinfeld SB, Myerson MS: Interdigital neuritis: Diagnosis and treatment. *J Am Acad Orthop Surg* 1996;4:328-335.

# Section 5

## Arthritic Disorders

Section Editor:
Bruce E. Cohen, MD

# Chapter 15

# Arthritis of the Ankle and Hindfoot

Arthur K. Walling, MD

## Introduction

Degeneration of the ankle and hindfoot joints is most commonly a result of posttraumatic or inflammatory arthritis. Successful management requires a thorough knowledge of the anatomy and biomechanics of the foot and ankle coupled with a thorough medical history, physical examination, and appropriate imaging studies. Treatment options include a variety of nonsurgical and surgical options. Pain relief and function may be obtained through the use of shoe modification, orthoses, or anti-inflammatory drugs. Should these methods fail, surgical treatment may be beneficial. Surgical goals include pain relief, correction or prevention of deformity, and restoration or preservation of function.

## Ankle and Hindfoot Anatomy

The ankle is a modified hinge joint consisting of three bones (tibia, fibula, and talus) and their connecting ligaments. The primary motions of this single, functional unit are dorsiflexion and plantar flexion, with small amounts of inversion and eversion and minimal rotation.

The tibial plafond is the distal articular surface of the tibia. It is concave from anterior to posterior and slightly concave from medial to lateral. It is also wider anteriorly than posteriorly and longer laterally than medially. The tibial plafond is contiguous with the medial malleolus, which is the most distal projection of the tibia.

The distal extension of the fibula is called the lateral malleolus, and its broad medial surface articulates with the lateral surface of the talus and provides key lateral support to the ankle. The distal fibula typically extends approximately 1 cm distal and posterior to the medial malleolus.

The talus articulates with the tibia above, the calcaneus below, the fibula laterally, and the medial malleolus medially; the talar head articulates distally with the navicular. The articular cartilage that covers the talus superiorly mirrors the configuration of the tibial plafond and is also wider anteriorly than posteriorly. Medially, where it articulates with the medial malleolus, the surface of the talus is comma-shaped and curvilinear. The lateral articulation of the talus with the fibula is almost triangular.

In addition to the bony support provided by the fibula, the articular surfaces are maintained by strong ligamentous support. Medial support is provided by the deltoid ligament, which is divided into superficial and deep portions. The lateral collateral ligament is made up of three components: the anterior talofibular ligament, the calcaneofibular ligament, and the posterior talofibular ligament.

The subtalar joint is made up of three articular facets (anterior, medial, and posterior) through which the talus articulates with the calcaneus, permitting inversion and eversion of the foot. In addition to its inherent bony stability, the subtalar joint is stabilized by the talocalcaneal interosseous ligament, which is synovial lined and lies within the sinus tarsi and capsular structures around the individual facets.

The talonavicular and calcaneocuboid joints have adapted to fulfill their functional roles in their respective columns of the foot. The talonavicular joint is part of the more mobile medial column. It has a condyloid shape and is supported by the talonavicular ligament and the adjacent superior medial and lateral calcaneonavicular ligaments. The calcaneocuboid joint is more inherently stable and forms the more rigid lateral column of the foot. It is saddle shaped and is stabilized by the calcaneocuboid ligaments. These two joints function as a unit and, together with the subtalar joint, allow inversion, eversion, and rotation of the hindfoot.

## Types of Arthritis and Related Disorders
### Traumatic Arthritis

In distinct contrast to the hip and knee, trauma remains the most common cause of ankle and hindfoot arthritis. Posttraumatic arthritis of the ankle can develop after fractures of the ankle, tibial pilon (plafond), talus, or combinations of these injuries. Fractures of the talus, calcaneus, or both are the main source of posttraumatic arthritis in the subtalar joint. Despite the ability of open reduction and internal fixation (ORIF) to better restore articular congruity, the resulting injury to the articular cartilage often predisposes patients with these intra-articular injuries to posttraumatic arthrosis.

Although anatomic restoration of the joint surfaces remains the ideal goal of treatment, the complexity of pilon, talar, and calcaneal fractures makes this difficult to achieve. In addition, because of the soft-tissue injury occurring with tibial pilon fractures and subsequent wound healing complications following ORIF, there has been a recent trend to accept less than perfect anatomic reduction of the joint in an attempt to reduce secondary wound complications. Although this trend has led to a decreased incidence of subsequent amputations, it may also be leading to an increase in posttraumatic arthritis. Talar fractures continue to be particularly problematic because of the increased incidence of traumatic arthritis of both the ankle and subtalar joints; if complicated by the development of osteonecrosis, the difficulty of performing reconstructive options greatly increases.

### Inflammatory Arthritis

The many causes of inflammatory arthropathies can be grouped according to their underlying pathophysiology. Synovial inflammatory causes include both seropositive (rheumatoid arthritis) and seronegative (Reiter's syndrome, psoriatic arthritis, and ankylosing spondylitis) disorders. The seronegative arthropathies are characterized by the absence of a positive rheumatoid factor and the more common symptom of enthesopathy. The characteristic erosions seen on radiographs at the insertions of ligaments, tendons, and other soft-tissue insertional sites are a key to the correct diagnosis. Other causes include crystal deposition disease (gout and pseudogout) and connective tissue disorders (systemic lupus erythematosus and mixed connective tissue disease) as well as inflammatory bowel disease (Crohn's disease or ulcerative colitis).

Rheumatoid arthritis is characterized as a symmetric polyarthropathy estimated to affect 1% to 2% of the general population and is more common in women. Although rheumatoid arthritis can occur at any age, its peak incidence is during the third through fifth decades. The ankle and hindfoot are not affected until later in the disease process and are usually involved less frequently than the forefoot. Ankle joint involvement is primarily manifested as synovitis and, as a rule, does not result in significant deformity.

Complaints of ankle pain often are mistakenly attributed to ankle joint disease when the real source of the pain is in the surrounding subtalar or transverse tarsal joints. Destruction of the supportive soft-tissue structures of the subtalar and midtarsal joints results in hindfoot deformity, which leads to the progressive development of a pes planovalgus deformity. This deformity, in turn, can lead to impingement on the fibula with subsequent pain

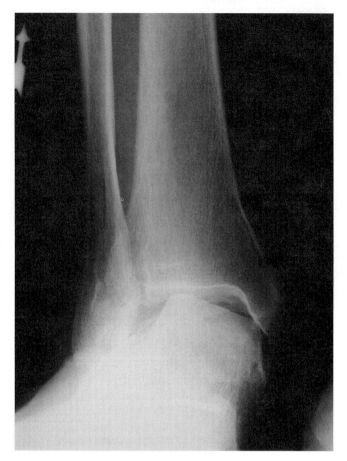

**Figure 1** AP ankle radiograph showing valgus tilt in the ankle mortise secondary to severe pes planovalgus of the hindfoot.

or even fracture. The development of severe valgus of the hindfoot can produce severe concomitant valgus of the ankle (Fig. 1); malalignment of the ankle and hindfoot makes this condition more difficult to treat.

Patients with Reiter's syndrome complain of foot pain more often than those with psoriatic arthritis or ankylosing spondylitis. Reiter's syndrome is associated with the triad of conjunctivitis, urethritis, and asymmetric arthritis. The condition has been expanded to include the symptoms of mucosal ulceration, balanitis circinata, and keratoderma blennorrhagicum (a pustular lesion seen on the sole of the foot in approximately 10% of patients). Although the cause of Reiter's syndrome is unknown, an infectious etiology is suspected. However, an immunologic predisposition is also suspected based on the presence of a positive HLA-B27 antigen in 60% to 80% of patients.

Psoriatic arthritis is an asymmetric polyarthritis and is often associated with characteristic skin and nail changes. In the foot, it is characterized by fusiform enlargement and erythema of a lesser toe, usually the third or fourth toe, that is not associated with trauma (sausage toe). The toe is nontender or mildly tender. Positive HLA-B27 antigen is found in 20% of patients with psoriatic arthritis (50% of patients with sacroiliitis).

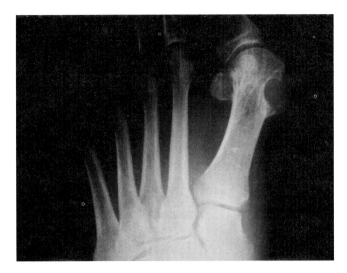

**Figure 2** Erosion of the extra-articular surface of the first metatarsal with preservation of the articular cartilage in a patient with gout. Note the overhanging edge sign.

Ankylosing spondylitis has a strong association with positive HLA-B27 antigen (75% to 100% of patients). It is more common in males than females (4:1 ratio) and has a strong familial tendency. Foot and ankle symptoms are uncommon. Seronegative arthritides may also be associated with both human immunodeficiency virus and acquired immunodeficiency syndrome.

Crystal-induced arthropathies result from the deposition of crystalline material within the soft tissues and bone, which produces a secondary inflammatory response. The crystals responsible for causing gout and pseudogout are monosodium urate and calcium pyrophosphate dihydrate, respectively. Both gout and pseudogout most commonly affect the first metatarsophalangeal joints, but the hindfoot or ankle also can be affected. In the late stages of gout, a characteristic radiographic finding called the overhanging edge sign develops, in which the articular space remains but an elevated margin of bone around the erosions appears to overhang the tophaceous deposit (Fig. 2). In contrast to the characteristic presence of erosive lesions located somewhat remotely from the articular surface seen in gout, pseudogout is comparable to osteoarthritis in that patients with either condition can have progressive joint narrowing, osteophytes, and degenerative cysts.

## Osteoarthritis

The exact causes of osteoarthritis are unknown. Both biochemical and histologic changes cause a distortion of the articular surface. Increased water content and decreased compliance of the articular cartilage lead to alterations in the collagen molecules and an increase in proteoglycan breakdown. The biochemically altered cartilage transfers greater loads to the subchondral bone, resulting in biomechanical alterations caused by repetitive injury. Radiographs of patients with osteoarthritis demonstrate diminished articular cartilage, subchondral sclerosis, subchondral cyst formation, and proliferative bone formation at the periphery of the joint. Joint inflammation is uncommon with osteoarthritis; therefore, periarticular osteoporosis is also rare.

## Infectious Arthritis

Both septic arthritis and osteomyelitis continue to account for a significant percentage of ankle and hindfoot arthritis and deformity. In developed countries, factors that contribute to the increased incidence of septic arthritis and osteomyelitis include immunosuppressed patients receiving organ transplants and the increased survival rate of hospitalized patients. Unusual etiologies, such as tuberculosis, should also be considered as causative factors. Treatment usually requires eradication of the infection first, followed by treatment of the sequelae. Another unusual cause of possible ankle and hindfoot arthritis is Lyme disease, the most common arthropodborne infectious disease diagnosed in the United States. Chronic arthritis may develop in 10% of patients, usually late in the disease process. Diagnosis requires a high degree of suspicion and may be confirmed by serologic or indirect fluorescent antibody tests.

## Neuropathy and Arthropathy

Neuroarthropathy is common in both the ankle and hindfoot. The most common cause of Charcot neuropathy is diabetes, but it can also occur as a result of other peripheral neuropathies. Although the stages of neuropathic arthropathy are well described, many patients are initially misdiagnosed as having an infection during the initial inflammatory stage of the process (Fig. 3). Surgery is more often indicated to treat the resulting deformity and subsequent skin breakdown than the arthritis.

## Synovial Abnormalities

Certain pathologic synovial conditions can also produce arthritic changes of both the ankle and hindfoot. Pigmented villonodular synovitis typically results in recurrent effusions with bloody aspiration of the affected joint and can cause arthritic changes even after repeated synovectomy. Synovial chondromatosis can cause progressive articular surface damage secondary to the mechanical effect of the intra-articular loose bodies disgorged into the joint. These partially calcified cartilage lesions can often be seen on radiographs of the affected joint (Fig. 4).

# History and Physical Examination

A thorough medical history and physical examination will usually lead to an accurate diagnosis and localization of the problem. A history of previous trauma and subsequent surgery should raise suspicion regarding possible posttraumatic disorders. Symmetric, multiple joint involvement and seropositivity confirms the presence of

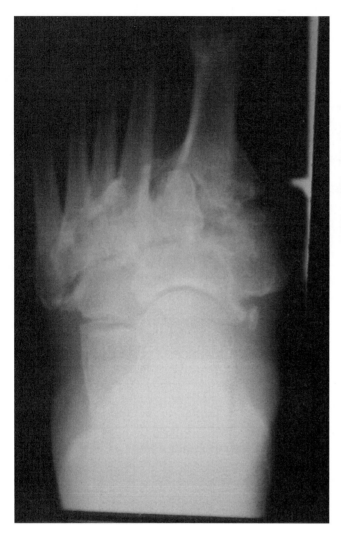

Figure 3 Charcot collapse secondary to diabetes that was initially misdiagnosed as infection during the early inflammatory stage.

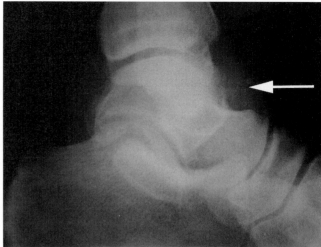

Figure 4 Lateral radiograph of the ankle showing partially calcified loose bodies (arrow) produced in synovial chondromatosis.

rheumatoid arthritis. Seronegative causes are usually more difficult to confirm, and appropriate examination for skin lesions, enthesopathies, conjunctivitis, and urethritis will help to establish the diagnosis, as will patient reports of fever, night sweats, swelling, and neurologic sensory or motor neurologic changes. The determination of the onset and duration of symptoms, aggravating factors, and the presence or absence of night pain is also important. Information on the patient's response to previous attempts at treatment can be helpful, as can identification of concurrent medical problems and medications being taken. In addition, a family history to confirm hereditary diseases or tendencies should be obtained. It is especially important to be aware of a history of tobacco use in patients with ankle and hindfoot arthrosis because a history of tobacco use can impact treatment options and increase the risk of nonunion (ie, slower fusion and more frequent nonunion in smokers).

Physical examination of the ankle and hindfoot requires observation of both lower extremities when the patient is standing and walking. Significant deformity can be missed if the patient is examined only while not bearing weight or while sitting. Inspection should include not only the ankle and hindfoot, but also the knee and hip. Range of motion, swelling, pain, alignment, ligament stability, and motor strength should be assessed. Weight-bearing alignment of the ankle and hindfoot from behind will help to detect varus or valgus malalignment. Single-stance heel rise with terminal inversion of the heel should be performed to assess posterior tibial tendon function. It is important to check for Achilles tendon contracture with the hindfoot corrected. The appearance of the skin, including the presence or absence of hypertrophic callus formation, should be noted. Vascular sufficiency testing and monofilament sensory testing should also be done. With multiple joint involvement, selective injection of a local anesthetic may help to identify the most symptomatic joint.

## Imaging

Relying on non–weight-bearing radiographs to evaluate ankle and hindfoot pathology can significantly underestimate the amount of deformity or joint involvement. Therefore, radiographic evaluation should include weight-bearing AP, mortise, and lateral views of the ankle as well as AP and lateral weight-bearing views of the foot. Special views, including oblique, Broden's, axial heel, and Cobey's, may all be helpful.

More sophisticated imaging tests include the use of technetium Tc 99m bone scanning, CT, MRI, and occasionally fluoroscopic evaluation. Bone scanning can be helpful in identifying stress reactions, occult fractures, arthritis, and specific activity in the hindfoot complex. CT can provide additional two-dimensional or even three-dimensional information that can be especially useful when assessing the magnitude of a deformity. MRI is superior in providing soft-tissue detail as well as multiplanar orientation. Fluoroscopy is particularly helpful in assessing nonunions by detecting minimal amounts of motion.

## Nonsurgical Treatment

It is unusual for arthritis, whatever the cause, to leave the affected joint or joints anatomically aligned. In the ankle and hindfoot, valgus or varus malalignment are frequently encountered. In the ankle, especially after pilon injuries, there may also be anterior as well as superior translation of the talus in the ankle mortise. In the hindfoot, there may be accompanying forefoot abduction or adduction as well as supination or pronation. All of these potential malalignments need to be considered when deciding on appropriate treatment.

### Anti-inflammatory Drugs

Symptomatic treatment of arthritic conditions of the foot and ankle should include nonsteroidal anti-inflammatory drugs (NSAIDs), which block the cyclooxygenase (COX) pathway in the production of prostaglandins and can provide significant relief of inflammation and pain. Recently, the COX-1 isoenzyme was found to exist constitutively in many tissues (where it is necessary for several homeostatic and physiologic functions, particularly in the stomach), whereas the COX-2 isoenzyme was found to be expressed locally in states of inflammation. This discovery led to the development of new NSAIDs, COX-2 inhibitors. Although COX-2 inhibitors have not been shown to be more effective in relieving symptoms of inflammatory arthritis than COX-1 inhibitors, they do not produce the platelet and gastrointestinal adverse effects associated with COX-1 inhibitors.

### Mechanical Aids

A variety of braces, shoe modifications, and orthoses are available for nonsurgical treatment. An ankle-foot orthosis (AFO) of molded, lined polyurethane that is worn inside a shoe or a double-bar caliper brace, especially when accompanied with a rocker-bottom shoe, can provide relief by limiting joint motion in the ankle or hindfoot. A patellar tendon–bearing modification to the AFO can provide further offloading, particularly at the tibiotalar joint. A soft-molded ankle corset, which can be worn in a standard lace-up shoe, allows more motion but may be better tolerated than the more rigid AFO.

Shoe modifications for hindfoot arthritis depend on the amount of rigidity, type and degree of deformity present, and whether the patient's main problem is pain from the arthritic joint or pressure from the deformity. Attempts to correct fixed deformity usually fail and are poorly tolerated by the patient. If the problem is primarily pain from the bony deformity, successful accommodation of the deformity and cushioning is best achieved by varying densities of polyethylene blown foam with soft rubber liners. If there is a flexible component to the deformity, use of a corrective orthosis, such as a lined University of California Biomechanics Laboratory (UCBL) orthosis, may decrease the deformity and provide pain relief.

Intra-articular steroid injections can provide temporary pain relief. In general, this type of nonsurgical treatment is more likely to modify than alleviate a patient's symptoms. Therefore, it should be used judiciously before surgical options are considered.

## Surgical Treatment of the Ankle

### Synovectomy

Synovectomy of the ankle joint is primarily indicated for the treatment of pathologic conditions of the synovium, such as pigmented villonodular synovitis and synovial chondromatoses. Although a complete synovectomy is unrealistic, the goal is to remove as much of the diseased synovium as possible using arthroscopic or open synovectomy, or a combination of both methods. Despite surgical intervention, local recurrences are common, and repeated surgical intervention is required in an attempt to prevent the eventual arthritic changes that accompany these recurrences. As a result, the role of synovectomy in managing inflammatory synovitis remains controversial.

### Débridement

Patients sometimes have anterior osteophytes of the distal tibia and/or dorsal talus, resulting in a bony impingement. These patients may experience anterior ankle pain with restricted dorsiflexion. However, radiographic evidence of osteophytes that do not cause any impingement and are not the source of the patient's pain or symptoms is a more common occurrence. Fluoroscopy or radiographs of the ankle in maximal dorsiflexion may help document the presence of impingement. If impingement is present, arthroscopic or open débridement of the impinging osteophytes can help improve symptoms and increase range of motion. The débridement of anterior osteophytes that do not result in impingement usually does nothing to improve symptoms or range of motion.

### Osteotomies

Although technically demanding, corrective osteotomies for fracture malunion are an effective treatment that can improve quality of life and eliminate or at least delay the need for salvage procedures such as arthrodesis or arthroplasty. Indications for late reconstruction are pain or diminished activity and a malunited ankle fracture.

The most common malunion of the ankle involves shortening and lateral (external) rotation of the distal fibula, producing widening of the ankle mortise and lateral tilt of the talus. Associated malunions of the medial malleolus or the posterior malleolus may complicate the situation. The surgical technique involves fibular osteotomy, lengthening, and internal rotation of the distal fragment followed by internal fixation. If there is obstruction between the talus and medial malleolus, medial arthrotomy with resection of any interposed fibrous tissue is necessary. If malunion or nonunion of the medial malleolus is also present, osteotomy or osteosynthesis of the medial malleolus may be required to eliminate obstruction between the talus and medial malleolus.

Varus or valgus deformities of the ankle also can be corrected by secondary reconstruction with opening, closing, or combined wedge osteotomies of the tibia. More commonly, deformities in the supramalleolar or intermalleolar area are multiplanar deformities requiring careful preoperative planning to correct the sagittal, coronal, and axial planes. In younger patients, arthritic changes are well tolerated if there is perfect alignment.

All components of the malunion need to be corrected, with the goal being full restoration of normal anatomy. Neither the interval between the injury and secondary reconstruction, the presence of arthritis, nor the age of the patient alone or in combination are absolute contraindications to attempted reconstruction. The end result does not depend necessarily on the severity of malunion or on preexisting arthritic changes. Consequently, especially in younger patients, secondary reconstruction should be the first step in the treatment of a malunited ankle fracture, and salvage procedures should be considered only if this fails.

### Ankle Arthrodesis

Until there is a total ankle replacement that stands the test of time, ankle arthrodesis continues to be the gold standard for surgical treatment of the arthritic ankle joint. It enables the surgeon to create a painless, stable, plantigrade foot and is used most commonly to correct a painful joint secondary to any form of arthritis. This procedure provides stability to the ankle and corrects deformity at or near the ankle joint. In contrast to the hip and knee, by far the most common cause of ankle arthrodesis is posttraumatic arthritis.

Arthrodesis can provide significant improvement in both pain and function, but it places increased stress on the surrounding joints of the foot. Patients with isolated posttraumatic arthritis who undergo ankle fusion often show, in long-term radiographic follow-up studies, secondary arthritic changes in the ipsilateral subtalar, talonavicular, calcaneocuboid, naviculocuneiform, tarsometatarsal, and first metatarsophalangeal joints. However, the knee is usually not affected. Although these secondary radiographic findings are troublesome, their correlation with clinical symptoms requires further evaluation. Radiographic changes often precede functional complaints and arthritis, pain, and dysfunction in the surrounding joints eventually follow. It is important to assess the flexibility of the hindfoot joints before ankle arthrodesis. The stiffer

the surrounding joints, the less capable they are of dissipating the additional stresses from the ankle fusion and the greater their potential for developing arthrosis.

Final alignment and position of the arthrodesis are critical. The preferred alignment is neutral plantar flexion–dorsiflexion, hindfoot valgus of approximately 5°, external rotation similar to the uninvolved extremity (usually 5° to 10°), and neutral to slight posterior translation of the talus in relation to the tibia. This ideal alignment, however, is not always obtainable. Occasionally, the position of fusion must be individualized depending on any deformity that may be present above or below the ankle. Optimal positioning may require some compromise of the final position to achieve the best functional result. It may even require additional surgical procedures or osteotomies done either simultaneously or as staged procedures to obtain the desired result. When ankle arthrodesis is done, the hindfoot must be aligned in mild valgus to the weight-bearing longitudinal axis of the lower extremity, and the forefoot must be aligned to the hindfoot to create a plantigrade foot.

Many techniques for ankle arthrodesis have been described since Albert's initial description more than a century ago. Multiple surgical approaches have likewise been proposed that range from single to combined incisions to allow intra-articular, extra-articular, or transmalleollar fusions. External fixation is done primarily to treat septic arthritis, and internal fixation using intra-articular compression has become the most widely accepted method of achieving stability and compression at the fusion site. A variety of fixation options exists, including the use of screws, plates, combinations of both, and intramedullary nails. Standard fusion principles include an attempt to create broad congruent cancellous surfaces that can be placed into close apposition and stabilization of the arthrodesis site with rigid internal fixation. The supplemental use of bone graft or bone-graft substitute shows no clear consensus and should be used on a case-by-case basis.

Arthroscopic and mini-open techniques represent valid alternatives to traditional open techniques. Reported advantages include less soft-tissue dissection, decreased postoperative pain, and shorter time to union. However, these procedures are indicated only in patients with little or no deformity. Significant malalignment requires open techniques. Also, it should not be assumed that arthroscopic procedures require less fixation to obtain fusion.

Successful arthrodesis is much more difficult to achieve when associated with avascularity of the talus, Charcot neuropathies, high-grade open fractures that result in significant bone loss, failed ankle arthroplasty, neuromuscular disease, nonunions of previous ankle arthrodeses, extended hindfoot arthrodesis, and pyarthrosis. When attempting arthrodesis, it is important to identify these conditions because they require additional considerations and methods of fixation, and the patient

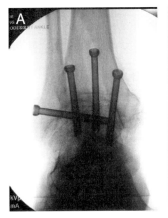 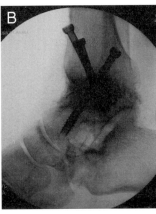

**Figure 5** **A,** AP intraoperative fluoroscopy of an ankle arthrodesis using multiple compression screws. Supplemental fixation (such as an anterior plate) is used for more complex fusions. **B,** Lateral intraoperative fluoroscopy of the same ankle.

should be carefully informed of the increased difficulty in obtaining successful arthrodesis.

Clinical satisfaction after ankle arthrodesis remains high, with most patients indicating significant improvement in postoperative pain. Union rates with internal compression techniques for low-risk patients approach 90%, and radiographic fusion usually takes place within 12 weeks (Fig. 5). Studies show that gait analysis after ankle arthrodesis demonstrated near-normal walking velocity and cadence despite a shortened stride. Patients continued to display decreased time in single-stance phase. Sagittal plane movement of the hindfoot was significantly decreased in the foot of patients who had ankle arthrodesis compared with normal subjects. Sagittal plane movement of the forefoot and transverse plane movements in the hindfoot and forefoot increased in patients who had arthrodesis compared with control patients.

The most frequent complications after ankle arthrodesis include nonunion, malunion, wound complications, and infection. Higher rates of nonunion are associated with diabetes, renal failure, smoking history, and alcohol consumption. Other causes of increased nonunion rates include infection, failure of or inadequate fixation, inadequate bone preparation, poor bone stock, and inadequate immobilization after surgery. Transmalleolar approaches, especially those that discard the fibula, medial malleolus, or both, are associated with higher malunion or nonunion rates. When using the transfibular approach, it is prudent to replace and stabilize the fibula as part of the arthrodesis. The high-risk groups identified earlier are much more difficult to successfully treat and have higher rates of all complications.

## Total Ankle Arthroplasty
Introduced in the 1970s, the first-generation total ankle arthroplasty (TAA) designs had unacceptably high complication and failure rates compared with arthrodesis. However, because longer-term results of ankle arthrodesis have

confirmed radiographic arthritic changes in adjacent joints and patient dissatisfaction (especially from a functional standpoint) with extended hindfoot fusions (ankle plus subtalar or pantalar), interest in joint preservation and enthusiasm for TAA has again emerged. In addition, results from improved implant designs and fixation (bone ingrowth rather than cement) have been encouraging. This optimism for second-generation TAA remains tempered by the satisfactory early results reported with first-generation devices, the difficulty of the actual surgical technique, and the difficulty of revision or salvage.

Indications for TAA are still evolving because the follow-up periods for all current TAA prostheses are at best intermediate term. As with other joint replacements, the optimal patient is older and has fewer functional demands. Particularly, patients with concomitant arthritis in the hindfoot or midfoot may benefit from TAA. Patients with posttraumatic ankle arthrosis, especially younger patients, have poorer reported outcomes and are more likely to require revision with TAA than from other causes of arthrosis. TAA performed for rheumatoid arthritis and osteoarthritis have similar outcomes, although some authors have suggested that higher subsidence rates occur among patients with rheumatoid arthritis. Prospective, peer-reviewed reports of large numbers of comparatively matched cohorts with long-term follow-up from multiple trial centers using similar surgical techniques and prosthetic components are not available.

Absolute contraindications for TAA include active infection, talar necrosis, Charcot neuropathy, absence of muscle function in the lower extremity, previous ankle arthrodesis with removal of the malleoli or insufficiency of the medial and lateral ligaments, tibiotalar malposition of more than 35°, peripheral vascular disease, or inadequate soft-tissue envelope about the ankle. Relative contraindications include previous infection, severe osteoporosis, and very aggressive arthritis (such as destructive uncontrolled psoriatic arthritis).

Although second-generation TAA implants have shown encouraging intermediate results, the optimal articulation configuration is unknown. Mobile-bearing designs offer theoretically less wear and potential for loosening because of full conformity and minimal restraint. Newer fixed-bearing designs avoid bearing dislocation and the potential for added wear from a second articulation. Prospective trials and long-term follow-up are still needed to provide objective and controlled data to replace anecdotal experience with TAA.

## Tibiotalocalcaneal Arthrodesis
Tibiotalocalcaneal arthrodesis is an effective salvage procedure in arthritic conditions that affect both the ankle and subtalar joint. Indications also include failed TAA, osteonecrosis of the talus, and unbraceable deformity secondary to neuromuscular disease or neuropathy. As with all fusions that involve more than one joint, it is harder to

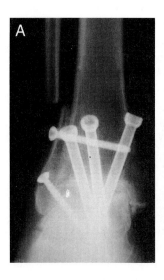
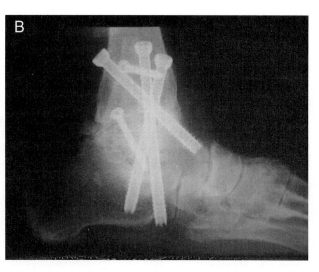

**Figure 6** AP (**A**) and lateral (**B**) radiographs of a tibiotalocalcaneal arthrodesis performed through a lateral approach by osteotomizing the fibula. It is important to decorticate and replace the fibula so that valgus drift does not occur. A second medial approach is also used to denude the joints. Although this example uses only compression screws to obtain fixation, supplementation with anterior plate fixation is often necessary.

achieve union of a tibiotalocalcaneal arthrodesis than ankle or subtalar arthrodesis alone. The ankle is more likely to be the site of nonunion than the subtalar joint. Transarticular compression screw techniques are not as effective as for ankle arthrodesis and subtalar fusion alone. Satisfactory fusion usually requires additional fixation and combinations of screws and plates (Fig. 6). Second-generation intramedullary revision nails allow compression and the ability to apply fixation in 90° configurations. Biomechanical studies also show superior strength with the use of intramedullary nail fixation over that of conventional cross-screw techniques. Other methods of fixation include the use of a blade plate or external fixation.

Surgical approaches use combined medial and lateral incisions or a posterior incision with the patient prone. Regardless of the approach or method of fixation, this type of arthrodesis requires rigid internal fixation and often substantial amounts of bone graft. Accurate alignment and position of the hindfoot and ankle are essential because of the loss of accommodation through both the ankle and subtalar joints.

The short-term results of tibiotalocalcaneal arthrodesis have proved acceptable in terms of pain relief. However, the functional limitations are significant, and satisfaction reported by patients may be because the only other treatment option is amputation. The long-term concern regarding compensatory arthritis and pain developing in the transverse tarsal joints is real, and some of these patients may require additional fusion or amputation despite early reports of satisfaction.

### Tibiocalcaneal Arthrodesis
Tibiocalcaneal arthrodesis is done primarily when the talar body is absent or not salvageable. Indications include osteonecrosis of the talus, failed TAA, severe rheumatoid hindfoot involvement, or severe Charcot deformity. When possible, sparing the talar head increases vascularity to the region, increases the surface area of the fusion, and

preserves the transverse tarsal joint. Fixation devices include screws, revision intramedullary nails, blade plates, or a combination of these. Intramedullary fixation becomes more difficult because of diminished bone stock for adequate purchase solely in the calcaneus. Alignment remains crucial. Complications include shortening of the extremity, malleolar prominences, and arthrosis of the transverse tarsal joints.

## Surgical Treatment of the Hindfoot
### Subtalar Arthrodesis
An isolated subtalar arthrodesis can produce satisfactory correction of deformity and pain relief for a variety of hindfoot conditions. The most common indication is for posttraumatic arthrosis after calcaneal fractures, but subtalar arthrodesis is also useful for posttraumatic arthritis after talar fractures. Other arthritic conditions, talocalcaneal coalition, posterior tibial insufficiency, muscle imbalance, or neuromuscular disease may also benefit from subtalar fusion (Fig. 7). Although subtalar arthrodesis can achieve excellent results, it should still be considered a salvage procedure. If the deformity can be corrected by

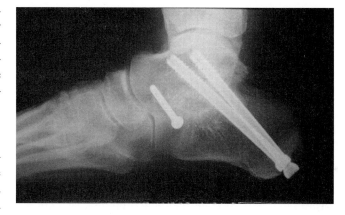

**Figure 7** Subtalar arthrodesis using traditional compression screws and a transverse lag screw.

osteotomy instead of fusion, osteotomy is preferable. The subtalar joint should be considered an essential joint, and fusion increases the likelihood of and decreases the time to development of compensatory arthritis in the surrounding joints. However, an isolated subtalar arthrodesis produces a superior result with less stress on the ankle joint than a triple arthrodesis.

The position of the subtalar joint influences the mobility of the transverse tarsal joints. It is, therefore, imperative that a subtalar fusion be positioned in about 5° to 7° of valgus to permit mobility of the transverse tarsal joints. If placed in varus, the transverse tarsal joint is locked, and the patient will tend to walk on the lateral border of the foot. The position of the forefoot also needs to be considered. If there is more than 10° to 12° of fixed forefoot varus (supination) after a subtalar arthrodesis, the patient will not be able to compensate and will increase weight bearing on the lateral border of the foot, placing inversion stress on the lateral ankle ligaments.

Surgical exposure of the subtalar joint is through either a straight lateral or a modified Ollier incision. Deformities can be corrected by appropriate osteotomy or grafting. Compression screws are generally used for fixation and may be placed from talus to calcaneus or calcaneus to talus. The use of two screws is preferred because this eliminates rotation through the subtalar joint. Nonunion is uncommon.

### Arthrosis After Intra-articular Calcaneal Fractures

Posttraumatic arthritis secondary to calcaneal fracture deserves special consideration. Nonsurgical treatment of calcaneal fractures can result in significant subtalar arthrosis and malalignment. These fractures result in increased heel width, loss of calcaneal height, peroneal impingement and subluxation, calcaneofibular impingement, anterior ankle impingement secondary to loss of the normal talar declination angle, and sural neuritis. Classification schemes for calcaneal malunions are helpful in deciding which surgical procedures are indicated and when to do them. Depending on what is actually producing the patient's symptoms, lateral wall exostectomy, peroneal tenosynovectomy, sural neurectomy, or osteotomy may be more appropriate than arthrodesis. When significant arthritis occurs, subtalar arthrodesis is indicated, but it may require any or all of the above-mentioned procedures as well. When ankle impingement occurs, distraction bone block arthrodesis may be necessary (Fig. 8). This procedure is associated with resultant varus malunion, and attention to detail is critical to restoring talar inclination without subsequent varus. Debate regarding the indications for open reduction and primary subtalar arthrodesis for highly comminuted intra-articular calcaneal fractures continues.

### Talonavicular Arthrodesis

Isolated arthritis of the talonavicular joint is uncommon and usually either posttraumatic or secondary to rheu-

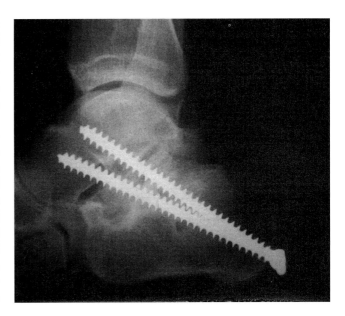

**Figure 8** Subtalar arthrodesis using an interpositional bone block to restore hindfoot height as well as talar inclination following the development of posttraumatic arthritis caused by a calcaneal fracture. Fully threaded screws are used to prevent collapse.

matoid arthritis. Older reports caution against solitary arthrodesis of the talonavicular joint, except in low-demand patients, and recommend double or triple arthrodesis. However, newer data support satisfactory long-term success with isolated talonavicular fusion. Although arthrodesis of the talonavicular joint involves only a single joint, it is an essential joint, and its loss results in almost complete loss of motion in the subtalar and transverse tarsal joints. This motion is lost because the navicular must rotate over the talar head in order for the subtalar joint to invert.

Successful fusion will alleviate talonavicular pain, but development of adjacent compensatory arthritis is common in the subtalar, calcaneocuboid, or navicular-cuneiform joints. In addition to using it to treat arthritis, some authors have proposed talonavicular arthrodesis for correction of adult acquired flatfoot secondary to posterior tibial insufficiency and spring ligament rupture. This method of reconstruction limits hindfoot motion, and controversy regarding the advantages of single, double, or triple arthrodesis in patients with posterior tibial insufficiency remains.

### Calcaneocuboid Arthrodesis

Although arthritis involving only the calcaneocuboid joint is rare, evidence of radiographic involvement of the calcaneocuboid joint after calcaneal fractures is fairly common. However, it is rarely clinically symptomatic enough to require fusion. Calcaneocuboid arthrodesis is more commonly done with correction of an acquired flatfoot deformity. The use of calcaneocuboid arthrodesis to obtain lateral column lengthening has been advocated by

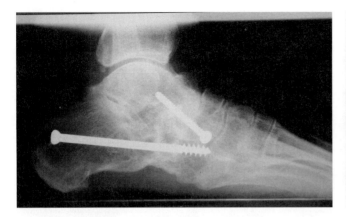

**Figure 9** Double arthrodesis (talonavicular and calcaneocuboid) for correction of adult acquired flatfoot.

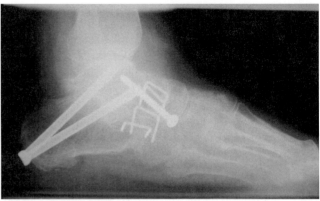

**Figure 10** Triple arthrodesis for stage III adult acquired flatfoot with fixed deformity and hindfoot arthritis.

some authors as preferable to lengthening through the calcaneus (Evans procedure). Of the hindfoot joints, calcaneocuboid fusion results in the least amount of restriction of hindfoot motion (60% to 80% of hindfoot motion remains). Unfortunately, this flexibility probably contributes to its troublesome nonunion rate. Considerable attention to detail is required to obtain a successful union. The joint surfaces must be well prepared and fixation must be solid and durable.

### Double Arthrodesis

Double arthrodesis refers to the simultaneous fusions of the talonavicular and calcaneocuboid joints (Fig. 9). It is used most commonly for malalignment associated with posterior tibial insufficiency and associated adult acquired flatfoot when the patient is not a candidate for tendon transfer and realignment. In these situations, the subtalar joint must be flexible and without arthritis. In addition, the major deformity is a fixed forefoot varus (supination) with abduction of the transverse tarsal joints. A fusion of the talonavicular and calcaneocuboid joints should allow for correction of the deformity without including the subtalar joint. A midtarsal arthrodesis results in minimal subtalar motion. If arthrosis or deformity exists in the subtalar joint, triple arthrodesis would be more appropriate. It was previously believed that there was no functional difference between double and triple arthrodesis, but recent studies show that approximately 25% of subtalar motion remains after double arthrodesis. Whether or not this is clinically significant is unknown.

### Triple Arthrodesis

Surgical fusion of the subtalar, talonavicular, and calcaneocuboid joints historically evolved for the treatment of paralytic deformities, primarily poliomyelitis, in patients who often had significant bony deformities that required the removal of large bone wedges to place the foot in a plantigrade position. Today, triple arthrodesis is most commonly done to treat posttraumatic arthritis or rheu-

matoid arthritis in adults, or for salvage of adult acquired flatfoot with arthritis and fixed deformity (Fig. 10).

Triple arthrodesis is a technically demanding procedure, and the position of the fusion is critical to success. Once the foot is in a fixed position, it can no longer accommodate to the ground. It is essential, therefore, to place the hindfoot in 5° to 7° of valgus, the transverse tarsal joints in 5° to 10° of abduction, and the forefoot in less neutral rotation in the axial plane. Obtaining a satisfactory union requires meticulous joint preparation, judicious bone graft or bone graft substitute, and rigid internal stabilization.

When proper position, alignment, and union are obtained, predictable and significant improvement in symptoms occurs, but the resultant loss of hindfoot motion is not without consequence. Long-term follow-up shows progressive compensatory arthritis in the ankle and midfoot both radiographically and clinically. Despite these long-term consequences, triple arthrodesis, when used for the appropriate indications, has stood the test of time. Improvement in a patient's symptoms and function remains gratifying to both the patient and surgeon.

### Pantalar and Extended Hindfoot Arthrodesis

Pantalar arthrodesis refers to simultaneous fusions of the tibiotalar, subtalar, and talonavicular joints (Fig. 11). Extended hindfoot fusions include the calcaneocuboid joint in addition to the other three. These salvage procedures are most commonly used to treat patients with posttraumatic arthritis and those with severe rheumatoid disease, neuropathic conditions, or compensatory arthritis following previous ankle or hindfoot fusions. Both pantalar and extended hindfoot arthrodesis can be done as single or staged procedures. Although pain relief is the primary benefit of these procedures, function is extremely limited. These fusions are technically demanding and have higher complication rates than isolated ankle or hindfoot fusions. Nonunion rates are higher, with the most common site of nonunion being in the ankle component of the fusion.

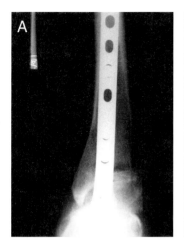
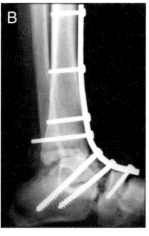

**Figure 11** AP (**A**) and lateral (**B**) radiographs of a pantalar arthrodesis performed for complete traumatic extrusion of the talus. An interpositional tricortical bone graft was used to restore height.

Complications or dissatisfaction after these procedures may require amputation as the only other treatment option.

## Summary

Arthritic disorders of the ankle and hindfoot account for considerable pain, disability, and functional impairment. Nonsurgical and surgical management can significantly improve the quality of life for patients with these disorders. The use of appropriate bracing and orthoses provides not only pain relief, but may also delay or prevent surgical intervention and the long-term consequences of salvage procedures. When assessing surgical options, it is imperative to search for possible reconstructive procedures that, although they may not eliminate arthritis, may delay the need for salvage procedures. Fusions, either in isolation or combination, represent the gold standard for the treatment of advanced arthritis of the ankle and hindfoot. These procedures provide significant pain relief, allow for correction of deformity, and restore function when properly used.

## Annotated Bibliography

### Arthritis

Coughlin MJ: Arthritides, in Coughlin MJ, Mann RA (eds): *Surgery of the Foot and Ankle*, ed 7. St. Louis, MO, Mosby, 1999, pp 560-650.

This is a comprehensive review of the arthritides that are most commonly encountered in foot and ankle surgery, and both nonsurgical and surgical recommendations for treatment are provided.

### Surgical Treatment of the Ankle

Chou LB, Mann RA, Yaszay B, et al: Tibiotalocalcaneal arthrodesis. *Foot Ankle Int* 2000;21:804-808.

The authors of this multicenter, retrospective study of 55 patients undergoing simultaneous tibiotalocalcaneal arthrode-

sis found that the most common complication was nonunion at the ankle.

Coester LM, Saltzman CL, Leupold J, Pontarelli W: Long-term results following ankle arthrodesis for post-traumatic arthritis. *J Bone Joint Surg Am* 2001;83:219-228.

The authors of this study report long-term results of patients undergoing an isolated ankle arthrodesis for posttraumatic arthritis. Although arthrodesis resulted in good early pain relief, it was associated with premature deterioration of other joints, resulting in arthritis, pain, and dysfunction.

Cooper PS: Complications of ankle and tibiotalocalcaneal arthrodesis. *Clin Orthop* 2001;391:33-44.

Algorithms for the treatment of the most frequent complications of ankle and tibiotalocalcaneal fusions are presented.

Easley ME, Vertullo CJ, Urban WC, Nunley JA: Total ankle arthroplasty. *J Am Acad Orthop Surg* 2002;10:157-167.

The authors of this article discuss four second-generation total ankle designs and their intermediate results.

Gould JS, Alvine FG, Mann RA, Sanders RW, Walling AK: Total ankle replacement: A surgical discussion. Part I: Replacement systems, indications, and contraindications. *Am J Orthop* 2000;29:604-609.

Panelists review the development of total ankle replacement, current system availability, and indications and contraindications for the procedure.

Gould JS, Alvine FG, Mann RA, Sanders RW, Walling AK: Total ankle replacement: A surgical discussion. Part II: The clinical and surgical experience. *Am J Orthop* 2000;29:675-682.

Panelists address such issues as deformities, laxities, malalignments, and late complications.

Mann RA: Arthrodesis of the foot and ankle, in Coughlin MJ, Mann RA (eds): *Surgery of the Foot and Ankle*, ed 7. St. Louis, MO, Mosby, 1999, pp 651-699.

This is an extensive review of the types and techniques of arthrodesis in the foot and ankle used to treat arthritic conditions. Technical considerations as well as surgical principles and complications of specific arthrodeses are presented.

### Surgical Treatment of the Hindfoot

Bibbo C, Anderson RB, Davis WH: Complications of midfoot and hindfoot arthrodesis. *Clin Orthop* 2001;391: 45-58.

The authors describe the major complications associated with midfoot and hindfoot fusions and discuss prevention and treatment.

Easley ME, Trnka HJ, Schon LC, Myerson MS: Isolated subtalar arthrodesis. *J Bone Joint Surg Am* 2000;82:613-624.

In this retrospective review of 174 consecutive isolated subtalar arthrodeses, less favorable results were found compared with previous reports. Increased nonunion rates were attributed to smoking, avascular bone at the arthrodesis site, and previous failure of attempted subtalar arthrodesis.

Flemister AS Jr, Infante AF, Sanders RW, Walling AK: Subtalar arthrodesis for complications of intra-articular calcaneal fractures. *Foot Ankle Int* 2000;21:392-399.

The authors of this study compared three groups of patients (ie, those with calcaneal malunions, failed ORIF, and primary subtalar fusions) for union rates, clinical results, and length of hospitalization.

Saltzman CL, Fehrle MJ, Cooper RR, Spencer EC, Ponseti IV: Triple arthrodesis: Twenty-five and forty-four-year average follow-up of the same patients. *J Bone Joint Surg Am* 1999;81:1391-1402.

The authors of this retrospective review of young patients undergoing triple arthrodesis report that despite progressive symptoms and radiographic degeneration in the joints of the ankle and midfoot, 54 patients (95%) were satisfied with the results of the operation.

Walling AK: Section I: Symposium adult acquired flatfoot-symposium. *Clin Orthop* 1999;365:2-99.

This is an updated symposium with contributing authors discussing the etiology, staging, and nonsurgical and surgical alternatives for treatment of the adult acquired flatfoot (multiple articles).

Wulker N, Stukenborg C, Savory KM, Alfke D: Hindfoot motion after isolated and combined arthrodeses: Measurements in anatomic specimens. *Foot Ankle Int* 2000; 21:921-927.

The authors calculated passive motion in the hindfoot after all feasible combinations of fusions were performed. It was believed that the key articulation is the talonavicular joint.

## Classic Bibliography

Fogel GR, Katoh Y, Rand JA, Chao EY: Talonavicular arthrodesis for isolated arthrosis: 9.5-year results and gait analysis. *Foot Ankle* 1982;3:105-113.

Gellman H, Lenihan M, Halikis N, Botte MJ, Giordani M, Perry J: Selective tarsal arthrodesis: An in vitro analysis of the effect on foot motion. *Foot Ankle* 1987;8:127-133.

Marti RK, Raaymakers EL, Nolte PA: Malunited ankle fractures: The late results of reconstruction. *J Bone Joint Surg Br* 1990;72:709-713.

Methods and follow-up statistics on ankle arthrodesis: Symposium. *Clin Orthop* 1991;268:1-111.

Papa JA, Myerson MS: Pantalar and tibiotalocalcaneal arthrodesis for post-traumatic osteoarthrosis of the ankle and hindfoot. *J Bone Joint Surg Am* 1992;74:1042-1049.

Walling AK, Padrta BJ: Ankle arthrodesis, in Asnis SE, Kyle RF (eds): *Cannulated Screw Fixation: Principles and Operative Techniques.* New York, NY, Springer, 1996, pp 260-267.

Weber BG, Simpson LA: Corrective lengthening osteotomy of the fibula. *Clin Orthop* 1985;199:61-67.

# Chapter 16

# Arthritis of the Midfoot and Forefoot

Paul J. Juliano, MD

## Introduction

Midfoot and forefoot arthritis may be quite mild and require little treatment. However, even moderate involvement of the apical arch, metatarsal-cuneiform joints, or the metatarsophalangeal (MTP) joints of the forefoot can limit function depending on the extent of involvement. This chapter addresses the most common types of inflammatory arthritides involving the midfoot and forefoot, their pathophysiology, and nonsurgical and surgical treatment options.

## Midfoot

Painless function of the foot depends on the complex biomechanical interaction of numerous small bones and joints. In osteoarthritis, commonly characterized by the deterioration of articular cartilage with secondary mechanical joint surface destruction, periarticular osteophytes develop in an attempted repair process. This pathologic process is particularly debilitating to the midfoot because it interferes with the complex architectural relationship of small bones and joints in this mechanically vulnerable area, which undergoes loading during each gait cycle. Once the degenerative process of osteoarthritis develops, it follows a relentless, albeit variable, course.

### Anatomy

The midfoot has three distinct articular columns: medial, containing the first metatarsal-cuneiform joint; central, containing the second and third metatarsal-cuneiform joints and the intercuneiform joints; and lateral, containing the cuboid fourth and fifth metatarsal joints. In addition, a complex and variable ligament configuration consisting of dorsal, plantar, and interosseous ligaments provides a stout soft-tissue envelope. The three cuneiforms and cuboid form the transverse arch with the apex at the third metatarsal-cuneiform articulation. The columnar division is based on stability, structural rigidity, and movements of each, which vary markedly. The fourth and fifth metatarsals have considerably more motion in both the sagittal and horizontal planes; however, even with ra-diographic evidence of arthritis, the metatarsal cuboid articulation is the least likely to be symptomatic. Conversely, the second metatarsal moves the least, the third metatarsal moves slightly more than the second, and these two articulations are the most likely sources of painful arthritis. The rigidity at the apex of the medial central longitudinal arch supports weight bearing through thousands of gait cycles a day. Cumulative stress across the intercuneiform and metatarsal joints can cause damage, particularly once an inflammatory, traumatic, or degenerative process begins.

The second metatarsal base is recessed between the medial and lateral cuneiforms by approximately 1 to 4 mm. A strong, oblique interosseous ligament (Lisfranc ligament) connects the second metatarsal base with the medial cuneiform. This ligament, approximately 8 to 10 mm long and 5 to 6 mm thick, is the largest in the tarsometatarsal complex. A separate plantar ligament, traversing from the medial cuneiform to the second and third metatarsal bases, adds stability. Strong plantar ligaments provide the primary stabilization of the apex of the longitudinal arch of the midfoot. The first metatarsal-cuneiform joint is stabilized during weight bearing primarily by its plantar ligament. Clinical studies show that in an asymptomatic foot, first metatarsal-cuneiform joint motion averages 4.37° in the sagittal plane, and if the patient has thumb hypermobility, the first tarsometatarsal joint motion is also increased. Multiple variables, including intermetatarsal angle, sex, age, elbow and knee hyperextension, and distal medial cuneiform articular configuration, do not correlate with first metatarsal medial cuneiform motion. The morphology of this joint is variable, and description has been based on medial inclination, lateral radiographic slope, and type of articular facet with the second metatarsal.

### Presenting Complaints and Physical Examination

Patients with midfoot arthritis usually describe a deep, aching pain aggravated by prolonged standing and walking. A bony prominence (also known as a boss) may be present dorsally at the apex of the arch, and local pressure symptoms from laced shoes may be a source of pain.

The deep peroneal nerve, the medial dorsal cutaneous branch of the superficial peroneal nerve, or the saphenous nerve may become irritated as they traverse these bony prominences. This neuritic pain frequently radiates toward the hallux and first web space. Pain with motion of the toes may indicate inflammation of the extensor tendons, which can also be aggravated by dorsal osteophytes. Occasionally, a collapse deformity of the arch with abduction of the forefoot is present, and painful calluses, medial and plantar, develop at the apex of this deformity. Pain is the most common presenting complaint. Deformity may cause problems with shoe wear and bracing because of pressure against bony prominences.

An examination with the patient standing (frontal and lateral) is important to determine the degree and apex of the deformity. The examination of both of the feet with the patient sitting allows determination of flexibility of the deformity and heel cord contractures, as well as motion, neurovascular, and skin assessment. It is very important to carefully palpate each metatarsal-cuneiform joint in turn, medial to lateral. Because it is very easy to overlook subtle radiographic or clinical osteoarthritis of the second and third metatarsal-cuneiform joints, a measure of suspicion from a careful history will guide the examiner to individually palpate these joints during passive motion of the respective metatarsal in the sagittal plane. The midfoot can be stressed with the pronation-abduction maneuver.

### Radiographic Findings

Weight-bearing radiographs are usually needed to assess midfoot arthritis. The AP view may only show minimal narrowing of the metatarsal-cuneiform joint (second or third usually). On the non–weight-bearing oblique view, minimal subluxation of the medial sides of the metatarsal-cuneiform joints (again second and third most commonly) may be visible. Whether the earliest radiographic or clinical findings occur most commonly at the base of the second or third metatarsal-cuneiform joint is debatable and not crucial to formulating a treatment plan. The third metatarsal-lateral cuneiform articulation is believed to absorb the most stress during the stance phase of gait and therefore is the most likely part of the midfoot to show the earliest clinical and radiographic signs of osteoarthritis. Joint space narrowing, subchondral sclerosis, cysts, and marginal osteophytes are typically seen in the later stages of osteoarthritis.

When it is difficult to determine the extent of midfoot arthritis with physical examination and plain radiographs alone, bone scanning and CT can be useful, particularly if surgical intervention is being considered. (MRI is generally not as useful in the evaluation of arthritic conditions of the midfoot because it does not provide any additional information about bony destruction or joint space narrowing.) CT with three-dimensional reconstructions is helpful when the patient has a significant deformity. Selective injection of a local anesthetic into the involved joints guided by fluoroscopy or CT may also be helpful as a diagnostic tool, and pain relief with selective injection into the fourth and fifth tarsometatarsal joints has been shown to be a prognostic indicator of the potential success of resection arthroplasty of the lateral column. However, repeated physical examinations on different occasions can be more useful than radiographic imaging, CT, and bone scanning.

### Treatment

Nonsurgical treatment often includes anti-inflammatory medication and shoe modifications, including use of a rocker-bottom shoe with a rigid shank or an ankle-foot orthosis with a fixed ankle. These orthotic measures decrease the sagittal plane motion of the foot, partially unload the involved joints, and are usually all that is needed to successfully treat a compliant patient.

Three surgical options are available to treat midfoot arthritis: (1) fusion in situ, (2) fusion with corrective osteotomy, and (3) resectional arthroplasty. Fusion in situ (Fig. 1) is recommended for patients who have radiographic changes and arthritic symptoms in the same areas and have demonstrated compliance with nonsurgical treatment but in whom conservative therapy has failed to relieve symptoms. Normal or near-normal alignment should be present with the patient in the aligned weight-bearing position before an in situ fusion is chosen. An abducted forefoot (usually associated with some degree of medial arch collapse) is the most common deformity in patients with midfoot osteoarthritis (Fig. 2). Arthrodesis of the tarsometatarsal joints can be accomplished with a variety of internal fixation methods, including Kirschner wire (K-wire) and/or screw or plate fixation, screw fixation without bone grafting, and a dowel peg iliac crest bone graft with or without the addition of screw or wire fixation (Fig. 3).

The most troublesome technical pitfall of midfoot fusion when a corrective osteotomy is needed is unequal joint surface resection. When more bone is removed dorsally, dorsiflexion of the joint with joint surface compression and weight transfer to adjacent metatarsal heads occurs. Most authors agree that workers' compensation patients and those who have undergone fusion of the fourth and fifth tarsometatarsal joints have the worst outcomes. Midfoot fusion with corrective osteotomy is usually required to restore the alignment in the sagittal, frontal, and transverse planes as well as to reconstruct the longitudinal arch. The goal of this procedure is to restore the foot to a plantigrade position while restoring stability. A medial and plantar closing wedge osteotomy will correct the abduction and plantar flexion. A contoured plate placed inferiorly and medially will act as a tension band and will add significant stability to the medial column. An external fixator placed laterally will facilitate the correction of the abduction deformity. The fixator can be used

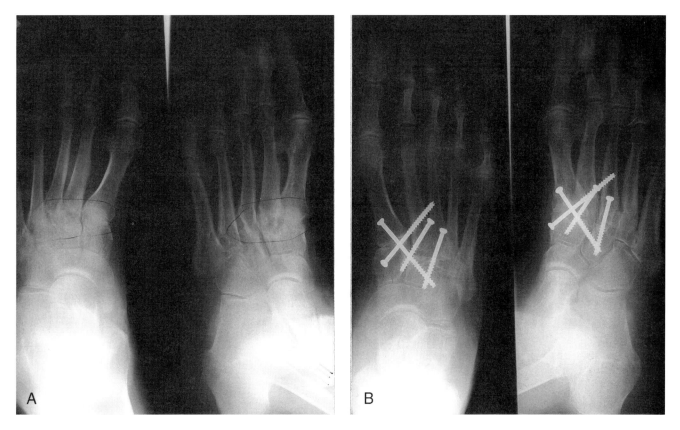

Figure 1  **A,** AP radiograph showing diffuse osteoarthritic involvement of the tarsometatarsal joints without deformity. **B,** Fusion in situ.

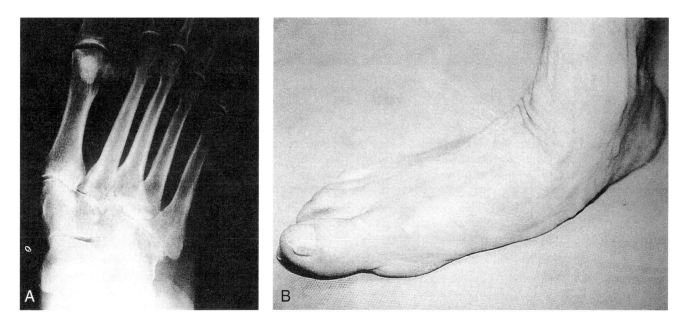

Figure 2  **A,** AP radiograph of abducted forefoot. **B,** Clinical photograph demonstrating the flatfoot appearance. (Reproduced from Beaman DN, Saltzman CL: Arthritis of the foot, in *Orthopaedic Knowledge Update: Foot and Ankle 2.* Rosemont, IL, American Academy of Orthopaedic Surgeons, 1998, pp 293-303.)

postoperatively in instances in which it is not prudent to place internal fixation on the medial side (for example, when an active medial ulcer or soft-tissue compromise is present). The intercuneiform complex should be included in the fusion when there are radiographic signs of disease or preoperative symptoms or at the discretion of the surgeon. The trend is to use more local bone graft (distal tibia, calcaneus) as well as allograft to improve the fusion rate.

Motion in the fourth and fifth metatarsals is so important in walking that arthrodesis of these joints is seldom

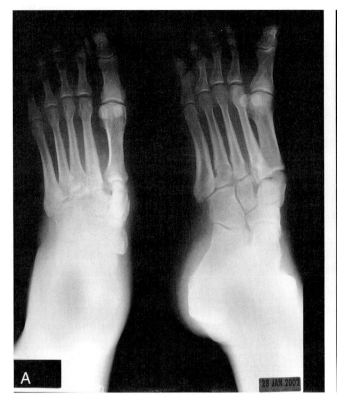
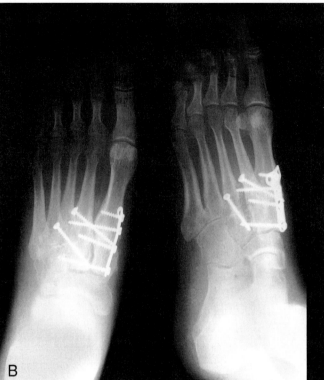

**Figure 3** **A,** AP radiograph showing osteoarthritic involvement of metatarsal-cuneiform joints one, two, and three. **B,** Plantar medial plate and correction of deformity.

recommended. An alternative method of surgical treatment is resection arthroplasty, usually the dorsal 40% to 50% of the fourth and fifth metatarsal base articular surface; however, complete resection of the base of the lateral two metatarsals with collagen tendon in interposition has been reported. In one recent study of eight patients who underwent resection-interposition arthroplasty, 75% reported satisfactory results at 25-month follow-up. Pain relief with preoperative injection of local anesthetic into the symptomatic areas was found to correlate well with the highest degree of patient satisfaction.

Some patients with midfoot arthritis have extensive erosion involving a large portion of the medial and central columns and extending into the naviculocuneiform articulation, which may be caused by osteoarthritis or a posttraumatic (Lisfranc) injury. Occasionally, there is also collapse of the lateral portion of the navicular, and the original injury may propagate through the cuboid metatarsal or cuboid calcaneal articulations involving the lateral column.

Treatment for these patients is complex because of the extent of articular involvement. In most instances, nonsurgical treatment is with an ankle-foot orthosis and a steel shank shoe or boot. Surgical treatment should include inlay or interpositional bone grafting and internal fixation. The inlay technique involves the creation of a medial or dorsal rectangular slot from the talus to the involved cuneiforms or metatarsal bases. This slot can be formed with a burr. The joints are then distracted, and a tricortical inlay graft is interposed. Distraction is released and internal fixation is inserted. The involved joints are not prepared separately but are spanned by the graft. In patients with osteopenic bone, supplementary external fixation may be useful in the early phases of graft incorporation, and weight bearing is not recommended until the inlay graft is incorporated, which may take many months.

## Complications

The most common complications associated with surgical treatment include wound healing, nerve injury, nonunions, malunions, implant complications, and late complications associated with progressive arthritis. Wound complications can be decreased with preoperative vascular assessment, smoking cessation, and discontinuing perioperative antibiotics. Halting the administration of immunosuppressive drugs may decrease wound complications, but this is unclear in the literature. Nerve complications include neuritis or complex regional pain syndrome (type I or II). Nonunions of the medial and middle columns of the midfoot have been reported to occur in 3% to 7% of patients, and nonunions of the lateral column have been reported to occur in more than 50%. There is some evidence to suggest that nonsteroidal antiinflammatory drugs contribute to nonunion. Malunions can be corrected with osteotomies in the sagittal or frontal plane, depending on the deformity. To assess frontal plane balance, the second toe should line up with the tibial tubercle. Because equinus contractures can contribute to midfoot breakdown and recurrence of the deformity, Achilles tendon lengthening or gastrocnemius slide procedures should be considered at the time of the initial surgery.

## Forefoot

### *Rheumatoid Forefoot Deformities*

Rheumatoid arthritis (RA) is a systemic, inflammatory disorder that primarily affects women, with a peak incidence at age 30 to 50 years. RA is often a severe chronic disorder that, even with early and aggressive intervention, often leads to joint erosions and progressive joint damage, functional limitations, and disability. In multiple populations, RA has a prevalence of 0.5% to 1.0%, which underscores the worldwide impact of this illness.

RA is diagnosed clinically, and symptoms usually include malaise, stiffness, and symmetric swelling and pain in the small joints of the hands and feet. The clinical diagnosis is supported by a positive rheumatoid factor and characteristic radiographic changes. The clinical course of the disease varies widely, and when first diagnosed, the clinical outcome for each patient is unpredictable.

The foot and/or ankle is the initial site of involvement in 16% of patients with RA, and the forefoot is the earliest and most frequently affected part of the foot. The hindfoot, consisting of the subtalar, talonavicular, and calcaneocuboid joints, is also frequently involved, and the talonavicular is the earliest and most frequently affected joint. The least frequently involved joint is the ankle, which is often secondarily affected as an adjacent segment following hindfoot fusion. Although severe deformities can be present in patients in whom medical management of their disease has been poor, the incidence of severe deformities is diminishing with appropriate medical care.

### *Pathophysiology*

RA results in a complex cascade of pathology involving both the cellular and humoral immune systems. Proliferative inflammatory synovium, which secretes catabolic enzymes, destroys articular cartilage and compromises the integrity of the periarticular soft tissues. In the foot, the end result is often one or more stiff, painful, and deformed joints; however, medical and surgical treatment may provide substantial benefits. In forefoot involvement, articular effusion and periarticular edema can loosen attachments of tendon, muscle, and ligaments mechanically and enzymatically (enthesopathy). This process leads to instability, subluxation, and dislocation of one or more metatarsal joints when weight-bearing forces are dissipated across the unstable joint(s), translating the toes dorsally on the metatarsal heads. The plantar fat pad subsequently migrates distally, uncovering the metatarsal heads. Because these bony prominences are covered only

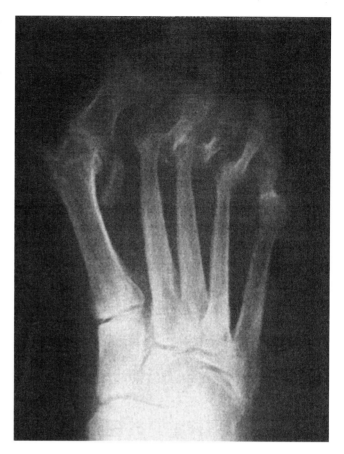

**Figure 4** AP radiograph of typical rheumatoid forefoot involvement. (Reproduced with permission from Graves SC, Winterton PW: Surgical management of the rheumatoid forefoot, hindfoot, and ankle. *Arthritis* 1999;4:223-234.)

by skin, calluses and bursae can form. If the patient also has a history of neuritic complaints at the level of the MTP joints, then vasculitis with neuropathy must be considered. Initially, deformities at the MTP and proximal interphalangeal joints in the forefoot are correctable passively but eventually become fixed.

The presentation and surgical management of juvenile RA differ from those of adult RA. In patients with juvenile RA, the foot and ankle are often spared early in the course of the disease, and the rheumatoid factor is usually negative. During initial examination, there may be swelling in only one ankle joint or across one metatarsus. Development of cavus deformity, thinner and shorter metatarsals and phalanges, and other growth disturbances may result from inflammatory physeal involvement.

### *Surgical Reconstruction: Indications/Options*

Surgical management of the rheumatoid forefoot is warranted when painful deformities and stiffness are refractory to conservative management (Fig. 4). However, all forefoot surgery in patients with RA is a compromise between the ideal and the unacceptable. The goals of surgery include restoring alignment and position of the great and lesser toes, relieving painful bones, removing plantar

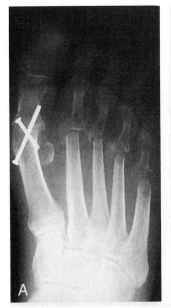
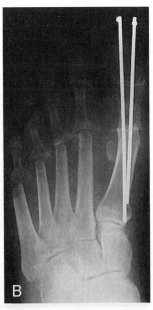
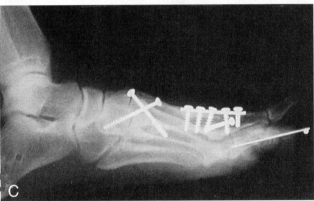

**Figure 5** **A,** AP radiograph of rheumatoid forefoot repair by resecting metatarsal heads two through five and hallux MTP fusion using crossed screws. **B,** AP radiograph of rheumatoid forefoot repair by resecting metatarsal heads two and three and hallux MTP joint fusion using threaded Steinmann pins. **C,** Lateral radiograph of rheumatoid forefoot repair using a dorsal plate for the hallux MTP joint fusion; medial column fusion is also illustrated. (Reproduced with permission from Graves SC, Winterton PW: Surgical management of the rheumatoid forefoot, hindfoot, and ankle. *Arthritis* 1999; 4:223-234.)

prominences, and restoring some degree of stability to the distal forefoot while maintaining enough flexibility (usually passive) to allow a less painful and more fluid gait.

Resection of the metatarsal heads, with resection of the head and neck of the proximal phalanx (when needed), is the most commonly used surgical procedure for the treatment of lesser toe deformities. The extent of bony resection (both metatarsal and phalangeal) as well as concomitant extensor tenotomy and/or lengthening depends on the severity of the frontal and sagittal deformity. Methods for preserving the anatomy of the distal forefoot and toes have been reported and usually include using metatarsal osteotomies, which shorten the bone, relieve soft-tissue contracture, and allow relocation of subluxated or distorted joints. However, these techniques are not com-

monly used. Use of Silastic total joint arthroplasty has been criticized because of associated adverse effects, including fragmentation of the implant, foreign body reactions, and periprosthetic osteolysis, that complicate future surgical reconstruction.

The most widely used surgical treatment for severe forefoot rheumatoid deformity is resection arthroplasty. Arthrodesis of the interphalangeal joint of the hallux and resection of the lesser metatarsal heads is a reasonable option (Fig. 5). When the interphalangeal joint of the hallux is unstable, a resection arthroplasty, arthrodesis of the interphalangeal joint of the hallux, and resection of the lesser metatarsal heads is a reasonable treatment option. The sesamoid apparatus should be mobilized to rest beneath the first metatarsal head or as close to that position as possible. However, arthrodesis of the first MTP joint is done whenever possible. The first metatarsal should not require an osteotomy to correct metatarsal varus, and sufficient distal lesser metatarsal resection should allow the toe to rest in a plantigrade position and not against the distal metatarsal remnant. Because the second metatarsal is the longest metatarsal and the fifth metatarsal is the shortest, a parabola must be established, and the bone must be beveled from dorsal distal to proximal plantar with an additional bevel for the fifth metatarsal made dorsal lateral distal to plantar medial proximal. Patient satisfaction is generally predictable when this reconstructive procedure is used. However, in patients with psoriatic forefoot deformities similar to those seen in RA, the level of patient satisfaction after surgical treatment is not quite as high.

Occasionally, a patient will present for surgery with some uninvolved rays and no hallucal deformity. As a general rule, forefoot arthroplasty should include all lesser MTP joints, even if one or two are not appreciably affected, because there is a high likelihood of symptoms and disease progression in these rays. Likewise, even though it is disconcerting to the patient and surgeon to recommend surgery on a normal or near-normal first MTP joint when resection of two or more lesser metatarsal heads is indicated, it is highly likely that another surgical procedure will be required if the entire reconstruction is not done initially. One recent clinical series reported failure of hallux preservation surgery in less than 24 months, and multiple clinical series have warned of this pitfall.

### Seronegative Inflammatory Arthritides
Psoriatic arthritis typically affects the distal interphalangeal joints of the toes and may cause erosion of proximal phalanges, leading to a "pencil and cup" appearance of the joints. The radiographic and clinical appearance may be striking (arthritis mutilans), with severe destruction of multiple joints. Distal phalangeal tuft erosion and pitting of the nails are also present. The MTP joints may or may not be involved. When the MTP, proximal inter-

phalangeal, and distal interphalangeal joints are involved, the deformities are rigid and resemble those seen in patients with RA. Deformities caused by Reiter's syndrome are clinically similar to those caused by psoriatic arthritis, but they are less often symmetric and have less interphalangeal joint involvement. Both disorders can cause diffuse fusiform enlargement (sausage digits), as well as erythematous cyanosis, which may be painless.

With respect to the forefoot, ankylosing spondylitis causes deformities similar to those seen in patients with RA, with involvement of the MTP joints. The inflammatory process of ankylosing spondylitis, however, is typically less severe than in RA. Joint ankylosis may occur secondary to intra-articular or capsular ossification. Clinical management should follow the same principles as those used to treat the rheumatoid patient.

Gout and pseudogout are crystalline deposit disorders that may affect the foot. Gout is characterized by the intra-articular presence of monosodium urate crystals, which are needle-shaped and negatively birefringent under a polarizing microscope. Gout is usually caused by a disorder of purine metabolism, but it also may be caused by medications that elevate serum uric acid levels. Gout occurs more frequently in men than women and typically presents as an acute arthritis or periarticular inflammatory reaction of the first MTP joint (podagra). This joint is involved in 50% to 75% of patients with early evidence of gout, and 90% of patients with gout will have involvement of this joint over time. Acute gout often occurs postoperatively, and symptoms include severe pain, swelling, erythema, and warmth about the involved joint that typically lasts for several days and then subsides. Diagnosis can often be made on a clinical basis and confirmed with crystal analysis of the joint fluid (sodium monourate crystals are strongly birefringent under polarized light). In the early stages, serum uric acid levels may be normal, and radiographs are typically normal; however, radiographs may later demonstrate periarticular erosions or lesions on both sides of the joint. Joint destruction may occur in chronic cases.

The acute gouty episode of the hallux is treated with rest, elevation, and the use of a stiff-soled, open-toed, postoperative shoe. Medical management involves the use of nonsteroidal anti-inflammatory drugs (typically indomethacin) or colchicine. Chronic tophaceous gout is rare, and management includes local débridement of symptomatic or draining deposits. Arthrodesis may be indicated in the presence of significant joint destruction. Perioperative complications can be minimized if the patient continues allopurinol therapy and is kept well hydrated in the perioperative period.

Pseudogout is caused by calcium pyrophosphate dihydrate crystal deposits in the joints or periarticular tissue that cause an inflammatory reaction. These crystals are of variable shape and have weak positive birefringence when examined under the polarizing microscope.

Radiographs may demonstrate fine intra-articular calcifications, but joint destruction is uncommon. The MTP joints are most commonly affected in the foot, and treatment is symptomatic and includes medical management of acute synovitis if severe joint involvement occurs. The disease process of pseudogout may be similar to that of degenerative arthritis or neuroarthropathy with bony fragmentation.

## Summary

Inflammatory arthritis of the midfoot is most commonly osteoarthritis, whereas the diffuse forefoot involvement is most commonly RA. Plantigrade alignment and stability of the arch are essential for a functional foot. Commonly, these two criteria can be met with nonsurgical treatment consisting of proper shoe wear, molded insoles, and/or braces. If surgical treatment is indicated, alignment and stability must be paramount in the preoperative planning, and the inflammatory component of the arthritides should be controlled as best as possible before surgery. Despite the recent advances in the medical treatment of arthritis, surgery remains an excellent option for patients when nonsurgical treatment has failed. Surgery can provide predictable pain relief for patients with midfoot and forefoot arthritis.

## Annotated Bibliography

*Midfoot*

Berlet GC, Hodges Davis W, Anderson RB: Tendon arthroplasty for basal fourth and fifth metatarsal arthritis. *Foot Ankle Int* 2002;23:440-446.

The authors retrospectively evaluated eight patients who underwent débridement of the fourth and fifth tarsometatarsal joints with tendon interposition. At mean 25-month follow-up, 75% reported satisfactory results. The authors concluded that relief from preoperative injection was prognostic of surgical results.

Bibbo C, Anderson RB, Davis WH: Complications of midfoot and hindfoot arthrodesis. *Clin Orthop* 2001;391: 45-58.

This study describes the major complications associated with midfoot and hindfoot fusions in adults and discusses the prevention and treatment of these complications.

Kuo RS, Tejwani NC, Digiovanni CW, et al: Outcome after open reduction and internal fixation of Lisfranc joint injuries. *J Bone Joint Surg Am* 2000;82:1609-1618.

The results of this study support the concept that stable anatomic reduction of fracture-dislocations of the Lisfranc joint leads to the best long-term outcomes because patients undergoing this treatment report less arthritis and better American Orthopaedic Foot and Ankle Society (AOFAS) midfoot scores.

Lin SS, Bono CM, Treuting R, Shereff MJ: Limited intertarsal arthrodesis using bone grafting and pin fixation. *Foot Ankle Int* 2000;21:742-748.

Sixteen patients with tarsometatarsal arthritis were treated with K-wire fixation and iliac crest bone grafting. At mean 36-month follow-up, AOFAS scores improved an average of 41 points, and 81% rated their result as good or excellent.

Myerson MS, Badekas A: Hypermobility of the first ray. *Foot Ankle Clin* 2000;5:469-484.

The authors recommend arthrodesis of the tarsometatarsal joint, exostectomy, capsulorrhaphy, and distal soft-tissue release to correct and stabilize the first metatarsal at the apex of the deformity. With this procedure, the authors found it unnecessary to include the base of the second metatarsal.

Park DS, Schram AJ, Stone NM: Isolated lateral tarsometatarsal joint arthrodesis: A case report. *J Foot Ankle Surg* 2000;39:239-243.

Revisional inlay bone grafting resulted in solid arthrodesis in this case report. The authors conclude that although there are some detrimental biomechanical effects of this procedure, they do not outweigh the need to alleviate debilitating symptoms associated with degenerative arthritis of the lateral tarsometatarsal joint.

Schon LC, Acevedo JI, Mann MR: Sliding wedge local bone graft for midfoot arthrodesis. *Foot Ankle Int* 1999; 20:340-341.

The authors describe a technique for midfoot arthrodesis using local bone in which a sliding wedge of bone is used to fill gaps and avoid shortening. Additionally, the need for autograft from an alternate site is avoided.

Solan MC, Moorman CT III, Miyamoto RG, Jasper LE, Belkoff SM: Ligamentous restraints of the second tarsometatarsal joint: A biomechanical evaluation. *Foot Ankle Int* 2001;22:637-641.

Twenty pairs of matched cadaver feet were tested with combinations of the plantar, dorsal, and Lisfranc ligaments sectioned. The authors found the Lisfranc ligament to be stronger than the plantar ligament and the plantar ligament to be stronger than the dorsal ligament.

Teng AL, Pinzur MS, Lomasney L, Mahoney L, Havey R: Functional outcome following anatomic restoration of tarsal-metatarsal fracture dislocation. *Foot Ankle Int* 2002;23:922-926.

Eleven patients with excellent radiographic results following surgical treatment of unilateral closed Lisfranc fracture-dislocation of the tarsometatarsal joint of the foot were evaluated at an average of 41.2 months following injury and surgery. Despite excellent radiographic results and a return to normal dynamic walking patterns, subjective patient outcomes were less than satisfactory.

## Forefoot

Belt EA, Kaarela K, Lehto MU: Destruction and arthroplasties of the metatarsophalangeal joints in seropositive rheumatoid arthritis: A 20-year follow-up study. *Scand J Rheumatol* 1998;27:194-196.

One hundred three patients with seropositive rheumatoid arthritis who experienced destruction of the interphalangeal and MTP joints and underwent arthroplasty were prospectively evaluated. The authors concluded that because erosive changes occur early in the MTP joints and their grade of destruction is high, these factors should be included in radiographic criteria and scores.

Coughlin MJ: Rheumatoid forefoot reconstruction: A long-term follow-up study. *J Bone Joint Surg Am* 2000;82: 322-341.

Arthrodesis of the first MTP joint, resection arthroplasty of the lesser metatarsal heads, and repair of fixed hammer-toe deformities with intramedullary K-wire fixation resulted in a stable repair with a high percentage of successful results at a mean 6-year follow-up.

Davies MS, Saxby TS: Metatarsal neck osteotomy with rigid internal fixation for the treatment of lesser toe metatarsophalangeal joint pathology. *Foot Ankle Int* 1999;20: 630-635.

Forty-four feet in 39 patients with persistent pain from MTP joint instability and/or plantar callosity formation underwent oblique metatarsal neck osteotomy with screw fixation. Average shortening of the metatarsal was 4.1 mm. At follow-up, 33 patients were pain free, 6 had mild pain, and 2 had moderate pain.

Fuhrmann RA, Anders JO: The long-term results of resection arthroplasties of the first metatarsophalangeal joint in rheumatoid arthritis. *Int Orthop* 2001;25:312-316.

In this retrospective study of 188 patients (254 feet) with RA, the late results of the Keller procedure were compared with those of the Heuter-Mayo technique after 7.9 years. More than 60% of the Keller group and 30% of the Heuter-Mayo group reported persistent metatarsalgia (resulting from increased forefoot pressure) and pain around the great toe. Plantar callosities, recurrent hallux valgus deformity, lack of plantar flexion, and weakened push-off were more frequent after the Keller procedure.

Myerson MS, Schon LC, McGuigan FX, Oznur A: Result of arthrodesis of the hallux metatarsophalangeal joint using bone graft for restoration of length. *Foot Ankle Int* 2000;21:297-306.

Of 24 patients who underwent arthrodesis of the first MTP joint with bone graft to restore length, fusion occurred in 19 (average lengthening: 13 mm); 3 of 5 nonunions required a second surgical procedure, and AOFAS scores improved from 39 to 79 points.

Shi K, Hyashida K, Tomita T, Tanabe M, Ochi T: Surgical treatment of hallux valgus deformity in rheumatoid arthritis: Clinical and radiographic evaluation of modified Lapidus technique. *J Foot Ankle Surg* 2000;39:376-382.

A modified Lapidus technique was used to treat 21 rheumatoid hallux valgus deformities. Fifteen patients were satisfied or satisfied with some reservations. The authors concluded that this modified Lapidus technique is a useful method for treating rheumatoid hallux valgus deformity while preserving the first MTP joint.

Thordarson DB, Aval S, Krieger L: Failure of hallux MP preservation surgery for rheumatoid arthritis. *Foot Ankle Int* 2002;23:486-490.

Eight patients (15 feet) underwent surgery for rheumatoid forefoot problems. Although patients with rheumatoid forefoot disease may have a well-preserved hallux MTP joint with minimal or no deformity and no active inflammation, when severe lesser toe involvement is present, these authors conclude that most surgical procedures that do not involve fusion of the hallux MTP joint will not produce successful outcomes.

Trnka HJ: Arthrodesis procedures for salvage of the hallux metatarsophalangeal joint. *Foot Ankle Clin* 2000;5: 673-686.

Although first MTP joint fusion has been recommended as a means to salvage various great toe deformities, a variety of complications, such as hallux varus, first MTP joint instability, infection, recurrent hallux valgus, and osteonecrosis of the first metatarsal head can develop from procedures used to treat hallux valgus deformity.

Vandeputte G, Steenwerckx A, Mulier T, Peeraer L, Dereymaeker G: Forefoot reconstruction in rheumatoid arthritis patients: Keller-Lelievre-Hoffmann versus arthrodesis MTP1-Hoffmann. *Foot Ankle Int* 1999;20:438-443.

Thirty-eight patients with RA who underwent Keller-Lelievre arthroplasty were compared with 48 who underwent first MTP joint arthrodesis. Both groups underwent Hoffman resection of the lesser metatarsal heads. Ten arthrodeses were performed for failed arthroplasties. Satisfactory results were reported by 93% of the arthroplasty group and 87% of the arthrodesis group.

## Classic Bibliography

Bitzan P, Giurea A, Wanivenhaus A: Plantar pressure distribution after resection of the metatarsal heads in rheumatoid arthritis. *Foot Ankle Int* 1997;18:391-397.

Clayton ML: Surgery of the forefoot in rheumatoid arthritis. *Clin Orthop* 1960;16:136-151.

Coughlin MJ: Arthrodesis of the first metatarsophalangeal joint. *Orthop Rev* 1990;19:177-186.

Fu F, Scranton PE Jr: Forefoot arthroplasty in rheumatoid arthritis: Clinical appraisal and force plate analysis. *Orthopedics* 1982;5:163-168.

Guerra J, Resnick D: Arthritides affecting the foot: Radiographic-pathological correlation. *Foot Ankle* 1982; 2:325-331.

Hanyu T, Yamazaki H, Murasawa A, Tohyama C: Arthroplasty for rheumatoid forefoot deformities by a shortening oblique osteotomy. *Clin Orthop* 1997;338:131-138.

Kates A, Kessel L, Kay A: Arthroplasty of the forefoot. *J Bone Joint Surg Br* 1967;49:552-557.

Komenda GA, Myerson MS, Biddinger KR: Results of arthrodesis of the tarsometatarsal joints after traumatic injury. *J Bone Joint Surg Am* 1996;78:1665-1676.

Mann RA, Prieskorn D, Sobel M: Mid-tarsal and tarsometatarsal arthrodesis for primary degenerative osteoarthrosis or osteoarthrosis after trauma. *J Bone Joint Surg Am* 1996;78:1376-1385.

Mann RA, Thompson FM: Arthrodesis of the first metatarsophalangeal joint for hallux valgus in rheumatoid arthritis. *J Bone Joint Surg Am* 1984;66:687-692.

Michelson J, Easley M, Wigley FM, Hellmann D: Foot and ankle problems in rheumatoid arthritis. *Foot Ankle Int* 1994;15:608-613.

Ouzounian TJ, Shereff MJ: In vitro determination of midfoot motion. *Foot Ankle Int* 1989;10:140-146.

# Section 6

# General Foot and Ankle Topics

Section Editor:
Kathleen A. McHale, MD, FACS

# Chapter 17

# Imaging of the Foot and Ankle

Susan N. Ishikawa, MD

## Introduction

After history taking and physical examination, radiographic imaging is usually the next step in the diagnosis of diseases of the foot and ankle. Plain radiographs are usually the first choice in the diagnostic algorithm. More advanced imaging techniques are available, including tenography, ultrasound, scintigraphy, CT, and MRI.

## Plain Radiographs

Routine views of the foot include weight-bearing AP, oblique, and lateral views. The routine ankle views are the AP, mortise, and lateral views. To be more cost-effective, it has been suggested that only the AP and lateral views be taken. A recent study has shown, however, that the oblique view clarified or changed the diagnosis in 4.3% of ankle examinations and 5.8% of foot examinations after acute trauma. In addition to the standard views, special views may be necessary because a fracture fragment may be missed or its size underestimated with standard views alone. A 50° external rotation view of the ankle has been recommended to more clearly outline posterior malleolar fractures (Fig. 1). The oblique anteromedial impingement view may show an anteromedial tibial osteophyte that would not be seen on a standard lateral view (which primarily shows anterolateral osteophytes). The oblique anteromedial impingement view is obtained with the leg in 30° of external rotation and the x-ray beam tilted 45° in a craniocaudal direction (Fig. 2).

Varus stress views have long been used to evaluate the stability of the lateral collateral complex of the ankle; however, their utility is somewhat controversial. Valgus stress views may be used to evaluate suspected deltoid injuries and can be considered positive if there is an absolute value of more than 2° of tilt or more than 2° of difference from the contralateral uninjured side. Stress views can also be helpful in diagnosing Lisfranc injuries. With abduction stress, the medial column line, which is a line drawn from the medial aspect of the navicular to the medial aspect of the medial cuneiform, should intersect the base of the first metatarsal in a normal foot but will lie medial to the first metatarsal in a foot with a Lisfranc

injury (Fig. 3). Care must be taken when obtaining stress views, however, because internal rotation can create a false-positive result.

Radiographs are often taken intraoperatively to evaluate bony alignment and ensure proper hardware placement. When placing a screw across the talar neck from posterior to anterior for talar neck fractures, the convexity of the talar head may make it difficult to determine whether a screw is intra-articular. A cadaveric study has shown that in addition to AP and lateral views, lateral oblique and medial oblique views may be necessary to assess screw penetration in the inferior quadrants of the talar head. For assessment of fixation of a medial malleolar fracture, the AP view has been shown to be best for evaluating intra-articular penetration of the hardware. The mortise view may falsely imply that screws are in the joint. For tibial plafond fractures, the lateral radiograph may be compromised by an external fixator. The AP view cannot always be relied on to confirm adequate reduction because the AP view shows primarily the anterior plafond and a malreduction of the posterior plafond will not be seen.

### Radiographic Measurements

Various radiographic measurements have been described to evaluate injuries of the foot and ankle. For ankle injuries, the bimalleolar angle, talocrural angle, tibiofibular overlap, medial clear space, and displacement of the lateral malleolus, medial malleolus, and posterior malleolus have been found to be reliable measurements. The tibiofibular clear space, however, cannot be measured reliably. Although measurements of the tibiofibular overlap and the medial clear space have been found to be affected by rotation of the ankle, the tibiofibular clear space is not. In most injuries to the ankle that are severe enough to require fixation, widening of the ankle mortise is obvious. However, if routine AP and mortise views are not conclusive, stress radiographs, particularly when the medial injury is to the deltoid ligament and not the medial malleolus, remain the only method to definitively diagnose ankle mortise instability.

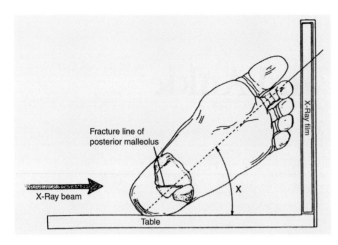

**Figure 1** Illustration of the position of the foot and ankle, the location of the x-ray film, and the direction of the x-ray beam while obtaining a 50° external rotation lateral view of the ankle. *(Reproduced with permission from Ebraheim NA, Mekhail AO, Haman SP: External rotation: Lateral view of the ankle in the assessment of the posterior malleolus. Foot Ankle Int 1999;20:379-383.)*

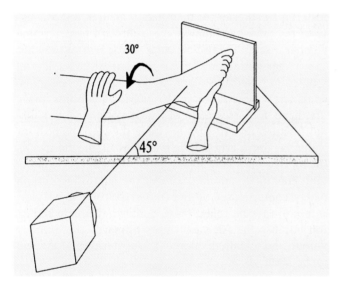

**Figure 2** Illustration of the position of the foot and ankle relative to the x-ray beam while obtaining an oblique anteromedial impingement view. Starting from a standard lateral view, the x-ray beam is tilted to a 45° craniocaudal position with the foot in 30° of external rotation. The patient is asked to place the foot in the maximal plantar flexed position. *(Reproduced with permission from van Dijk CN, Wessel RN, Tol JL, Maas M: Oblique radiograph for the detection of bone spurs in anterior ankle impingement. Skeletal Radiol 2002;31:214-221.)*

The accuracy of radiographic measurements in hallux valgus is controversial. The hallux valgus angle (HVA) and the first-second intermetatarsal angle ($IMA_{1-2}$) can be measured with a high intraobserver and interobserver reliability. However, measurement of the distal metatarsal articular angle and determination of congruency are less reliable. Because the anatomy becomes altered after surgery for hallux valgus correction, it is difficult to choose landmarks on which to base measurements. Depending on the method used to choose landmarks, the postoperative HVA and $IMA_{1-2}$ can have a range of al-

most 12°, which makes it difficult to evaluate postoperative correction and to compare studies. Because of these difficulties, an ad hoc committee of the American Orthopaedic Foot and Ankle Society has made several recommendations regarding the measurement of angles in hallux valgus. The first metatarsal axis should be drawn by choosing two points in the center of the shaft 1 to 2 cm from the distal and proximal articular surfaces. The second metatarsal axis should be drawn in the same manner. The axis of the proximal phalanx should be drawn by determining the two points that bisect the shaft 0.5 to 1 cm from the articular surfaces and connecting them. Postoperatively, the first metatarsal axis should be determined by dual measurements as measured preoperatively and also from a point 1 to 2 cm distal to the proximal articular surface and a point that is the center of the metatarsal head, which is determined by the use of Mose spheres. Another study recommended that sesamoid subluxation should be determined from the tangential sesamoid view and not from the AP view of the foot because first metatarsal rotation may make the sesamoids appear to be subluxated on the weight-bearing AP view when they remain anatomically in their respective facets.

## Tenography

Plain radiographs have a limited ability to evaluate soft tissues such as tendons. Tenography is a cost-effective way to examine the tendons; however, it is an invasive procedure. Abnormal findings include sacculations of the tendon sheath (indicative of tenosynovits), blockage of the dye (indicative of stenosing tenosynovitis), or rupture of the tendons. When coupled with steroid injections that are administered in the absence of partial or complete tendon tears, the procedure can provide relief of symptoms in 46% of patients with posterior tibial tendinitis or peroneal tendinitis. Reported complications include posterior tibial tendon (PTT) rupture in 0.89%, skin discoloration in 13%, and paresthesia at the injection site in 0.9%.

## Ultrasound

Ultrasound is another cost-effective method of evaluating soft tissues. It is more advantageous than other diagnostic imaging modalities because it provides dynamic studies, is not limited to predetermined scanning planes, involves no ionizing radiation, and localizes intratendinous pathology. The disadvantages of ultrasound include operator-dependence to reduce artifacts, the inability to visualize bone, the inability to be used when the patient is in a cast, and the inability to demonstrate landmarks that can help surgeons localize pathology intraoperatively. Newer, higher frequency transducers provide better resolution but are limited in their depth of penetration to 5 cm. Nevertheless, higher frequency transducers are better at showing structures in the foot and ankle, which are

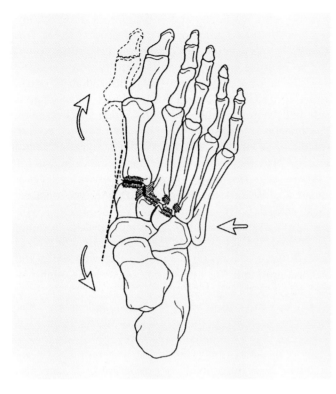

**Figure 3** Illustration showing that abduction stress displaces the forefoot lateral to the medial column line when the dorsal and Lisfranc ligaments are disrupted. *(Reproduced with permission from Coss HS, Manos RE, Buoncristiani A, Mills WJ: Abduction stress and AP weightbearing radiography of purely ligamentous injury to the tarsometatarsal joint.* Foot Ankle Int *1998;19:537-541.)*

relatively subcutaneous.

Normal tendons viewed on ultrasound have fine, parallel, echoic lines, indicative of the linearly arranged collagen when studied in the longitudinal axis. In the transverse axis, the normal tendon has echoic dots in an oval or round configuration. Ultrasound has been found to provide an accurate diagnosis of tendon degeneration by demonstrating a hypoechoic line from the periphery into the tendon substance, thickening of the tendon with a hypoechoic area within the tendon, a hypoechoic signal around the tendon (>1 cm in length), and a lack of gliding of the tendon within the sheath. Ultrasound can also provide an accurate diagnosis of peritendinitis by identifying a target sign, with a hyperechoic area centrally and a hypoechoic halo. Complete rupture is indicated on ultrasound by the presence of an empty groove. In one study, ultrasound was found to be more sensitive and accurate than MRI in evaluating tendon pathology because chronic fibrotic changes of the tendon may not be detectable on MRI, whereas ultrasound will demonstrate these changes as disruption of the fibrillar arrangement of collagen within the tendon.

Ultrasound can also be used to detect lateral ligament tears of the ankle with a sensitivity and specificity comparable to that of MRI and to evaluate masses and abscesses, which can then be aspirated or biopsied using ultrasound imaging. Additionally, ultrasound may be

helpful in determining the recurrence of an interdigital neuroma when physical examination is equivocal. Moreover, it has been shown to be useful in evaluating subtalar instability, which is difficult to evaluate otherwise. For this purpose, the fibulotrochlear angle has been described. When the ratio of this angle in the neutral position to the angle under stress is greater than 1.6, subtalar instability is indicated. Ultrasound may also be helpful in detecting the presence of wooden foreign bodies that cannot be seen on plain radiographs.

## Nuclear Medicine

Scintigraphy visualizes physiologic and biochemical processes and can provide functional information, such as degree of bone turnover. For nuclear medicine studies, a radioactive tracer is administered to the patient by injection and a gamma camera acquires the images at time intervals determined by the type of tracer used.

In conventional bone scanning, technetium 99m methylene diphosphonate ($^{99m}$Tc MDP) is used because it binds to hydroxyapatite crystals during bone formation. Because bone formation is usually associated with bone destruction, it is an indirect marker of bone destruction. There are three and sometimes four phases of image acquisition in conventional bone scanning. The first phase is the blood flow phase in which images are obtained immediately (up to 1 minute) after the administration of the tracer. The second phase is the blood pool phase in which images are obtained approximately 5 minutes after the administration of the tracer; the third and fourth phases are bone turnover phases and images are obtained at approximately 4 hours and 24 hours after tracer administration, respectively. The utility of bone scanning in the detection of malignant lesions, occult fractures, and various other conditions involving bone turnover has long been documented.

Leukocytes may be obtained by drawing blood from the patient, labeling the white blood cells with radioactive tracer, and then reinjecting the labeled cells into the patient to accumulate in areas of infection. The white blood cells may be labeled with Tc 99m hexamethylpropyleneamineoxime ($^{99m}$Tc HMPAO) or indium$^{111}$ oxime. $^{99m}$Tc HMPAO is advantageous in that imaging occurs approximately 4 hours after its administration versus 24 hours for indium$^{111}$, and it requires a smaller radiation dose. Antibodies or antibody fragments may also be labeled with radioactive tracer and reinjected into the patient for later imaging.

$^{99m}$Tc sulfur colloid is used for marrow scanning because it is taken up by the reticuloendothelial system. Imaging usually is done in three phases: (1) the vascular phase is obtained within the first 3 minutes, (2) the blood pool phase is obtained within 5 to 10 minutes, and (3) the static delayed image is obtained within 30 to 60 minutes after injection of the tracer. A study that is positive for osteomyelitis shows more uptake in the static delayed image than the blood pool image. Marrow scanning can be done in conjunction with a leukocyte-labeled study and is positive for osteomyelitis when there is incongruence; that is, when the leukocyte-labeled study is positive in one area and the marrow scan is negative in that same area.

Most of the recent studies involving scintigraphy of the foot and ankle focus on the diagnosis of osteomyelitis in the diabetic foot, especially in the presence of Charcot arthropathy, which can confuse the clinical picture. Triple-phase bone scanning alone is not helpful in this instance because it shows increased uptake in both infection and Charcot arthropathy. Four-phase bone scanning may improve the specificity of the study. A leukocyte-labeled study used in conjunction with bone scanning can improve the accuracy of the study and has been shown to be better than MRI in the midfoot and hindfoot, where Charcot changes usually occur. In the forefoot, however, MRI may be a better study for identifying infection because Charcot changes rarely occur in this area. Antibody-labeled scans are not as helpful because they do not differentiate between soft-tissue infections and osteomyelitis. Bone marrow scanning has also been shown to be useful in detecting infection, either alone or in conjunction with leukocyte-labeled studies, and it may have better sensitivity and specificity than MRI or combination bone scanning/leukocyte-labeled scanning.

Nuclear medicine imaging may also be useful for the detection of arterial perfusion in the lower extremities of diabetic patients who often have calcified vessels, which can falsely elevate indices of perfusion, such as the ankle-brachial index. Lower extremity scanning with thallium 201, which is used in myocardial studies, has been shown to detect perfusion abnormalities in asymptomatic diabetic patients with a normal Doppler ankle-brachial index. Breaking the first blood flow phase of a $^{99m}$Tc bone scan into arterial (20 to 40 seconds after injection) and capillary (20 to 120 seconds after injection) phases may give information about the appropriate level of amputation to allow healing. Poor blood flow in the capillary phase can indicate areas where necrosis will occur if amputation is done there.

Scintigraphy has also been used in the evaluation of frostbite injuries. In severe cases of frostbite, bone scanning done approximately 2 days after injury and rewarming can determine the level of amputation if there is no uptake in the distal portion of the digit. Bone scanning of areas of low uptake approximately 8 days after injury can help determine whether amputation is necessary. In less severe frostbite injuries, areas of no uptake may not necessarily lead to gangrene and the need for amputation; rather, the digit may become fibrotic.

## Computed Tomography

CT is especially useful in evaluating fractures involving a joint or areas with complex anatomy, such as the tibial

plafond, talus, calcaneus, and tarsometatarsal joints. Care must be taken to obtain images in the proper planes. This involves proper patient positioning and the use of scout views. CT uses ionizing radiation, a gantry with a rotating x-ray tube, a moving patient table, and radiation detectors. During CT, a cross-sectional radiographic image is obtained; then the table moves to obtain the next slice. The images are subsequently processed by a computer. Axial and coronal images are obtained, and sagittal images are provided by reconstructions. Spiral or helical CT scanning requires less study time and provides quicker image acquisition and improved three-dimensional reconstructions; however, it may increase the artifact resulting from metallic implants. Cast immobilization does not interfere with CT, but it may make positioning of the patient difficult. CT requires that the patient remain still because motion artifact may interfere with the quality of the images.

CT can provide more detail than plain radiographs. For example, it can demonstrate diastasis of the syndesmosis that may be undetectable radiographically, and with Lisfranc injuries, subluxation may be seen on CT before it can be measured on plain radiographs. CT can also show fractures in a Lisfranc injury that cannot be seen radiographically and for this type of injury generally provides as much information as MRI regarding bony injury. For subtalar dislocations, CT can demonstrate additional injury not seen radiographically that may affect treatment. In a study comparing radiographic and CT stress examinations of the subtalar joint using the same method of providing stress, increased tilt seen radiographically could not be demonstrated by CT. This suggests that the tilt seen on plain radiographs may not be truly indicative of subtalar instability but may be the result of looking at three-dimensional motion in a two-dimensional plane.

## Magnetic Resonance Imaging

After plain radiography, MRI is the most commonly used diagnostic imaging modality. MRI provides images by aligning proton nuclei in a magnetic field; radiofrequency is then applied to displace the nuclei, which subsequently regress to their original positions. The relaxation time is measured, and different types of tissues have different relaxation times. MRI can be used to evaluate pathology in tendons and ligaments, osteochondral and chondral injuries, soft-tissue masses, osteonecrosis, infection, arthritis, chronic regional pain syndrome, tarsal coalition, stress fractures, physeal plate injuries, and tarsal tunnel syndrome. Its advantages include better visualization of the internal architecture of structures such as tendons, ligaments, and bone marrow (osteonecrosis, bone bruises, osteochondral defects) and the absence of ionizing radiation. Different MRI sequences can be used to provide more information than other diagnostic imaging modalities. The disadvantages of MRI include (1) patients may become claustrophobic during imaging, (2) patients must remain in one position to minimize motion artifact, and (3) MRI does not provide good bony detail. In addition, MRI cannot be used in patients with pacemakers, intracerebral aneurysm clips, automatic defibrillators, biostimulators, implanted infusion devices, internal hearing aids, metallic orbital foreign bodies, or metal external fixation devices. Patients with prosthetic heart valves and metallic implants can undergo MRI scanning, although ferrous metals can create local artifacts. False-positive results can be created by the magic angle effect in which an intratendinous artifact is seen when a tendon curves at a 55° angle. Magnetic resonance arthrography can increase the sensitivity of detecting ankle ligament injury, anterolateral ankle soft-tissue impingement, and the extent of cartilaginous injury in osteochondral lesions of the talus.

Smaller coils provide better resolution of foot and ankle structures. Ligament injuries are demonstrated by partial or complete disruption, high-signal intensity within the ligament, thickening, or a change in contour of the ligament. The anterior talofibular ligament (ATFL) is usually best seen on axial images at the level where the lateral malleolus is crescentic. The optimal position for imaging of this ligament is 20° of plantar flexion. The calcaneofibular ligament (CFL) is best seen in the oblique-coronal plane with the foot in 20° of plantar flexion and 20° of inversion. The posterior talofibular ligament, which is rarely injured, has a more striated appearance, and, like the ATFL, is best seen on axial images at the level where the lateral malleolus is crescentic. The syndesmotic ligaments are best seen on the axial images at or just above the level of the talar dome. The deep deltoid ligament has a striated appearance and is depicted on the coronal images. The superficial deltoid is more band-like and is seen on multiple coronal or axial images. The talocalcaneal interosseous ligament can be seen on coronal images. The peroneal tendons are best seen on axial and sagittal T2-weighted sequences or oblique axial images. If the foot is dorsiflexed, there may appear to be an anomalous muscle or low-lying belly of the peroneus brevis. The brevis tendon is subject to the magic angle effect, which can be minimized by placement of the foot in plantar flexion; the optimal angle is 20° of plantar flexion and 20° of inversion. The PTT can also be seen best on axial and sagittal T2-weighted images. It is twice the size of the flexor digitorum longus, is oval on cross-section, and can have an intermediate signal at its insertion. Injury usually occurs behind the medial malleolus. The Achilles tendon is also seen on axial and sagittal T2-weighted images. It is shaped like a kidney bean, with an anterior concavity.

## Normal Variants

Many normal variants may mimic pathology on MRI. A heterogeneous signal at the insertion of the PTT can be normal. Fat present between the planes of the Achilles tendon can appear to be intratendinous degeneration; if

the tendon is normal in shape and size, this is a false-positive finding. The soleus tendon may join the distal Achilles, appearing as a thickening or a partial tear. The flexor hallucis longus tendon can often have fluid in the sheath because this sheath often communicates with the ankle joint. Increased fluid also may be present around this tendon at Henry's knot. Medial subluxation of the peroneus brevis may be normal. Accessory muscles that can be seen on MRI include the accessory soleus, accessory flexor digitorum longus, tibiocalcaneus internus, peroneocalcaneus internus, and peroneus quartus. The os sustentaculi, which may not be visible on plain radiographs, may be seen on MRI medial to the sustentaculum. A pseudocoalition of the middle facet may be seen on coronal images; this will appear normal on sagittal images. A pseudocoalition of the calcaneonavicular area may appear on sagittal images but not on axial and coronal images. A pseudo-osteochondral lesion of the posterior tibial plafond may be seen on coronal images but will not be seen on other sequences. Heterogeneous signal of the posterior talofibular ligament, the posterior talotibial band of the deltoid, or the anterior tibiofibular ligament may be normal if there is no change in the morphology of the ligament. A prearticular fat pad medial to the talar neck can mimic an avulsion fracture. Some findings seen on MRIs of physically active asymptomatic individuals include low-grade changes in the Achilles tendon, fluid in the retrocalcaneal bursa, tendon sheath fluid, and joint effusions.

## Imaging of Pathology

Achilles tendinopathy is seen on MRI as thickening of the tendon with intratendinous signal changes. Complete rupture is seen as a discontinuity of the tendon, and the proximity of the torn ends can be determined. MRI with gadolinium contrast has been shown to demonstrate a larger area of abnormality than ultrasound, with the ultrasound appearing normal in areas that were proved by biopsy to be pathologic. In addition, MRI allows evaluation of the retrocalcaneal bursa (Fig. 4). This structure is pathologic if it is larger than 1 mm in the AP dimension, 11 mm on the transverse cut, and 7 mm from inferior to superior. MRI after surgical or nonsurgical treatment of an Achilles tendon rupture cannot be relied upon to correlate with the clinical outcome. Thickening or heterogeneity of the tendon seen 1 year after the injury is not predictive of muscle strength, endurance, or range of motion.

MRI accurately demonstrates PTT degeneration, which usually occurs behind the medial malleolus (Fig. 5). Tendon thickening with normal signal may indicate tendinosis or an old tear. Thickened tendons with increased signal in a portion of the tendon signify an acute partial tear. Complete tears have high signal intensity fluid between the torn tendon ends. Some secondary signs of PTT dysfunction include fluid within the sheath, tibial

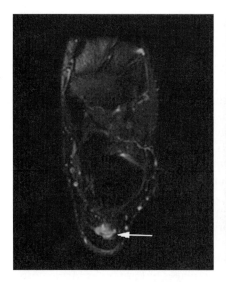

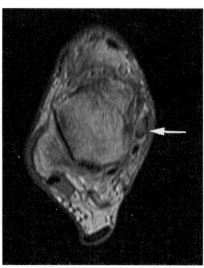

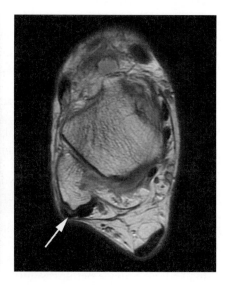

**Figure 4** MRI showing enlarged retrocalcaneus bursa anterior to the Achilles tendon (arrow).

**Figure 5** MRI showing posterior tibial tendon degeneration (arrow).

**Figure 6** MRI showing chevron-shaped peroneus brevis tendon indicating a tear (arrow).

spurring, and medial uncovering of the talar head. The spring ligament is often involved in PTT dysfunction but can be difficult to visualize on MRI. The medial portion of the ligament can be seen on axial images and is abnormal if it is thickened or if there is increased signal heterogeneity. The plantar portion of the ligament, which is more difficult to image, may be seen on sagittal oblique images.

MRI is less accurate in the depiction of pathology of the peroneus longus tendon because it can show more severe pathology than what is actually seen during surgery. In several studies, tears of the peroneus longus most often occurred at the cuboid notch, followed by the lateral calcaneal process. Additionally, peroneus brevis pathology was associated with tears of the longus in one third of patients and were more commonly found at or near the superior peroneal retinaculum. MRI findings associated with a longitudinal tear of the peroneus brevis include a chevron-shaped tendon (Fig. 6), bony changes, a flat peroneal groove, abnormal lateral ligaments, and a lateral fibular spur. Subluxation of the peroneal tendons may be difficult to diagnose by routine MRI if the tendons are not in the subluxated position. Dynamic MRI may more easily confirm the diagnosis because the ability to move the foot and ankle during the study may make the tendons move out of the retromalleolar groove and into the subluxated position.

MRI can be helpful in the evaluation of flexor hallucis longus tendinopathy, but only if clinical information is available for the interpretation of the study. Findings may include intratendinous degeneration, longitudinal tears, hypertrophied muscle distally, and pseudocyst of the tendon.

MRI has been shown to be accurate in demonstrating tears of the ATFL after an acute sprain (as confirmed surgically) but can underestimate injury to the CFL. MRI findings after an acute ankle sprain, such as ATFL or CFL injury, tendon sheath fluid, effusion, soft-tissue swelling, or bone bruises, have not been consistently predictive of clinical outcome. Most lateral ligament tears have been shown to be healed on follow-up MRI. MRI used in the evaluation of lateral ligament injuries has the added benefit of demonstrating additional pathology that may contribute to the patients' symptomatology, such as osteochondral lesions of the talus or peroneal tendon pathology.

Close to one half of patients will have an abnormal signal in the sinus tarsi after an ankle sprain. Injury to the interosseous talocalcaneal, cervical, or deltoid ligaments has been shown to correlate with giving way on clinical follow-up. Other abnormalities seen in the sinus tarsi can include signal changes consistent with fibrosis, synovitis or inflammatory changes, or synovial cysts (Fig. 7).

Of the several components of the deltoid ligament, the most easily imaged are the posterior tibiotalar and tibiocalcaneal ligaments. The former demonstrates a heterogeneous signal, and the latter demonstrates lower signal intensity. Injury can be seen as signal changes or discontinuity of the ligaments.

While CT may show the associated fractures better, MRI can delineate ruptures of the two different components of the Lisfranc ligament (the plantar and dorsal bands) or chondral injuries of the tarsometatarsal joints. This is helpful when radiographic findings are equivocal and more information about the degree of injury to the Lisfranc ligament is needed to determine treatment.

MRI is known to be accurate in the depiction of osteochondral lesions of the talus. These lesions appear as well-demarcated areas of low-signal intensity on axial and coronal images. Signs of instability of the fragment in-

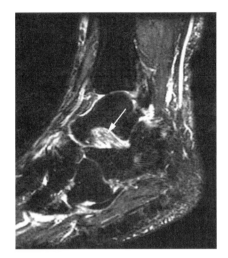

Figure 7  MRI showing signal change in the sinus tarsi (arrow).

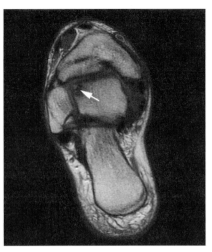

Figure 8  MRI showing osteochondral lesion of the talus (white arrow).

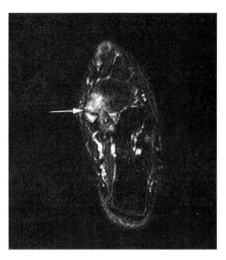

Figure 9  MRI showing accessory navicular with bony changes (arrow).

clude a thin line of high-signal intensity between the lesion and bone; a discrete, round, homogeneous area of high-signal intensity beneath the fragment; a focal defect in the articular surface of the lesion; and a high-signal intensity line through the articular cartilage and subchondral bone into the lesion (Fig. 8). MRI can also be useful in monitoring the degree of healing after surgical intervention. Signs of healing include reduction in the area of low-signal intensity on T1-weighted images and the disappearance of high-signal rims on T2-weighted images.

MRI changes in patients with osteonecrosis can be correlated with the stage of involvement. In stage 0, diffuse, decreased signal intensity is visible on both T1- and T2-weighted images. Stage I involves a necrotic zone of normal intensity, with a surrounding area of increased signal on T1-weighted images and decreased signal on T2-weighted images. In stages III and IV, the necrotic zone has normal to mixed intensity, new bone has decreased signal intensity on both T1- and T2-weighted images, and hyperemic areas have a decreased signal on T1-weighted images and increased signal on T2-weighted images. Stage V has the same features as stage II but with subchondral fracture. The double-line sign is a rim of low signal around the lesion on T1-weighted images of which the inner aspect increases on T2-weighted images. This may indicate healing potential and is more commonly seen when the osteonecrosis is secondary to a systemic disease as opposed to a posttraumatic cause. MRI provides the earliest detection of avascular changes.

Although fractures can be evaluated by MRI, CT provides better bony detail. MRI may not show the fracture line, but it will detect marrow edema associated with the fracture on both T1- and T2-weighted images. MRI can be helpful in the detection of occult fractures (most commonly seen in the navicular, talus, and calcaneus) because of marrow changes. Bone bruises that represent trabecu-

lar disruption without cortical break can be seen on short tau inversion recovery and T2-weighted images, but they may be difficult to visualize on T1-weighted images. MRI can also provide information on accessory bones such as the os trigonum or accessory navicular. Injury can be seen as signal changes in the bone and synchondroses (Fig. 9).

## Summary

Plain radiography remains the most useful imaging technique for examination of the foot and ankle, especially bony anatomy. Soft tissues are better evaluated with tenography or ultrasound. More advanced modalities, such as bone scanning, CT, and MRI, can provide additional information. Combinations of imaging techniques can provide a complete picture of foot and ankle disorders to allow selection of appropriate treatment.

## Annotated Bibliography

### Plain Radiographs

Brage ME, Bennett CR, Whitehurst JB, Getty PJ, Toledano A: Observer reliability in ankle radiographic measurements. *Foot Ankle Int* 1997;18:324-329.

In evaluating the radiographs of 50 normal ankles and 50 ankles with fractures, these researchers identified the parameters that could be reliably measured, including the tibiofibular overlap, medial clear space, bimalleolar angle, talocrural angle, and displacement of the medial malleolar fragment, lateral malleolar fragment, and posterior malleolar fragment.

Coss HS, Manos RE, Buoncristiani A, Mills WJ: Abduction stress and AP weightbearing radiography of purely ligamentous injury in the tarsometatarsal joint. *Foot Ankle Int* 1998;19:537-541.

Abduction stress radiography was performed on volunteer controls (40 feet) and cadavers (9 feet) that had undergone sectioning of tarsometatarsal ligaments. A medial column line was described, which, if a Lisfranc injury is present, will lie medial to the base of the first metatarsal.

Coughlin MJ, Saltzman CL, Nunley JA II: Angular measurements in the evaluation of hallux valgus deformities: A report of the ad hoc committee of the American Orthopaedic Foot & Ankle Society on angular measurements. *Foot Ankle Int* 2002;23:68-74.

Standard reference points and techniques for radiographic measurements of hallux valgus deformities are described.

Ebraheim NA, Mekhail AO, Haman SP: External rotation-lateral view of the ankle in the assessment of the posterior malleolus. *Foot Ankle Int* 1999;20:379-383.

This cadaveric study describes a radiographic view that visualizes a fracture of the posterior mallleolus that cannot be seen on standard radiographs.

Ebraheim N, Sabry FF, Mehalik JN: Intraoperative imaging of the tibial plafond fracture: A potential pitfall. *Foot Ankle Int* 2000;21:67-72.

Using a cadaveric tibial plafond fracture model, these authors found that although the AP view of the ankle shows the anterior part of the joint, a malreduction in the posterior part of the joint may be missed if a lateral view is not also taken or is obscured by an external fixator.

Gourineni PV, Knuth AE, Nuber GF: Radiographic evaluation of the position of implants in the medial malleolus in relation to the ankle joint space: Anteroposterior compared with mortise radiographs. *J Bone Joint Surg Am* 1999;81:364-369.

In this cadaveric study, the AP view of the ankle was better than the mortise view to evaluate for intra-articular penetration of hardware when placing screws for a fracture of the medial malleolus.

Schneider W, Knahr K: Metatarsophalangeal and intermetatarsal angle: Different values and interpretation of postoperative results dependent on the technique of measurement. *Foot Ankle Int* 1998;19:532-536.

Five different methods of measurements were used to measure HVA and $IMA_{1-2}$ both preoperatively and postoperatively. The biggest differences were seen in the postoperative measurements, with mean HVA ranging from 8.6° to 20.3° and mean $IMA_{1-2}$ ranging from 5.2° to 16.7°.

van Dijk CN, Wessel RN, Tol JL, Maas M: Oblique radiograph for the detection of bone spurs in anterior ankle impingement. *Skeletal Radiol* 2002;31:214-221.

A cadaveric study was performed and followed by confirmation in 25 patients to describe a radiographic view to visualize anteromedial distal tibial osteophytes. Anterolateral osteophytes are visualized using the standard lateral radiograph.

## Tenography

Jaffee NW, Gilula LA, Wissman RD, Johnson JE: Diagnostic and therapeutic ankle tenography: Outcomes and complications. *AJR Am J Roentgenol* 2001;176:365-371.

Results and complications in 111 patients who underwent tenography are reported.

## Ultrasound

Hsu TC, Wang CL, Wang TG, Chiang IP, Hsieh FJ: Ultrasonographic examination of the posterior tibial tendon. *Foot Ankle Int* 1997;18:34-38.

Sixteen patients with posterior tibial tendon dysfunction and 10 control patients underwent ultrasound examination. Findings consistent with tendon degeneration, peritendinitis, and tendon rupture are described.

Rockett MS, Waitches G, Sudakoff G, Brage M: Use of ultrasonography versus magnetic resonance imaging for tendon abnormalities around the ankle. *Foot Ankle Int* 1998;19:604-612.

Findings on ultrasound and MRI of tendons in 28 patients were compared with surgical findings. Ultrasound had a sensitivity, specificity, and accuracy of 100%, 89.9%, and 94.4%, respectively, versus 23.4%, 100%, and 65.8%, respectively, on MRI for the detection of intrasubstance or complete tears of tendons around the ankle.

Waldecker U, Blatter G: Sonographic measurement of instability of the subtalar joint. *Foot Ankle Int* 2001;22:42-46.

Measurement of subtalar instability with ultrasound was first shown to be feasible in a cadaveric model. This was then confirmed in 15 patients. A high correlation between radiographic subtalar instability and that seen with ultrasound was identified.

## Nuclear Medicine

Cauchy E, Chetaille E, Lefevre M, Kerelou E, Marsigny B: The role of bone scanning in severe frostbite of the extremities: A retrospective study of 88 cases. *Eur J Nucl Med* 2000;27:497-502.

This study reports that bone scans performed approximately 2 days after a severe frostbite injury and rewarming show no uptake can indicate the appropriate level of amputation. Areas of low uptake can be evaluated approximately 8 days after the injury to determine whether amputation is necessary.

Jay PR, Michelson JD, Mizel MS, Magid D, Le T: Efficacy of three-phase bone scans in evaluating diabetic foot ulcers. *Foot Ankle Int* 1999;20:347-355.

The authors found that the amputation rates for diabetic foot ulcers did not correlate with a confirmatory, indeterminate, or nonconfirmatory bone scan for osteomyelitis.

Lipman BT, Collier BD, Carrera GF, et al: Detection of osteomyelitis in the neuropathic foot: Nuclear medicine,

MRI and conventional radiography. *Clin Nucl Med* 1998; 23:77-82.

The authors found that combined three-phase bone scintigraphy and indium-111 labeled white blood cell scintigraphy was more specific for detecting osteomyelitis in the setting of Charcot arthropathy than conventional radiography or MRI; however, MRI was better in depicting the presence of osteomyelitis in the forefoot, where Charcot changes are rare.

### Computed Tomography

Bibbo C, Lin SS, Abidi N, et al: Missed and associated injuries after subtalar dislocation: The role of CT. *Foot Ankle Int* 2001;22:324-328.

In 9 patients with a subtalar dislocation, CT scans demonstrated injuries not seen on plain radiographs in 100% of patients; these injuries changed the management in 44% of these patients.

Preidler KW, Peicha G, Lajtai G, et al: Conventional radiography, CT, and MR imaging in patients with hyperflexion injuries of the foot: Diagnostic accuracy in the detection of bony and ligamentous changes. *AJR Am J Roentgenol* 1999;173:1673-1677.

In 49 patients with hyperflexion injuries of the foot, CT demonstrated more fractures and malalignment than plain radiography. MRI did not provide any additional information regarding fractures and malalignment.

van Hellemondt FJ, Louwerens JW, Sijbrandij ES, van Gils AP: Stress radiography and stress examination of the talocrural and subtalar joint on helical computed tomography. *Foot Ankle Int* 1997;18:482-488.

Positive stress radiographs of the subtalar joint that show lateral opening could not be confirmed with CT. This suggests that imaging three-dimensional motion in a two-dimensional plane may not provide a true indicator of instability.

### Magnetic Resonance Imaging

Higashiyama I, Kumai T, Takakura Y, Tamail S: Follow-up study of MRI for osteochondral lesion of the talus. *Foot Ankle Int* 2000;21:127-133.

These authors examined 21 patients with osteochondral lesions of the talus who had MRI performed both preoperatively and postoperatively. Findings on MRI that suggest healing of the lesion are outlined.

Rosenberg ZS, Bencardino J, Mellado JM: Normal variants and pitfalls in magnetic resonance imaging of the ankle and foot. *Top Magn Reson Imaging* 1998;9:262-272.

This article provides an excellent review of normal entities that may be read as falsely positive for pathology.

Schweitzer ME, Eid ME, Deely D, Wapner K, Hecht P: Using MR imaging to differentiate peroneal splits from other peroneal disorders. *AJR Am J Roentgenol* 1997;168: 129-133.

Findings on MRI that correlated with surgically confirmed tears of the peroneal tendons included a bisected tendon, convex or flat fibular groove, and a posterolateral fibular spur; however, fluid in the sheath, increased intratendinous signal, and tendon subluxation did not correlate with tendon tears.

Schweitzer ME, Haims AH, Morrison WB: MR imaging of ankle marrow. *Foot Ankle Clin* 2000;5:63-82.

MRI findings of ankle marrow disorders, including fractures, osteonecrosis, arthritis, and infection, are reviewed.

Timins ME: MR imaging of the foot and ankle. *Foot Ankle Clin* 2000;5:83-101.

In this review article, the use of MRI to identify disorders of the tendons, ligaments, soft tissues, and bones of the foot and ankle is discussed.

Zanetti M, De Simoni C, Wetz HH, Zollinger H, Hodler J: Magnetic resonance imaging of injuries to the ankle joint: Can it predict clinical outcome? *Skeletal Radiol* 1997;26:82-88.

Findings on MRI after an acute ankle sprain did not correlate with clinical outcome in 29 patients.

## Classic Bibliography

Astrom M, Gentz CF, Nilsson P, Rausing A, Sjoberg S, Westlin N: Imaging in chronic Achilles' tendinopathy: A comparison of ultrasonography, magnetic resonance imaging and surgical findings in 27 histologically verified cases. *Skeletal Radiol* 1996;25:615-620.

Bluemke DA, Zerhouni EA: MRI of avascular necrosis of bone. *Top Magn Reson Imaging* 1996;8:231-246.

Cardone BW, Erickson SJ, Den Hartog BD, Carrera GF: MRI of injury to the lateral collateral ligamentous complex of the ankle. *J Comput Assist Tomogr* 1993;17:102-107.

Chandnani VP, Harper MT, Ficke JR, et al: Chronic ankle instability: Evaluation with MR arthrography, MR imaging, and stress radiography. *Radiology* 1994;192:189-194.

De Smet AA, Ilahi OA, Graf BK: Reassessment of the MR criteria for stability of osteochondritis dissecans in the knee and ankle. *Skeletal Radiol* 1996;25:159-163.

Khoury NJ, el-Khoury GY, Saltzman CL, Brandser EA: MR imaging of posterior tibial tendon dysfunction. *AJR Am J Roentgenol* 1996;167:675-682.

Kirsch MD, Erickson SJ: Normal magnetic resonance imaging anatomy of the ankle and foot. *Magn Reson Imaging Clin N Am* 1994;2:1-21.

Klein MA: MR imaging of the ankle: Normal and abnormal findings in the medial collateral ligament. *AJR Am J Roentgenol* 1994;162:377-383.

Klein MA, Spreitzer AM: MR imaging of the tarsal sinus and canal: Normal anatomy, pathologic findings, and features of the sinus tarsi syndrome. *Radiology* 1993;186:233-240.

Miller TT, Staron RB, Feldman F, Parisien M, Glucksman WJ, Gandolfo LH: The symptomatic accessory tarsal navicular bone: Assessment with MR imaging. *Radiology* 1995;195:849-853.

Wakeley CJ, Johnson DP, Watt I: The value of MR imaging in the diagnosis of the os trigonum syndrome. *Skeletal Radiol* 1996;25:133-136.

Zeiss J, Saddemi SR, Ebraheim NA: MR imaging of the peroneal tunnel. *J Comput Assist Tomogr* 1989;13:840-844.

# Chapter 18

# Tumors

Johnny T.C. Lau, MD, MSc, FRCSC

Peter C. Ferguson, MD, MSc, FRCSC

Jay S. Wunder, MD, MSc, FRCSC

## Introduction

Foot and ankle tumors are rare in comparison with other common traumatic and overuse foot and ankle disorders. Soft-tissue lesions are much more common than osseous lesions, and benign bone tumors are more common than malignant bone tumors.

A delayed or incorrect diagnosis or inappropriate surgery for a malignant tumor can produce devastating results and may make limb salvage impossible. It is important for surgeons to investigate suspicious lesions and to adequately rule out malignancy before proceeding with definitive treatment.

## Patient Assessment

The differential diagnosis in more than 90% of patients is based on patient history, physical examination, and plain radiographs. Symptoms can include a soft-tissue mass, a bony mass, an incidental finding on radiographs following trauma, a painful lesion, or a pathologic fracture. The history must include an assessment of duration of symptoms and those factors that relieve or aggravate symptoms, pain at rest or at night, history of prior malignancy or systemic disease, antecedent trauma, and family history.

Pain may be caused by bone destruction and resultant mechanical instability, intraosseous and soft-tissue pressure caused by rapid tumor expansion and malignant tumor cell proliferation, or, in some tumors, proteinases that stimulate pain fibers. Nerve irritation caused by an enlarging primary nerve tumor or secondary neural compression from an enlarging mass can also produce pain. Pain during rest or at night that is not related to activity is suggestive of a tumor; pain of this nature should be investigated carefully, especially in patients in whom treatment for a traumatic or overuse syndrome of the foot and ankle is unsuccessful.

A complete physical examination should be performed with careful attention to local tenderness, nodules or masses, skin changes (for example, hemangioma or café au lait spots), and adenopathy. In older patients, metastatic disease is more likely; therefore, a detailed physical examination is essential to rule out a primary lesion, such as lung, thyroid, breast, renal, or prostate cancer.

Dorsal lesions become painful with shoe wear, whereas plantar lesions are painful with weight bearing. The important features of a mass include its size, location, depth, history of growth, and pain. Regional adenopathy is rare for soft-tissue sarcomas. If nodal metastasis is present, then rhabdomyosarcoma, synovial sarcoma, and epithelioid sarcoma are the most likely diagnoses. Soft-tissue masses larger than 5 cm that are deep to fascia and actively growing should be biopsied.

Laboratory testing (complete blood cell count [CBC], erythrocyte sedimentation rate, C-reactive protein, blood cultures), along with metastatic workup (calcium, phosphate, prostate-specific antigen, liver function, coagulation tests, protein immunoelectrophoresis, and alkaline phosphatase) are useful for ruling out infection and primary hematologic malignancies. L-lactate dehydrogenase may be elevated in the presence of some lymphomas, Ewing's sarcoma, and osteosarcoma. Serum alkaline phosphatase may be elevated in patients with osteosarcoma.

Plain radiographs must be carefully reviewed to determine the location and size of the lesion, the interface between the tumor and bone, the effect of the tumor on bone (lysis, sclerosis, and periosteal reaction), and the presence of matrix, cortical erosion, or soft-tissue mass. The bone involved and the location of the lesion in bone are the most important factors in determining a differential diagnosis.

The radiographic appearance of a mature matrix reflects the biology of the lesion. Fibrous dysplasia produces a ground glass pattern from the small trabeculae of woven bone scattered through the fibrous stroma. When compared with bony lesions, cartilage lesions produce a more disorganized pattern of punctate calcification or arc-ring patterns. Metastatic disease such as breast and prostate cancer, as well as lymphoma, can produce a marked sclerotic response.

Cross-sectional imaging is important to clearly delineate the local extent of the tumor. CT is useful for defining the area of cortical destruction and is as useful as MRI

**TABLE 1 | Principles for Performing Open Biopsy**

An extensile biopsy incision that can be incorporated into the definitive resection should be used.

Soft-tissue dissection and development of tissue planes should be kept at a minimum to avoid contamination of normal tissue.

Exposure of major nerves and blood vessels should be avoided.

For bone tumors, a biopsy of any associated soft-tissue mass should be performed.

Deflation of tourniquet prior to wound closure and maintenance of meticulous hemostasis should be done to avoid a postoperative hematoma.

A drain should be used to avoid postoperative hematoma—the drain should be brought out at the distal end of the incision to incorporate the drain site into the definitive resection or so that the longest stump possible can be maintained if amputation is necessary.

in assessing bone destruction. MRI is most useful for assessing the intraosseous extent of tumor and the margin of the soft-tissue mass and normal tissue. A technetium bone scan is used to evaluate the extent of skeletal involvement. However, in patients with multiple myeloma, the technetium bone scan will be cold and a skeletal survey is required to determine the extent of disease. A gallium scan is used predominantly to evaluate the extent of lymphoma in extraosseous sites.

## Biologic Potential of Bone Lesions

Tumors are best classified according to the biology of lesions: benign latent, benign active, benign aggressive, and malignant. Benign lesions generally have no potential to metastasize, whereas malignant lesions metastasize. Benign latent lesions are asymptomatic and are common incidental findings on radiographs. Benign active lesions are symptomatic but tend not to demonstrate significant bone destruction, whereas benign aggressive lesions demonstrate bony destruction and a wider zone of transition from tumor to normal bony architecture. Malignant lesions have poorly defined margins, cortical erosion, malignant matrix formation, and a soft-tissue mass.

In general, benign lesions are slow-growing lesions. They are smaller than malignant lesions and have a narrow zone of transition between the tumor and bone and an organized cortical thickening. Malignant lesions are larger than benign lesions, with a wide zone of transition between the tumor and bone and a poorly organized cortical response (such as Codman's triangle, sunburst appearance, onion skinning). Cortical erosion or a soft-tissue mass extending through the cortex suggests an aggressive or malignant lesion. Aggressive lesions (benign or malignant) can destroy the cortex and produce a soft-tissue mass, whereas malignant lesions may grow through the haversian canal system, leaving the cortex intact. However, cortical destruction, a soft-tissue mass, and periosteal reaction are suggestive of malignancy.

## Biopsy

Before planning any biopsy of a musculoskeletal tumor, it is essential that the surgeon take into account the clinical history, physical examination, laboratory investigations, and radiographic imaging to formulate provisional and differential diagnoses of the presenting lesion. For a lesion that is asymptomatic and clearly benign on imaging, a biopsy is usually not necessary and the lesion can simply be observed. If, however, the surgeon cannot confirm that the lesion is not a primary malignancy, it is advisable to refer the patient to a musculoskeletal oncologist for biopsy. Poorly planned and executed biopsies may result in errors in diagnosis or may make limb salvage surgery difficult or impossible. In the foot and ankle, because of the close proximity of neurovascular structures and the small compartments, a poorly performed biopsy may result in an amputation for an otherwise previously resectable tumor. Therefore, for benign aggressive bone tumors and primary malignant bone or soft-tissue tumors, it is recommended that the same surgeon perform both the biopsy and the definitive surgery. It has been documented that patients undergoing biopsy in centers not specializing in musculoskeletal oncology have a higher complication rate during subsequent treatment.

The technique of biopsy chosen depends on several factors, including the size of the lesion, location (intraosseous or soft tissue), proximity to vital neurovascular structures, and the patient's ability to endure local, regional, or general anesthesia. For these reasons, MRI should be done before biopsy to assess the presence of a soft-tissue mass and the intraosseous extent of the tumor. In the foot and ankle, most soft-tissue tumors or bone tumors with large soft-tissue masses are readily palpable, and percutaneous needle biopsy is sufficient. The method of needle biopsy depends on the degree of specialization of the pathologist. In centers where cytologic examination is available and is adequate for diagnosis, fine needle aspiration may be appropriate. Otherwise, a core biopsy that allows examination of the tissue architecture is preferable. Contraindications to a needle or core biopsy are an inability to clearly ascertain the location of the lesion clinically and an inability to enter the lesion without traversing, and therefore contaminating, essential neurovascular structures.

For tumors that are completely intraosseous or when a previous needle biopsy has failed to produce diagnostic tissue, an open biopsy is usually indicated. It is essential that the surgeon be familiar with the planned incision for definitive resection, either limb salvage or amputation; if the surgeon is unsure of this incision, then the biopsy must not be done and the patient should be assessed by a musculoskeletal oncologist familiar with the appropriate incision. The basic principles of open biopsy are outlined in Table 1. Adherence to these principles should result in excellent diagnostic accuracy of the procedure with a minimal complication rate and should not jeopardize future limb salvage surgery.

## Staging

Staging of musculoskeletal tumors is important for prediction of patient outcome and for decision making on appropriate treatment. Staging refers to the assessment of the extent of a lesion and is divided into local staging and systemic staging. Local staging applies to both benign and malignant tumors and is best accomplished with MRI, which allows for accurate assessment of the size and location of the lesion with respect to the deep fascia in the extremity, an important prognostic factor for soft-tissue sarcomas. For bone tumors, local staging provides information on the extent of intramedullary involvement, including the presence of skip metastases, and whether the lesion has extended outside its compartment. Systemic staging applies to malignant tumors and is used to assess the presence of metastatic disease. In soft-tissue sarcomas, more than 95% of metastases occur in the lungs. For this reason, a chest CT is adequate to systemically stage the tumor. Although most bone sarcomas also metastasize to the lungs, 5% to 10% also metastasize to other skeletal sites, and both a chest CT and total body bone scan are used for systemic staging. Should a patient with a sarcoma have pain or a mass in any other body region, that region should be imaged using plain radiographs or MRI to assess the presence of a possible unusual metastasis.

The final aspect of staging is the assessment of the degree of malignancy of the tumor, as determined from the biopsy material. This measure of malignancy, or histologic grade, is extremely important in predicting biologic behavior of the tumor and is believed to be the best predictor of the development of metastatic disease for both bone and soft-tissue tumors.

The surgeon must combine information obtained from local and systemic studies to assign a stage to the tumor, which correlates with patient prognosis. For bone tumors, the stage is based on three factors: histologic grade, local extent of the tumor outside the involved bone, and the presence of metastatic disease. In the surgical staging system of the Musculoskeletal Tumor Society, tumors are assigned a score of I if low grade (< 15% chance of metastasis) or II if high grade (> 15% chance of metastasis) and a score of A if contained to its osseous compartment or B if outside this compartment. These progressive stages of IA, IB, IIA, and IIB have increasing risk of developing metastatic disease. Therefore, stage I tumors are often treated with surgical resection alone, whereas stage II lesions are generally treated with combined chemotherapy and surgical resection. With stage III lesions, the patient has metastatic disease and invariably has a poor prognosis.

For soft-tissue tumors, the three most important factors that predict metastatic disease are (1) histologic grade, (2) the size of the lesion (with lesions > 5 cm having higher risk), and (3) the relation of the tumor to the fascia of the extremity (with lesions deep to the fascia having higher risk). Various staging systems have been proposed using this information, but none has been shown to be clearly more predictive of patient outcome than the others. The more individual poor prognostic factors a patient has (high grade, large, deep tumor), the more likely the patient is to develop metastatic disease. As in patients with bone tumors, patients with metastatic disease have a very poor prognosis.

## Primary Benign Bone Tumors

Overall, bone tumors are less common than soft-tissue tumors in the foot and ankle and are more frequently benign than malignant. Chondroblastoma, a rare tumor, occurs more frequently in the tarsal bones than some other more common benign tumors. The most common primary malignancy is osteosarcoma, whereas chondrosarcoma and Ewing's sarcoma occur less frequently. Metastases to the foot are extremely rare, with the lung being the most common primary site.

### Giant Cell Tumor

This benign aggressive tumor occurs fairly frequently in the distal tibial epiphyseal-metaphyseal region and less commonly in the metatarsals and tarsal bones. It is characterized by a lytic appearance on plain radiographs, with or without a sclerotic border (Fig. 1). Typically, a rim of periosteal new bone formation, or neocortex, surrounds the accompanying soft-tissue mass. Although the etiology of this tumor has long been a mystery, recent evidence suggests the cell of origin is of fibro-osteoblastic lineage and that several genetic mutations seen in giant cell tumor are also found in osteosarcoma. Treatment is generally by intralesional curettage, with the completeness of the curettage dictating the risk of subsequent local recurrence. Use of a high-speed burr on the periphery of the lesion is recommended. Other studies have shown benefits from phenol or liquid nitrogen as adjuvants. The resultant defect is packed with bone graft or bone cement.

### Osteochondroma and Subungual Exostosis

Osteochondromas occur frequently in the distal tibia and metatarsals. They may be solitary or multiple, as seen in hereditary multiple exostoses, an autosomal dominant condition. Mutations in the *EXT1* or *EXT2* genes are responsible for this condition. Osteochondromas often present as a growing mass in adolescents, as the structure of the cartilage cap of the osteochondroma is similar to the physeal plate and responds to the same hormonal influences. Radiographically, osteochondromas appear as extrusions from the bone, with a key feature being continuity between the medullary canal of the underlying bone and the osteochondroma. Osteochondromas in the foot

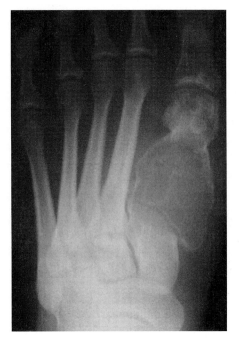

**Figure 1** AP radiograph depicting a giant cell tumor of the first metatarsal with aneurysmal dilatation of the bone.

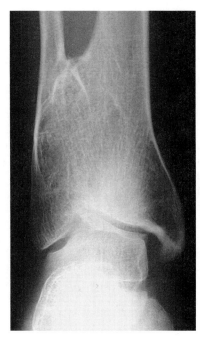

**Figure 2** AP radiograph of the ankle in a patient with a large sessile osteochondroma of the distal tibia, which resulted in limited range of motion and significant ankle valgus.

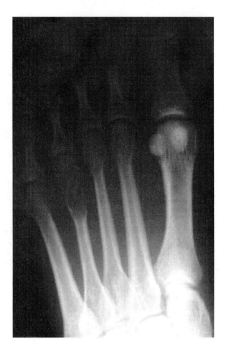

**Figure 3** A lytic lesion containing faint calcification is seen in the distal metadiaphyseal region of the fourth metatarsal, a common location for enchondroma.

and ankle can be particularly troublesome because they may cause angular deformities of the distal tibia or fibula or may limit range of motion of the ankle because of impingement in the syndesmosis (Fig. 2). Lesions at the distal tibiofibular syndesmosis may be sessile and resemble old syndesmotic trauma.

Subungual exostosis, which radiographically resembles osteochondroma, occurs on the distal phalanx and causes pain and nail deformity. Surgical excision of an osteochondroma is indicated if the lesion is painful, limits range of motion, impinges on neurovascular structures, or demonstrates growth after maturity. Growth after skeletal maturity may indicate malignant degeneration into a secondary chondrosarcoma, which occurs in approximately 1% of osteochondromas.

### Enchondroma

These lesions occur most frequently in the small bones of the hands but also occur in the feet. They are usually asymptomatic and often present as incidental findings on radiographs. Lesions in the hands and feet tend to appear more aggressive on radiographs than those situated elsewhere. Enchondromas typically are central in the affected bone and demonstrate calcification typical of chondroid matrix with endosteal erosion (Fig. 3). Histologically, these lesions are composed of hyaline cartilage, which may appear more cellular and therefore more aggressive than lesions located more centrally. However, despite their increased cellularity, these lesions rarely develop chondrosarcomatous changes. Treatment may be

necessary in two circumstances: to treat a pathologic fracture through an enchondroma or to investigate a lesion that is suspicious for low-grade chondrosarcoma. Pathologic fractures occur fairly frequently through the more aggressive-appearing lesions of the hands and feet and are usually treated initially by immobilization of the foot and ankle. Should the lesion continue to be symptomatic or if refracture occurs, curettage is usually done. It can be exceedingly difficult to differentiate between an enchondroma and a low-grade chondrosarcoma, even histologically. For lesions that demonstrate cortical erosion, soft-tissue mass formation, or bone expansion, a low-grade chondrosarcoma should be suspected. Although individual enchondromas rarely become malignant, patients with multiple enchondromas (Ollier's disease) have a 25% chance of developing a secondary chondrosarcoma. Patients with Ollier's disease often have significant problems with growth and angular deformities of the extremities.

### Osteoid Osteoma

Osteoid osteoma probably is not a neoplastic condition, but an inflammatory lesion that over time involutes and becomes asymptomatic. It most often affects patients in the second decade of life, and classic symptoms include constant dull pain that is most pronounced at night and is relieved by nonsteroidal anti-inflammatory drugs (NSAIDs). The biochemical basis for this pain relief is blockage of the cyclooxygenase pathway, which reduces production of prostaglandin $E_2$, thought to be the active substance in this lesion. Radiographically, osteoid osteoma appears as a small lytic nidus surrounded by a region of dense sclerotic bone or periosteal new bone formation in diaphyseal lesions. This nidus is often difficult to appreciate on radiographs because of the surrounding sclerosis, and a CT with fine (2 mm) cuts may be helpful in diagnosis. The nidus histologically is composed of fibrovascular stroma containing fine, immature osteoid. The first step in treatment is often NSAIDs, and long-term suppression of symptoms in this manner, rather than with surgical intervention, may be appealing to some patients. The traditional surgical treatment has been excision of the nidus, which is effective and associated with a low local recurrence rate, as long as the nidus is completely removed. Recently, radiofrequency ablation of the nidus using a probe passed percutaneously under CT guidance has been used with reasonable results.

### Osteoblastoma

Although osteoblastoma is an extremely rare lesion, the foot is the third most common site of its occurrence, usually in the talar neck. It typically occurs during the second decade of life, with symptoms similar to those of osteoid osteoma, including deep-seated pain in the region of the lesion. However, unlike osteoid osteoma, the pain is not typically nocturnal and not as effectively relieved by NSAIDs. These lesions appear similar to giant cell tumors radiographically; lysis is the dominant feature, although surrounding sclerosis can occur. Gross and histologic features of giant cell tumor, aneurysmal bone cyst, and osteoblastoma can often occur together in aggressive epiphyseal-metaphyseal tumors. Osteoblastoma often closely resembles osteoid osteoma histologically but is larger and may be more permeative. This feature causes difficulty in differentiating an aggressive osteoblastoma from osteosarcoma. The treatment of this tumor, like most benign aggressive tumors, is aggressive curettage and filling of the defect with bone graft or cement.

### Chondroblastoma

This unusual tumor occurs most often in the epiphysis or apophysis of long bones, but also occurs in the tarsal bones, especially in the hindfoot (Fig. 4). It commonly presents as a painful lesion that may produce a joint effusion as a result of synovitis or pathologic fracture caused by weakened subchondral bone. Chondroblastomas appear lytic with little or no matrix and can be very destructive. MRI usually shows intense edema in the marrow adjacent to a chondroblastoma. Histologically, they are often very cellular and demonstrate chicken-wire calcifications. Treatment is similar to that for other benign aggressive tumors, although extra attention must be paid to the adjacent joint. Contamination of the joint through accidental perforation of weakened subchondral bone should be avoided at all costs because it may increase the risk of local recurrence. Chondroblastoma, like giant cell tumor,

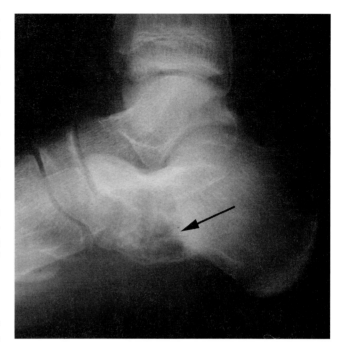

**Figure 4** Lateral radiograph of the hindfoot showing a lytic lesion in the anterior process of the calcaneus with arc-ring calcifications (arrow). Biopsy revealed a chondroblastoma.

can occasionally produce pulmonary metastases that appear to be histologically benign.

### Bizarre Parosteal Osteochondromatous Proliferation

This unusual lesion occurs most often in the tubular bones of the hands and feet in the second and third decades of life. The presenting complaint is usually a painful mass that may be enlarging, and there is frequently a history of trauma. The lesion appears as a sclerotic surface lesion, and the differential diagnosis must include osteochondroma and a parosteal osteosarcoma. Histologically, this lesion shows hypercellular cartilage maturing to trabecular bone, a process similar to enchondral ossification occurring in the physis. Surgical excision of the lesion is recommended despite a high local recurrence rate. Thorough investigation of this lesion is essential to differentiate it from a malignant lesion.

## Primary Malignant Bone Tumors

### Osteosarcoma

Osteosarcoma is the most common primary bone malignancy after myeloma, commonly occurring in the second and third decades of life. It most often occurs around the knee or proximal humerus. In the foot and ankle, the distal tibia is the most common site of occurrence, but lesions in the metatarsals and tarsal bones have been reported. Osteosarcoma usually presents as a painful mass that appears as a poorly defined destructive lesion with bony matrix on radiographs. A periosteal reaction and large soft-tissue mass are characteristic. Treatment of osteosarcomas in almost all bones once consisted of amputation, but long-term survival reached a maximum of only 20%, presumably because of micrometastases present at the time of diagnosis. The mainstay of current treatment of most osteosarcomas is neoadjuvant chemotherapy and surgical resection. Administration of chemotherapeutic agents including doxorubicin, high-dose methotrexate, cisplatin, and ifosfamide has raised the long-term survival to 60% to 70% in most studies. Although a clear benefit has not been shown in terms of survival, preoperative administration of chemotherapy allows for assessment of the response of the tumor to the agents, as well as facilitating resection by killing the cells at the periphery of the tumor. Wide resection is the ideal surgical management, which is often difficult in the foot and ankle because of the proximity of vital neurovascular structures, the difficulty of soft-tissue coverage, and limited bony reconstruction options. For this reason, foot and ankle osteosarcomas are still frequently treated by amputation.

### Chondrosarcoma

Malignant cartilage tumors typically occur in patients age 50 years or older. In the foot and ankle, these tumors are often found in patients who have an underlying predisposing condition such as Ollier's disease or multiple hereditary exostoses. They usually present as a slowly growing mass that may or may not be painful. These lesions appear primarily lytic with evidence of endosteal erosion and an arc-ring pattern of calcified matrix. MRI demonstrates high signal on T2 because of the high water content in the cartilage. Most chondrosarcomas are low grade, but higher-grade subtypes including dedifferentiated and mesenchymal chondrosarcomas may occur. For low-grade lesions, no adjuvant therapy is effective and surgical treatment alone is indicated. To obtain wide margins and limit the risk of local recurrence, some form of amputation is usually indicated. For higher grade lesions, chemotherapy is often used, similar to other high grade bone sarcomas, but appears less effective than in osteosarcomas.

Three recent studies of patients with chondrosarcomas indicate a 10-year survival rate of approximately 70%, with inadequate resection cited as the primary factor in poor outcome. In all three studies, only 1% to 3% of chondrosarcomas were located in the foot and ankle. In one study, better outcomes were found in patients with malignant tumors of the hand and foot (87% survival) than in those with malignant pelvic tumors (67% survival), whereas another study found that location within the body had no prognostic significance.

## Benign Soft-Tissue Tumors

### Lipoma

Lipomas consist of mature adipocytes. They can occur both superficial and deep to fascia, but in the foot and

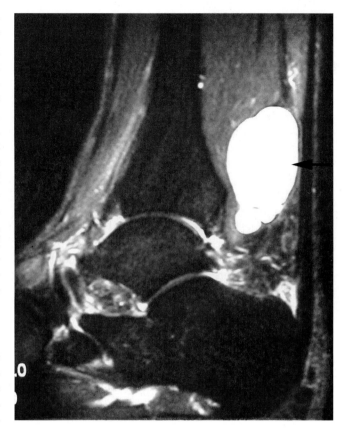

**Figure 5** Sagittal T2-weighted image showing a high-signal intensity lesion arising posterior to the tibiotalar joint (arrow). Aspiration produced clear fluid, confirming the diagnosis of a ganglion cyst.

hand, they usually are deep to fascia. Rarely, they occur within bone. They grow slowly and displace rather than invade adjacent soft-tissue structures. MRI demonstrates a homogeneous, bright, and well-circumscribed lesion on T1 images. Because fluid, hemorrhage, or necrosis may produce the same signal intensity, a fat suppression sequence is required to make the definitive diagnosis. Areas of lesser signal intensity within the lesion may indicate necrosis, different tissue differentiation, or rarely, malignant degeneration. In symptomatic lesions for which nonsurgical treatment has failed, marginal excision is required.

### Ganglion

Ganglions are believed to result from myxoid degeneration of connective tissues and are usually associated with inflammatory or degenerative arthritis. They can be found around joints, ligaments, menisci, tendons, nerves, periosteum, and within bone (Fig. 5). Foot and ankle ganglions account for up to 11% of all ganglions and may be the most common soft-tissue tumor in the region. Cysts can cause mechanical pain or nerve compression. Treatment begins with aspiration of the ganglion and injection of steroids. If this fails, excision of the ganglion, including the stalk and a portion of the joint capsule or tendon sheath, is required to prevent recurrence. In one series of 40 patients treated with surgical excision, 86% were satisfied, and the recurrence rate was 10%. Patients who underwent revision surgery had poorer results; therefore, care must be taken to trace the stalk of the ganglion to its origin. The use of a tourniquet to obtain a bloodless surgical field and magnifying loupes or an operating microscope are recommended to ensure adequate excision and reduce the chance of recurrence.

### Plantar Fibromatosis

Plantar fibromatosis is generally found in patients in their 20s, 30s, and 40s and can be associated with Dupuytren's contracture, or Peyronie's disease in more severe cases. It can occur as a solitary lesion or as multiple lesions and is bilateral in up to 50% of patients. The pathology is identical to that of Dupuytren's contracture. The lesion is usually fixed to the medial aspect of the plantar fascia and can grow to 2 cm in diameter. It is usually asymptomatic, but it can be painful with weight bearing or during an initial inflammatory phase that usually resolves in a few weeks to a few months.

Nonsurgical treatment with shoe modifications and NSAIDs is recommended. Excision of the plantar fibromatosis is generally discouraged because of the high risk of complications. Wide excision of the lesion can decrease the risk of recurrence, but it can be complicated by skin necrosis, delayed wound healing, and a reduced medial arch height. Marginal excision of the lesion will result in recurrence.

### Schwannoma

Schwannomas or neurilemmomas are benign nerve sheath tumors derived from the Schwann cell. Most are solitary lesions, but 20% of patients have multiple lesions associated with neurofibromatosis. These are slow-growing lesions within the epineurium of the nerve. They are encapsulated by a fibrous connective tissue layer and have no neural elements within the lesion. As these lesions enlarge, the surrounding nerve fibers are displaced. Unlike neurofibromas, schwannomas do not undergo malignant degeneration.

Patients present with a mass that may be painful, but usually there is little pain or neurologic impairment. A positive Tinel's sign is elicited in the nerve with the lesion. A malignant nerve tumor is more likely in patients with night pain and severe motor weakness. MRI demonstrates the relationship between the lesion and the nerve from which it arose (Fig. 6). Recurrence is rare after surgical excision, and nerve function is preserved because the well-encapsulated lesion has no neural elements and can be easily dissected free of neural elements.

### Neurofibromas

Neurofibromas are benign tumors of peripheral nerves consisting of a variety of cells. They occur as solitary le-

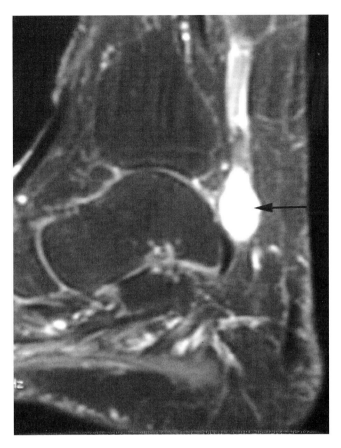

**Figure 6** Sagittal T2-weighted image delineates a small high-signal intensity lesion in continuity with the posterior tibial nerve (arrow). Surgical exploration revealed a schwannoma of the tibial nerve.

sions in 90% of patients and as multiple lesions in 10%. Multiple lesions are called neurofibromatosis (von Recklinghausen's disease). There are two types of neurofibromatosis: type I, involving peripheral nerves; and type II, involving acoustic nerves. Solitary neurofibromas are firm, nontender, and well-circumscribed masses that usually arise from small cutaneous nerves. Neurofibromatosis is characterized by multiple cutaneous lesions. Rapid growth of a lesion suggests malignant transformation and occurs in 5% of patients; 50% of all neurofibrosarcomas result from malignant transformation of neurofibromas.

Solitary neurofibromas resemble schwannomas in some respects, but significant differences alter their treatment and outcome. The MRI scans of a solitary neurofibroma and a schwannoma are similar, but unlike schwannomas, neurofibromas are not well circumscribed, do not have a distinct capsule, and infiltrate surrounding nerve fibers. Microscopically, the nerve fibers are seen entering the neurofibroma proximally and exiting it distally, which makes excision of the lesion impossible without sacrificing some neural function.

The treatment of symptomatic lesions is surgical excision. For lesions arising from small nerves whose loss has no functional consequence, complete en bloc excision of the lesion is recommended. For lesions arising from large nerves with significant neurologic function, incomplete excision of the lesion, which preserves some nerve fibers, gives a better functional result. The residual tissue rarely grows to its original size or becomes symptomatic.

## Malignant Soft-Tissue Tumors

### Soft-Tissue Sarcoma

Primary mesenchymal soft-tissue malignancies occur most often in the proximal extremities, but certain subtypes are more common in the foot and ankle. The most common soft-tissue sarcomas are malignant fibrous histiocytoma and leiomyosarcoma; these occur frequently in the calf or anterior leg but rarely in the foot. In contrast, clear cell sarcoma and synovial sarcoma are found frequently in the deep compartments of the foot. Soft-tissue sarcomas may present as painless masses, but pain may occur with extension to or destruction of adjacent bone, joint, or neurologic structures. Plain radiographs may show bone erosion and the lesion may be calcified, as in synovial sarcoma. An MRI is crucial to assess the local extent of the tumor and to assess whether the tumor is resectable. It is also imperative to assess the regional lymph nodes, because synovial sarcoma is one of few soft-tissue sarcomas that can metastasize via this route. Soft-tissue sarcomas are treated with a combination of radiation therapy and surgical excision, if possible. For larger tumors in the foot, it may be difficult if not impossible to achieve an acceptable margin while leaving a functional extremity, and amputation is often the only surgical option. For lesions that are resectable, radiation therapy can be administered preoperatively or postoperatively. A smaller dose is used preoperatively, which may be beneficial in the often-radiosensitive skin on the plantar aspect of the foot. This must be weighed, however, against the higher incidence of wound healing complications associated with preoperative irradiation.

## Summary

The most important factor in the treatment of foot and ankle tumors is accurate and early diagnosis, which is usually possible based on medical history, physical examination, and plain radiographs. CT, MRI, and biopsy can provide more information if the diagnosis is uncertain. Treatment ranges from curettage for nonaggressive benign lesions to amputation for some malignant lesions.

## Annotated Bibliography

### Staging

Agarwal S, Agarwal T, Agarwal R, Agarwal PK, Jain UK: Fine needle aspiration of bone tumors. *Cancer Detect Prev* 2000;24:602-609.

Two hundred twenty-six cases were reviewed to determine the effectiveness of fine needle aspiration in diagnosing bone tumors. The sensitivity was 86% and the specificity was 94.7%.

The positive predictive value was 99.4% and the negative predictive value was only 38.3%. The diagnosis of malignant tumors was more accurate.

Temple HT, Worman DS, Mnaymneh WA: Unplanned surgical excision of tumors of the foot and ankle. *Cancer Control* 2001;8:262-268.

In a retrospective review, 18 patients with malignant foot and ankle tumors treated with limb-sparing surgery following an unplanned surgical resection were assessed. When salvage was attempted, these patients had more complications, extensive surgical procedures, and were more likely to require adjuvant chemotherapy. However, there was no significant difference in recurrence or disease-free survival compared with 17 patients with planned surgical resection.

### Primary Benign Bone Tumors

Biscaglia R, Bacchini P, Bertoni F: Giant cell tumor of the bones of the hand and foot. *Cancer* 2000;88:2022-2032.

Giant cell tumors of the foot (21) and hand (8) were retrospectively reviewed. These tumors occurred more commonly in young females, and demonstrated a more aggressive behavior than giant cell tumors of large bones. No multicentricity or pulmonary metastases were observed.

Chin KR, Kharrazi FD, Miller BS, Mankin HJ, Gebhardt MC: Osteochondromas of the distal aspect of the tibia or fibula: Natural history and treatment. *J Bone Joint Surg Am* 2000;82:1269-1278.

Twenty-three patients with osteochondromas of the distal tibia and fibula were retrospectively reviewed. Most patients presented with a painful ankle mass at an average age of 16 years. Almost all patients had normal and symmetrical preoperative ankle motion, even though 11 had plastic deformation of the fibula from a large lesion. Following surgical excision, all patients had pain-free symmetrical ankle motion with partial remodeling of the tibia and fibula. Younger patients had more remodeling, but preexisting ankle deformity did not change significantly.

Donley BG, Philbin T, Rosenberg GA, Schils JP, Recht M: Percutaneous CT guided resection of osteoid osteoma of the tibial plafond. *Foot Ankle Int* 2000;21:596-598.

A case report of a juxta-articular osteoid osteoma of the tibial plafond treated by percutaneous CT guided excision.

Fiorenza F, Abudu A, Grimer RJ, et al: Risk factors for survival and local control in chondrosarcoma of bone. *J Bone Joint Surg Br* 2002;84:93-99.

In a study of 153 patients with nonmetastatic chondrosarcoma of bone, survival rates were 70% at 10 years and 63% at 15 years. Risk factors for local recurrence included inadequate surgical margins and tumor size of more than 10 cm. Location within the body, type of surgery, and duration of symptoms were not found to be of prognostic significance.

Mankin HJ, Fondren G, Hornicek FJ, Gebhardt MC, Rosenberg AE: The use of flow cytometry in assessing malignancy in bone and soft tissue tumors. *Clin Orthop* 2002;397:95-105.

Of 1,134 patients, 342 had verified malignant tumors of bone; only 2 of 15 (13%) with tumors of the hand or foot died, whereas 22 of 67 (33%) with pelvic tumors died. Flow cytometry did not appear useful in predicting risk of death for patients with osteosarcomas or chondrosarcomas; it did seem to be of value in patients with soft-tissue sarcomas and may help determine treatment.

Noonan KJ, Feinberg JR, Levenda A, Snead J, Wurtz LD: Natural history of multiple hereditary osteochondromatosis of the lower extremity and ankle. *J Pediatr Orthop* 2002;22:120-124.

A retrospective review of 38 patients was performed to document the natural history of the ankle joint in multiple hereditary osteochondromatosis. The average age was 42 years. Patients with osteoarthritis of the ankle had significantly more tibiotalar tilt and restricted motion compared to those without arthritis. Ankle pain interfered with vocation in 8% of patients, and with participation in sports in 32%. Correction or prevention of excessive ankle tilt may be warranted to improve outcome.

Ramappa AJ, Lee FY, Tang P, Carlson JR, Gebhardt MC, Mankin HJ: Chondroblastoma of bone. *J Bone Joint Surg Am* 2000;82:1140-1145.

Forty-three patients with chondroblastoma of bone were reviewed. Size of the lesion, age and gender of the patient, status of the growth plate, and an aneurysmal bone cyst component to the tumor had no significant effect on recurrence rate, but tumors around the hip were more likely to recur.

Rizzo M, Ghert MA, Harrelson JM, Scully SP: Chondrosarcoma of bone: Analysis of 108 cases and evaluation of predictors of outcome. *Clin Orthop* 2001;391:224-233.

In 108 patients with chondrosarcomas, a statistically significant association was found between positive surgical margins and local recurrence, metastasis, and death. Tumor grade was not predictive of outcome.

Shawen SB, McHale KA, Temple HT: Correction of ankle valgus deformity secondary to multiple hereditary osteochondral exostoses with Ilizarov. *Foot Ankle Int* 2000; 21:1019-1022.

A case report of an adult with multiple hereditary osteochondral exostoses and a symptomatic valgus ankle deformity caused by growth arrest and a shortened fibula was discussed. This patient was successfully treated with Ilizarov external fixation to correct the deformity.

Temple HT, Mizel MS, Murphey MD, Sweet DE: Osteoblastoma of the foot and ankle. *Foot Ankle Int* 1998;19: 698-704.

A total of 329 patients with osteoblastoma were retrospectively reviewed, of which 41 (12.5%) presented with tumors in the foot and ankle. The average age of patients was 22.5 years, with 85.4% being skeletally mature. Overall, pain was the most common presentation (97.2%). Eighteen (44%) of tumors in the foot and ankle were located in the hindfoot, of which 16 (89%) were in the talus. Two lesions in the metatarsals became sarcomas, while the rest remained benign.

Wu CT, Inwards CY, O'Laughlin S, Rock MG, Beabout JW, Unni KK: Chondromyxoid fibroma of bone: A clinicopathologic review of 278 cases. *Hum Pathol* 1998;29: 438-446.

The Mayo clinic experience with chondromyxoid fibroma was reviewed.

### Primary Malignant Bone Tumors

Biscaglia R, Gasbarrini A, Bohling T, Bacchini P, Bertoni F, Picci P: Osteosarcoma of the bones of the foot: An easily misdiagnosed malignant tumor. *Mayo Clin Proc* 1998; 73:842-847.

All the osteosarcomas of the foot treated at the Rizzoli Institute over an 80-year period were reviewed. Osteosarcoma of the foot was extremely rare (12 cases, 0.6% of all osteosarcomas). Late diagnosis and misdiagnosis (50%) were common. High-grade lesions were identified in seven patients, and four died of metastatic disease. Treatment consisted of amputation and chemotherapy. Because symptoms are relatively nonspecific, careful attention to this diagnosis is required for timely treatment of patients.

Bovee JV, van der Heul RO, Taminiau AH, Hogendoorn PC: Chondrosarcoma of the phalanx: A locally aggressive lesion with minimal metastatic potential: A report of 35 cases and a review of the literature. *Cancer* 1999;86:1724-1732.

A retrospective review of 35 patients with phalangeal chondrosarcoma was performed. Treatment was curettage or local excision in 16, and amputation in 19. Ten of 15 tumors recurred following local treatment and none in the amputation group. The median survival was 20.8 years, but no patients developed metastasis or died of the tumor. Local treatment, which is carefully followed, may be a treatment option when amputation significantly impairs function.

Choong PF, Qureshi AA, Sim FH, Unni KK: Osteosarcoma of the foot: A review of 52 patients at the Mayo Clinic. *Acta Orthop Scand* 1999;70:361-364.

Fifty-two patients with osteosarcoma of the foot were retrospectively reviewed. This was a rare tumor, which was more common in older patients. The most common site was the calcaneus, and the most common histology was a high grade, chondroblastic tumor. In many cases, amputation was required for treatment.

Hottya GA, Steinbach LS, Johnston JO, van Kuijk C, Genant HK: Chondrosarcoma of the foot: Imaging, surgical and pathological correlation of three new cases. *Skeletal Radiol* 1999;28:153-158.

The presentation, diagnosis, pathology, treatment, and follow-up of three patients with chondrosarcoma of the foot were presented. Limb salvage requires an early diagnosis with early tumor excision.

Natarajan MV, Annamalai K, Williams S, Selvaraj R, Rajagopal TS: Limb salvage in distal tibial osteosarcoma using a custom mega prosthesis. *Int Orthop* 2000;24:282-284.

Six patients with stage IIB distal tibial osteosarcoma were reviewed. A wide excision was possible in only three. At follow-up, three patients retained their prosthesis and the others required further surgery because of recurrence and flap necrosis with infection.

### Soft-Tissue Tumors

Beggs I, Gilmour HM, Davie RM: Diffuse neurofibroma of the ankle. *Clin Radiol* 1998;53:755-759.

Two cases of diffuse neurofibroma of the ankle were presented. The diagnosis was confirmed by a characteristic appearance on MRI on the postgadolinium T1-weighted images.

Brien EW, Mirra JM, Luck JV Jr: Benign and malignant cartilage tumors of bone and joint: Their anatomic and theoretical basis with an emphasis on radiology, pathology and clinical biology. II: Juxtacortical cartilage tumors. *Skeletal Radiol* 1999;28:1-20.

The authors emphasize the importance of the pathogenesis, in conjunction with radiographic and histologic findings, in choosing appropriate treatment.

Llauger J, Palmer J, Monill JM, Franquet T, Bague S, Roson N: MR imaging of benign soft-tissue masses of the foot and ankle. *Radiographics* 1998;18:1481-1498.

This review article correlates the clinical and pathologic features of benign tumors with MRI findings.

Marshall-Taylor C, Fanburg-Smith JC: Hemosiderotic fibrohistiocytic lipomatous lesion: Ten cases of a previously undescribed fatty lesion of the foot/ankle. *Mod Pathol* 2000;13:1192-1199.

The clinicopathologic features of a hemosiderotic fibrohistiocytic lipomatous lesion were presented. This lesion occurred mainly in the ankle region of middle-aged women, and most likely was a reactive process caused by prior trauma. After local therapy, there was a risk of recurrence, but not of metastasis.

Ogose A, Hotta T, Morita T, et al: Tumors of peripheral nerves: Correlation of symptoms, clinical signs, imaging features, and histologic diagnosis. *Skeletal Radiol* 1999;28:183-188.

Ninety-nine benign and 16 malignant tumors of peripheral nerves were retrospectively reviewed. Patients with malignant tumors were more likely to have severe motor weakness, pain at rest, and an invasive margin on CT or MRI.

Rozbruch SR, Chang V, Bohne WH, Deland JT: Ganglion cysts of the lower extremity: An analysis of 54 cases and review of the literature. *Orthopedics* 1998;21:141-148.

Fifty-four patients with ganglion cysts of the lower extremity were evaluated over a 12-year period retrospectively. These cysts were more common in women, patients in the fifth and sixth decades of life, and in the foot and ankle (67%). Forty patients were reviewed at an average of 5.9 years after surgery. Eighty-six percent of patients were satisfied, with recurrence in 10%. The only predictor of inferior results was revision surgery.

Sammarco GJ, Mangone PG: Classification and treatment of plantar fibromatosis. *Foot Ankle Int* 2000;21:563-569.

Eighteen patients with plantar fibromatosis undergoing subtotal plantar fasciectomy were reviewed. Preoperative and postoperative radiographs demonstrated decrease in height of the medial longitudinal arch following surgery. A surgical staging system was also presented. The stage of tumor correlated with postoperative wound healing, skin necrosis, and recurrence.

Vandeweyer E, Van Geertruyden J, de Fontaine S: Lipoma of the toe. *Foot Ankle Int* 1998;19:246-247.

This is the first case report of a lipoma on the plantar aspect of the toe.

## Classic Bibliography

Enneking WF, Spanier SS, Goodman MA: A system for the surgical staging of musculoskeletal sarcoma. *Clin Orthop* 1980;153:106-120.

Mankin HJ, Mankin CJ, Simon MA: The hazards of the biopsy, revisited: Members of the Musculoskeletal Tumor Society. *J Bone Joint Surg Am* 1996;78:656-663.

Ostrowski ML, Spjut HJ: Lesions of the bones of the hands and feet. *Am J Surg Pathol* 1997;21:676-690.

# Chapter 19

# Common Infections of the Foot

Steven M. Raikin, MD

## Introduction

Infections of the foot are much the same in etiology, diagnosis, and management as infections involving other areas of the body. Diabetes and peripheral vascular disease that involve the foot, however, add a unique dimension that can cause seemingly trivial infections to have disastrous effects, resulting in loss of function or limb and even death. Infections can involve the soft-tissue structures alone or invade joints and bone. They may be caused by bacteria, mycobacteria, fungi, or viruses and can be primary to the foot, or hematogenous spread from another site in the body can occur.

## Nondiabetic Infections

### Cellulitis

Cellulitis is a soft-tissue infection of the skin and subcutaneous tissue characterized by pain, erythema, swelling, and tenderness. Cellulitis may be acute or subacute and is rarely chronic. Trauma or breaks in the protective cutaneous skin layer may be a predisposing cause, but hematogenous and lymphatic dissemination can account for the sudden appearance of cellulitis in previously normal skin.

On physical examination of a leg with bacterial cellulitis, lymphangitis and local lymphadenopathy may be seen. A localized fluctuant area signifies abscess formation. Fever is uncommon and should prompt the physician to consider secondary bacteremia or systemic involvement. With local involvement, vital signs (other than a slight tachycardia) are usually normal. Unless there is systemic involvement, white blood cell counts are usually normal or mildly elevated.

The diagnosis of bacterial cellulitis is predominantly based on history and clinical findings. Bacterial cultures of blood or material obtained by direct needle aspiration are rarely conclusive when no purulence is present.

Radiographs and ultrasound of soft tissues may be useful to detect radiopaque foreign bodies, including glass, and the rare presence of air within the soft tissue, which signifies the presence of gas-forming organisms. CT or MRI are reserved for suspected deep space infections or abscesses.

For most localized infections in uncompromised hosts, no radiographic procedures are indicated.

*Staphylococcus aureus* and β-hemolytic *Streptococcus* are the most common organisms in uncompromised hosts. In community-acquired infections, these are usually responsive to first-generation oral cephalosporins, clindamycin, or ciprofloxacin. If parenteral antibiotics are required, broad-spectrum coverage is usually initially recommended using ampicillin-sulbactam or piperacillin-tazobactam.

Most patients with cellulitis respond to appropriate oral antimicrobial agents. Cellulitis in an area of edema resulting from a venous or lymphatic stasis is often difficult to manage and aggressive parenteral antibiotic therapy may be required. Trauma, puncture wounds, breaks in the skin, lymphatic or venous stasis, immunodeficiency, and the presence of foreign bodies all are predisposing factors and need to be considered in the management of cellulitis. β-hemolytic streptococcal cellulitis may be associated with a more virulent disease course that renders the patient systemically ill and progresses rapidly.

Cellulitis is often caused by puncture wounds, which are most frequent in children. Puncture wounds may be caused by metal (usually nails), wooden splinters, thorns, glass, or other objects. Penetration through a sneaker should always alert one to the possible presence of *Pseudomonas aeruginosa*.

If the patient is seen before any evidence of cellulitis has occurred, the area should be cleaned with an iodine-based solution and thoroughly irrigated, using a syringe for high-pressure irrigation. The penetration portal should be probed for retained material; if there is a possibility that foreign material is still present, radiographs with soft-tissue penetration are recommended. If radiographs are inconclusive, additional studies such as MRI or ultrasound may be useful in identifying foreign material and aiding in its removal. The use of antibiotics in these patients remains controversial. Penetration of a "clean" (uncontaminated) object probably does not require antibiotic coverage. However, if the area is contaminated in any way, administration of a first-generation cephalosporin (such as cephalexin) or clindamycin is recommended. The patient should be immunized against tetanus, and the area should be closely observed for development of any infection.

The delayed presentation of cellulitis after a puncture wound is usually caused by *Staphylococcus* or *Streptococcus* infection. Retained foreign material is often a nidus for infection and may cause persistent or delayed onset of an infection. Deep penetration may result in abscess formation or bone penetration. Osteomyelitis and septic arthritis occur in approximately 1.5% of patients with puncture wounds and may present as acute or late complications, often resulting from *Pseudomonas* infection.

### Abscess

*S aureus* infection of the pulp space of the distal phalanx of the toe is called a felon. Other organisms occasionally are responsible, usually in immunocompromised hosts. The infection is usually isolated to the complex septated area of the pulp space but may penetrate into the underlying bone, causing osteomyelitis. Presentation is usually characterized by severe pain in a tense erythematous pulp space, occasionally with pus draining from the adjacent nail fold.

Treatment requires surgical drainage through a semicircular incision extending from one side of the toe to the tip, with spreading of the soft tissues toward the far side of the pulp. The area should be left open to drain. Delayed primary closure can be done after 5 to 7 days of antibiotic treatment in uncompromised patients, or the wound can be allowed to heal without surgical closure.

### Necrotizing Fasciitis

Necrotizing fasciitis is an aggressive and rapidly extending soft-tissue infection usually caused by group A β-hemolytic *Streptococcus pyogenes*. It involves only the skin and underlying soft tissue, with muscle being spared. Presentation includes a rapid onset of ascending cellulitis that is unresponsive to antibiotic treatment. The limb is swollen and erythematous, bullous eruptions are common, and the patient usually has systemic symptoms indicative of sepsis. Septic shock and multiorgan failure can be fatal, particularly in immunocompromised hosts, such as patients with diabetes, a history of drug and alcohol abuse, connective tissue disease, or human immunodeficiency virus.

Emergency treatment should consist of aggressive surgical débridement combined with broad-spectrum antibiotic(s) and supportive care. Repeated débridement may be needed until the infection is under control. Rapid detection and treatment are essential in reducing morbidity and mortality.

### Deep Space Infection

Penetrating wounds may involve the deep fascial spaces of the foot, resulting in abscess formation. Deep space abscess formation is more likely after massive trauma, in

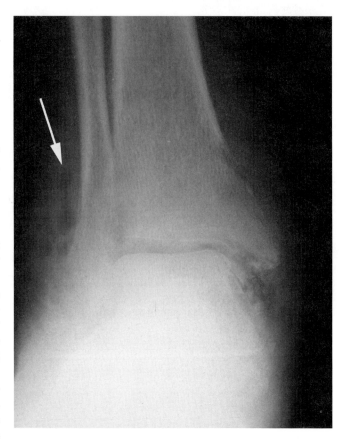

**Figure 1** Air seen in the soft tissue of an ankle radiograph (arrow) suggesting the presence of an infection from a gas-forming organism.

patients with diabetes, and in other immunocompromised hosts. A high level of clinical suspicion is essential for making a prompt diagnosis and initiating timely treatment.

The foot is swollen and often tense, painful, and fluctuant on palpation or squeezing of the compartments. Ascending cellulitis may be present and is usually not responsive to antibiotic treatment. Patients may be bacteremic and occasionally toxic, with fever, tachycardia, and a high white blood cell count, particularly if β-hemolytic *Streptococcus* is the primary pathogen. Radiographs may show air in the soft tissue in *Clostridium* and anaerobic streptococcal (gas gangrene) infections (Fig. 1). MRI with gadolinium contrast is the best method for confirming abscess formation and its location in the foot.

Treatment involves immediate surgical drainage and débridement of the abscess, communicating fascial planes, and tendon sheaths. Broad-spectrum intravenous antibiotic treatment should continue until the infectious organism and antibiotic sensitivities are identified. Whenever possible, initiation of antibiotic treatment should be delayed until surgical culture results can be obtained.

### Osteomyelitis

Infection of the bone may be acute or chronic and may develop through hematogenous spread of a distant infection or be secondary to involvement of an adjacent area. White blood cell count and erythrocyte sedimentation rate are usually elevated, and the diagnosis is confirmed on MRI (or CT if MRI is not available). MRI allows early diagnosis and the accurate anatomic localization of infection involving the bone and soft tissue. However, radiographic changes are not specific and can be mimicked by fracture healing and tumors. Plain radiographic changes do not develop for 7 to 10 days after the onset of osteomyelitis, and this diagnosis should not be excluded based on negative radiographs. If periosteal reaction and cortical disruption are seen on radiographs, this is a reliable diagnostic adjuvant. Additionally, a three-phase technetium bone scan will "light up" in the affected area before radiographic changes are visible. Diagnosis by bone biopsy and culture is definitive, but care must be used in interpreting aspiration performed through an infected cellulitic area.

Treatment of acute hematogenous osteomyelitis that is diagnosed early involves the use of intravenous antibiotics. In children, 2 weeks of intravenous antibiotics followed by 2 weeks of oral antibiotics is usually sufficient. Oral antibiotics have not been well studied in the treatment of osteomyelitis in adults, but treatment with oral ciprofloxacin has produced results comparable to intravenous antibiotics in some studies. In most instances, 4 weeks of intravenous antibiotics is recommended for adults with acute gram-positive infections and 6 weeks for gram-negative infections. Antibiotic choice is directed by cultures and sensitivities obtained from direct aspiration or blood cultures. In some patients, surgical débridement is required to drain an abscess.

Osteomyelitis in adults is usually caused by direct traumatic inoculation or contamination from an adjacent infection or during surgery. Although the location of osteomyelitis may be easier to determine in these patients, the diagnostic workup is the same as that described for hematogenous osteomyelitis. Treatment usually involves surgical débridement combined with parenteral antibiotics as previously described.

Chronic osteomyelitis may be more difficult to diagnose because of the absence of clinical symptoms such as fever and frequent false-positive results of technetium bone scans. White blood cell labeled indium-111 radionuclide scans may improve diagnostic accuracy and specificity. False-negative results can be caused by inadequate blood flow to the area or partial antibiotic therapy, and false-positive results can be caused by an associated fracture or malignant neoplasm. Gadolinium-enhanced MRI scans have been shown to be as good as or better than combined technetium-indium scans, with lower cost and better anatomic resolution (Fig. 2). Radiographs usually show cortical irregularity and cystic changes in the bone in patients with chronic osteomyelitis. Final diagnosis is confirmed with histologic analysis of the bone (via surgical or core biopsy) and culture. Aerobic, anaerobic, my-

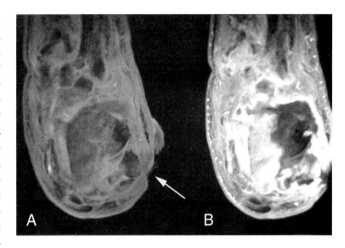

**Figure 2**  Pre- (**A**) and post- (**B**) gadolinium contrast enhancement MRI of the hindfoot showing increased signal in the bone following contrast consistent with osteomyelitis. Note the communicating lateral ulcer in the soft tissue (arrow).

cobacterial, and fungal cultures should always be obtained. Additionally, polymerase chain reaction can be done to identify organisms that may not grow during culture of the bone.

Treatment of chronic osteomyelitis usually involves surgical removal of the involved bone. In the foot, this often necessitates amputation of a digit or part of the foot combined with intravenous antibiotics chosen in accordance with culture analysis. Polymicrobial infections may require combination antibiotic therapy. Prolonged intravenous antibiotic therapy followed by treatment with chronic suppressive oral antibiotics may be required for infections in areas where surgical resection is not feasible.

## Diabetic Infections

Infection of the foot is one of the most common reasons for hospital admissions in diabetic patients. Among such patients, a seemingly minor infection may ultimately lead to partial foot or limb amputation. The incidence of amputation among diabetic patients is approximately 40 times higher than in the general population, with significant cost to the health care system and the economy.

Most foot infections in diabetic patients are preceded by ulceration. The etiology of ulceration and infections is multifactorial. Patients with chronic diabetes (of more than 10 years' duration), poor glucose control, and peripheral neuropathy are at high risk for developing ulceration. Structural foot changes resulting from Charcot neuroarthropathic fractures and collapse or motor neuropathies (often manifesting as Achilles contracture and/or toe clawing), combined with inadequate shoe wear, lead to additional prominences and an increased risk of ulceration. Inadequate blood flow (vascular disease) and localized edema also increase the risk of an ulcer not healing and becoming infected. When these factors are combined with the diminished immune response frequently found in patients with diabetes, infections often develop and may progress rapidly. Early detection of ulcers by frequent self-examination and immediate treatment are essential to prevent deep ulceration and progression to infection.

In most patients, diabetic foot infections are polymicrobial with three to five organisms commonly cultured. Superficial culturing of ulcers and sinuses are of little benefit, with poor correlation to deep tissue cultures. Infecting organisms can include gram-positive cocci (*S aureus* or *Staphylococcus epidermidis*, group B *Streptococcus*, and *Enterococcus*); gram-negative rods (*Proteus, Pseudomonas*, and *Escherichia coli*); and/or anaerobes (*Bacteroides*, anaerobic *Streptococcus*) in severe infections.

Diabetic foot infections can be classified as mild, moderate, or severe (limb or life threatening). Mild infections involve superficial ulceration with minimal cellulitis and no osteomyelitis. Moderate infections involve penetration of the ulcer into the deep tissue with purulent discharge, cellulitis, and the presence of some necrotic tissue, with or without osteomyelitis. These may become limb- or life-threatening if not adequately treated. Severe infections involve deep ulceration with marked necrosis or gangrene, purulent discharge, and systemic toxicity with bacteremia, with or without osteomyelitis. These infections are often life threatening and can lead to toxic shock and death if not treated emergently.

Diagnosis is based on a careful history and physical examination. Identification of or a history of ulceration precedes diabetic foot infections in over 80% of patients and should be carefully sought. Erythema around the ulcer and purulent drainage suggest an infection (malodorous drainage is suggestive of anaerobic infection). The ulcer should be probed under sterile conditions for its depth and the presence of a sinus that could reach bone. Exposed bone or an ulcer penetrating to bone is consistent with osteomyelitis in 80% of patients. In the absence of an ulcer, an acute neuroarthropathic (Charcot) process can easily be confused with an acute infection. An elevation test can be useful in distinguishing between these two pathologies. Swelling and erythema decrease markedly in the presence of an active neuroarthropathic process but only minimally in the presence of infection. The skin should also be palpated for crepitus indicative of gas within the soft tissue, suggesting anaerobic infection.

Results of baseline laboratory studies including a complete blood cell count, erythrocyte sedimentation rate, and C-reactive protein level may be normal, but these studies should be done to help determine progression or improvement in the infection with serial testing. As mentioned, superficial culture should be avoided to prevent inappropriate antibiotic choice. With the emergence of new broad-spectrum antibiotics, however, the importance of obtaining deep tissue for culture has diminished because culture-specific treatment has not been shown to improve outcomes compared with broad-

spectrum empiric treatment. Deep tissue culture or biopsies should be reserved for patients undergoing surgical treatment of their infections or with infections that are recalcitrant to treatment.

Imaging studies are indicated to detect abscess formation and osteomyelitis. Plain radiographs are of little benefit in the diagnosis of acute osteomyelitis. Bony changes are not seen radiographically until 10 to 21 days after the onset of bone infection and often even later in the vascularly compromised diabetic population. Abscess formation may be indicated by the presence of air within the soft tissue on plain radiographs of patients with anaerobic infections.

More sophisticated studies such as gadolinium-enhanced MRI or indium-111 labeled leukocyte scanning help confirm or exclude the presence of deep infection. MRI provides superior anatomic clarification of involvement of bone marrow (important in early osteomyelitis) and abscess formation, but it may not be able to differentiate infection from Charcot neuroarthropathic changes and may overstate the extent of the infectious involvement. Indium-111 labeled leukocyte scanning has a very low false-positive rate for infection, but is characterized by poor localization of the area and extent of involvement when infection is present.

An acute diabetic foot infection represents an orthopaedic emergency. Delay in treatment can result in cellulitis developing into an abscess or an area requiring débridement or even amputation. Overzealous interpretation of diagnostic studies should also be avoided. Most diabetic ulcers are not associated with cellulitis nor are they truly infected in a clinical sense. In addition, many neuroarthropathic fractures may mimic acute infections.

Mild infections often respond to first-generation oral cephalosporins, clindamycin, dicloxacillin sodium, or amoxicillin-clavulanic acid treatment. Close monitoring and frequent observation are recommended, and treatment is adjusted depending on the response. Treatment is usually continued for 14 to 21 days. Ulcers are managed with local care, débridement as needed, and protected weight bearing.

Moderate infections are usually polymicrobial and may be limb threatening. Intravenous, broad-spectrum antibiotics are usually required for treatment. Initial treatment usually involves the use of ticarcillin-clavulanate, ampicillin-sulbactam, or piperacillin-tazobactam. Vancomycin or clindamycin can be used for patients who are allergic to penicillin. This regimen should be continued for 4 to 6 weeks depending on the response. Any nonviable tissue or necrotic bone should be surgically débrided and any abscess drained. A partial foot amputation may be required to save more of the limb. Any vascular deficiency should be treated and appropriate consultations ordered to optimize healing.

Severe infections require early and aggressive surgical débridement or amputation of the infected area combined with supportive medical care. Powerful broad-spectrum antibiotics including imipenem-cilastatin; combinations of vancomycin, metronidazole, and aztreonam; or ampicillin-sulbactam with an aminoglycoside should be used in life-threatening situations.

Chronic osteomyelitis is commonly diagnosed in association with nonhealing, benign-appearing diabetic ulcers. Resection of the infected bone (which may be localized) combined with surgical débridement of the ulcer usually results in resolution of the osteomyelitis. An expanded discussion of the diabetic foot is presented in chapter 12.

### Amputations

Recent advances in antibiotic therapy, vascular surgery, and soft-tissue management have resulted in amputations for diabetic infections becoming less radical and partial foot amputations becoming more commonplace and successful. Partial foot amputations may allow the patient to walk without a prosthesis and have a less adverse effect on body image than above- or below-knee amputations. In addition, function is less impaired and less oxygen is required for ambulation.

The optimal level for an amputation must be determined by assessing the soft-tissue coverage, vascular status, and extent of the infection in the involved limb. In the presence of an acute infection, an open guillotine amputation is recommended. The guillotine amputation allows open drainage, removes all necrotic and most if not all of the infected tissue, and allows infections to be treated with antibiotics before definitive closure or revision amputation.

## Fungal Infections

Fungal infection of the toenails (tinea unguium or onychomycosis) is the most prevalent of nail and skin disorders, often involving all 10 toenails. Although painless and fairly benign, onychomycosis often causes concern and frustration because it responds poorly to most treatments. The infected nail has a yellowish white, opaque appearance on a thickened nail plate. Subungual debris may accumulate under the nail, giving the appearance of a double nail. The infection usually begins at the distal aspect of the nail plate and gradually spreads proximally to involve the nail matrix, nail bed, and entire nail plate. The most common infecting organisms are *Trichophyton rubrum* and *Trichophyton mentagrophytes,* although *Candida albicans* can often be cultured from moist subungual debris. Differential diagnoses include lichen planus, psoriatic nails, and posttraumatic nail dystrophy. Diagnosis can be confirmed by placing nail scrapings in a drop of potassium hydroxide on a glass slide, revealing the fungal hyphae coursing through the epidermal cells.

Short of removing the entire nail and nail matrix, definitive treatment for onychomycosis has not been identi-

fied. Palliation with periodic mechanical débridement is the treatment of choice unless too painful for patient tolerance, which is unusual. In early infections when the entire nail is not involved, topical antifungal treatment with miconazole, clotrimazole, ketoconazole, or terbinafine hydrochloride creams may be effective. Treatment with oral ketoconazole or griseofulvin has had limited success and is associated with a high risk of liver toxicity and blood dyscrasias with prolonged use. In addition, high recurrence rates have been reported after administration of these agents was discontinued. Newer oral antifungal agents have an improved safety profile and more clinical efficacy (90%). Itraconazole is effectively administered with a pulsed dosage of 200 mg twice daily for 7 days in each of 3 consecutive months. Drug interactions are potentially hazardous and must be considered when administering itraconazole. Terbinafine hydrochloride is effective only against dermatophytes and is administered for 90 days in single daily doses of 250 mg; however, taste disturbances, agranulocytosis, and liver toxicity have all been reported with treatment.

Permanent surgical removal of the nail (matricectomy) remains the only certain method of eradicating the mycotic nail with severe dystrophy of the nail plate. This procedure is not usually performed, however, unless the nail becomes symptomatic.

### Mycetoma

Mycetoma (or Madura foot) is a local, chronic, slowly progressive infection commonly seen in tropical or subtropical developing countries. It results from either bacterial (actinomycetoma) or fungal (eumycetoma) organisms. The infecting organism is usually *Nocardia*. Initial inoculation occurs via a puncture wound, and the infection spreads along fascial planes throughout the foot. Sinuses that extrude small sulfur granules within their exudates are the hallmark of the disease. These sulfur granules are formed by the coalescence of organisms within the fluid. The infection may invade bone, muscle, and nerve, and the area is prone to secondary bacterial infections. Initial treatment is with antibiotics or antifungal medications, but surgical débridement may be required. Amputation may be required for severe infections.

## Infection Associated With Open Fractures

Appropriate treatment is essential to prevent infection after open fractures. Infection risk depends on the velocity of the injury (amount of soft-tissue damage) and the degree of wound contamination. Débridement of devitalized tissue and irrigation, preferably pulsed irrigation lavage, are indicated in all cases. In all but the most minor wounds, 9 L of irrigation fluid is recommended to wash out any bacteria present in the wound. No benefit has been found in culturing open fracture wounds at the time of an initial washout, with a low correlation between cultured organisms and those found when an infection does develop. Repeated débridements with irrigation may be needed.

Uncontaminated open fractures should be treated prophylactically with first-generation cephalosporins for 24 to 48 hours. In contaminated wounds, the addition of an aminoglycoside or use of a third-generation cephalosporin is indicated. In farm- or soil-contaminated wounds (including lawnmower injuries), anaerobic coverage with penicillin or clindamycin is additionally used. Routine washouts with the patient under adequate anesthesia should be done every 48 hours until the wound is clean and all devitalized tissue has been removed. Antibiotic therapy should be continued for 48 hours following each washout.

Uncontaminated small "inside-out" fractures (Gustilo type I) can be treated with routine internal fixation after adequate irrigation and débridement. More contaminated wounds and those with soft-tissue loss (Gustilo types II and III) should be immobilized with an external fixator until a clean, stable wound is achieved; internal fixation then can be done as needed.

Development of infection associated with an open fracture should be treated with immediate drainage of the wound area, débridement of devitalized tissue, irrigation of the wound, and appropriate antibiotic treatment. Internal hardware usually should be removed. Stabilization with an external fixator may be required until adequate fracture healing occurs.

## Summary

Most foot infections, if diagnosed early, can be successfully treated with antibiotic or antifungal medications. Chronic or severe infection may require surgical drainage, débridement, or even amputation. Foot infections in patients with diabetes or peripheral vascular disease must be carefully monitored and aggressively treated to avoid limb- or life-threatening situations.

## Annotated Bibliography

### Nondiabetic Infections

Ledermann HP, Morrison WB, Schweitzer ME: Is soft-tissue inflammation in pedal infection contained by fascial planes? MR analysis of compartmental involvement in 115 feet. *AJR Am J Roentgenol* 2002;178:605-612.

This article presents a review of 115 contrast-enhanced MRI examinations of the foot in patients who underwent surgery for osteomyelitis. Soft-tissue inflammation of the forefoot tends to spread but hindfoot inflammation tends to stay confined to one compartment.

Ledermann HP, Morrison WB, Schweitzer ME, et al: Tendon involvement in pedal infection: MR analysis of frequency, distribution, and spread of infection. *AJR Am J Roentgenol* 2002;179:939-947.

MRI evidence of tendon infection is present in approximately half of the patients who require surgery for pedal infection. Evidence of spread of the infection along tendons is seen infrequently on MRI. Detection of a tendon infection could influence surgical therapy.

Lombardi CM, Silver LM, Lau KK, et al: Necrotizing fasciitis in the lower extremity: A review and case presentation. *J Foot Ankle Surg* 2000;39:244-248.

Necrotizing fasciitis is a rare but potentially fatal disease that is often confused with cellulitis. Emphasis is placed on the necessity of surgical débridement in combination with antibiotic therapy to minimize the possible morbidity associated with this condition.

### Diabetic Infections

Cunha BA: Antibiotic selection for diabetic foot infections: A review. *J Foot Ankle Surg* 2000;39:253-257.

Most soft-tissue diabetic foot infections are polymicrobial. Factors to consider in antibiotic selection include the severity of the infection, the presence of peripheral vascular disease, and the possibility of drug-resistant organisms. This review summarizes the clinical presentation and antimicrobial therapy of diabetic foot infections.

Diamantopoulos EJ, Haritos D, Yfandi G, et al: Management and outcome of severe diabetic foot infections. *Exp Clin Endocrinol Diabetes* 1998;106:346-352.

Unfavorable prognostic factors for diabetic foot infections are an ankle systolic blood pressure of < 50 mm Hg or toe systolic blood pressure of < 30 mm Hg and TcPo$_2$ < 20 mm Hg.

Eneroth M, Apelqvist J, Stenstrom A: Clinical characteristics and outcome in 223 diabetic patients with deep foot infections. *Foot Ankle Int* 1997;18:716-722.

This clinical review found that nearly all diabetic patients with a deep foot infection needed surgery and more than one third had a minor amputation before healing or death.

Lipsky BA, Berendt AR: Principles and practice of antibiotic therapy of diabetic foot infections. *Diabetes Metab Res Rev* 2000;16(suppl 1):S42-S46.

Antibiotic regimens are usually selected empirically, initially using broad-spectrum antibiotics and then modified depending on the results of culture and sensitivity tests and the patient's clinical response.

Mantey I, Hill RL, Foster AV, et al: Infection of foot ulcers with Staphylococcus aureus associated with increased mortality in diabetic patients. *Commun Dis Public Health* 2000;3:288-290.

Diabetic patients with foot ulceration have a poorer prognosis than those without ulceration. Infection with *S aureus* resulted in 52% mortality compared with 20% in those whose ulcers were not infected with *S aureus*.

Saltzman CL, Pedowitz WJ: Diabetic foot infections. *Instr Course Lect* 1999;48:317-320.

A detailed review of diabetic foot infection management is presented.

Shea KW: Antimicrobial therapy for diabetic foot infections: A practical approach. *Postgrad Med* 1999;106:85-86, 89-94.

Optimal management requires a multidisciplinary approach. Aggressive surgical débridement and wound management, carefully chosen antimicrobial therapy, and modification of host factors are recommended.

Snyder RJ, Cohen MM, Sun C, et al: Osteomyelitis in the diabetic patient: Diagnosis and treatment. Part 1: Overview, diagnosis, and microbiology. *Ostomy Wound Manage* 2001;47:18-22.

This article discusses the diagnosis and microbiology of osteomyelitis in the diabetic foot.

Snyder RJ, Cohen MM, Sun C, et al: Osteomyelitis in the diabetic patient: Diagnosis and treatment. Part 2: Medical, surgical, and alternative treatments. *Ostomy Wound Manage* 2001;47:24-30.

This article outlines the various medical, antibiotic, and surgical options available to the physician. Adjunctive and alternative therapies also are discussed.

Tennvall GR, Apelqvist J, Eneroth M: Costs of deep foot infections in patients with diabetes mellitus. *Pharmacoeconomics* 2000;18:225-238.

This article reports that topical treatment accounts for the largest proportion of total treatment costs and that the most important cost-driving factors are wound healing duration and repeated surgery. The cost of antibacterial treatment, however, should not be used as a factor when choosing between early amputation and conservative treatment.

### Fungal Infections

Bending A: Fungal nail infections: Far more than an aesthetic problem. *Br J Community Nurs* 2002;7:254-259.

This review article discusses the causes and types of onychomycosis and examines in detail the various treatments available.

Cribier BJ, Paul C: Long-term efficacy of antifungals in toenail onychomycosis: A critical review. *Br J Dermatol* 2001;145:446-452.

In this article, long-term efficacy achieved with the use of terbinafine hydrochloride is reported to be superior to that obtained with griseofulvin, ketoconazole, fluconazole, or itraconazole therapy.

Gupta AK: Types of onychomycosis. *Cutis* 2001;68(suppl 2):4-7.

Onychomycosis may be classified into several types: distal subungual, white superficial, proximal subungual, endonyx, and total dystrophic. Diagnosis and treatment are discussed.

## Classic Bibliography

Anger DM, Ledbetter BR, Stasikelis PJ, et al: Injuries of the foot related to the use of lawn mowers. *J Bone Joint Surg Am* 1995;77:719-725.

Fitzgerald RH Jr, Cowan JD: Puncture wounds of the foot. *Orthop Clin North Am* 1975;6:965-972.

Green NE, Bruno J III: Pseudomonas infections of the foot after puncture wounds. *South Med J* 1980;73:146-149.

Gustilo RB, Anderson JT: Prevention of infection in the treatment of one thousand and twenty-five open fractures of long bones: Retrospective and prospective analyses. *J Bone Joint Surg Am* 1976;58:453-458.

Loeffler RD Jr, Ballard A: Plantar fascial spaces of the foot and a proposed surgical approach. *Foot Ankle* 1980;1:11-14.

Riegler HF, Routson GW: Complications of deep puncture wounds of the foot. *J Trauma* 1979;19:18-22.

# Chapter 20

# Clinical Biomechanics of the Foot and Ankle

Vincent James Sammarco, MD

Jorge I. Acevedo, MD

## Introduction

The foot is a complex and dynamic structure that provides a stable base for standing, walking, and running on even or irregular surfaces. Its functions during weight bearing include balance, shock absorption, and propulsion. The study of biomechanics of the foot and ankle is integral to the understanding of their normal function and pathologies. The functions of the foot and ankle are interrelated in such a way that disruption of the normal mechanics of one structure often leads to significant dysfunction of the entire extremity. Alterations in muscle function resulting from weakness, spasticity, degeneration, or injury can directly affect the alignment of the foot during gait and standing, and such alterations can have profound effects on not only foot and ankle function, but also on the kinematics of the knees, hips, and spine. Similarly, abnormal bony architecture caused by congenital malformation, tarsal coalition, fracture, or arthritis can alter alignment and cause significant morbidity. The development of biomechanical models of the foot and ankle in normal and disease states, along with the development and improvement of various position and force-sensing devices, has led to an increased understanding of the biomechanics of the foot and ankle and provided insight into the structures involved with various disease states. This chapter reviews the mechanics and kinematics of the foot and ankle and relates them to the functional requirements of ambulation. Also included are clinical examples of how selected surgical procedures use these principles to improve biomechanical function.

## Gait

Normal walking speed averages 60 cycles per minute. The cycle begins and ends with subsequent heel strike of the same foot. Stride is the distance of one cycle in the same limb. The foot is in contact with the ground for approximately 60% of each cycle during the stance phase. The body is supported by both limbs during the initial 12% and final 12% of stance phase. Limb advancement occurs during the swing phase, which constitutes the final 40% of each cycle. Increased speed diminishes the period of double limb support, and running involves a float phase during which neither foot is in contact with the ground.

Three functions are completed in each cycle of gait: weight acceptance, single limb support, and advancement of the limb. Motions of the hip and knee are important in considering each of these functions, although an in-depth discussion is beyond the scope of this chapter. Coupled motions exist between the ankle and subtalar and transverse tarsal (talonavicular and calcaneocuboid) joints during the stance phase, and these motions change the shape and rigidity of the foot during weight acceptance and push-off. The functional anatomy of the plantar aponeurosis, the hallucal metatarsophalangeal (MTP) joint, and the lesser MTP joints is also important.

The extremity undergoes progressive internal rotation from the moment of heel strike to foot flat and then undergoes progressive external rotation as the contralateral limb swings to clear the ground and advance. Muscle and joint function can be considered in three intervals during the stance phase (Fig. 1).

The first interval occurs from heel strike to foot flat and is characterized by acceptance of impact forces and deceleration of the foot. At heel strike, ankle plantar flexion occurs. Following initial contact, rapid dorsiflexion of the ankle occurs as the momentum of the body's mass progresses forward. Active eccentric contraction of the anterior compartment muscles decelerates the foot as it rolls into foot flat. During this time, the posterior musculature is inactive. Progressive eversion of the subtalar joint in the first 15% of stance is coupled to ankle dorsiflexion and internal tibial rotation. Subtalar eversion brings the axis of the talonavicular and calcaneocuboid joints into parallel alignment, increasing the amount of motion that can occur through the midfoot for shock absorption. Anatomic structures important in weight acceptance during the first interval include the unique, septated fat pads of the heel; the glabrous plantar surface of the foot; and the viscoelastic properties of the plantar fascia and intertarsal ligaments that support the longitudinal arch.

The second interval occurs as the body's center of mass progresses over the foot, with the foot gradually ac-

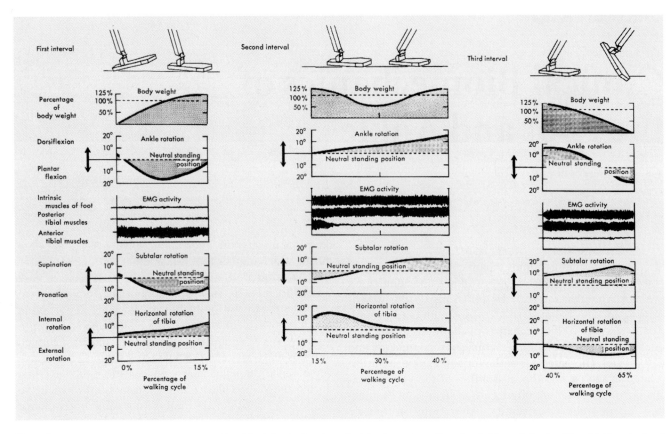

**Figure 1** Summary of kinematics and electromyographic activity during the three intervals of the stance phase. *(Reproduced with permission from Mann RA: Biomechanics of the foot and ankle, in Mann RA, Coughlin MJ (eds): Surgery of the Foot and Ankle, ed 6. St. Louis, MO, Mosby-Year Book, 1993, pp 29-31.)*

cepting more of the body's weight while beginning to translate that force into forward motion. Eccentric muscle contraction of the posterior compartments of the leg act to decelerate the tibia and stabilize the midfoot and ankle. Progressive dorsiflexion of the ankle occurs and maximal dorsiflexion is reached slightly after the heel lifts. External rotation of the tibia occurs as a result of swing from the contralateral limb. Subtalar inversion occurs progressively through coupled motions of tibial rotation, ankle dorsiflexion, and tightening of the plantar fascia. Contraction of the posterior tibialis and Achilles complex also acts to invert the subtalar joint, which locks the midfoot and creates a stable lever arm for push-off.

During the third interval, the ankle undergoes progressive, active plantar flexion. The posterior musculature contracts, pushing the body forward. The subtalar joint continues to invert in response to activity of the plantar flexors and posterior tibialis. Tightening of the plantar fascia through the windlass mechanism raises the arch, inverts the subtalar joint, and stabilizes the midfoot joints. The axis of the MTP break (the roll of the foot onto the metatarsal heads during the final phase of gait and toe-off) also contributes to foot supination. Posterior compartment muscle activity ceases at 50% of the gait cycle, and the anterior compartment begins to contract concentrically, clearing the foot from the ground as the foot enters the swing phase.

## Articular Anatomy and Kinematics
### Ankle
The ankle joint involves the tibiotalar, tibiofibular, and talofibular articulations, which function together to allow rotation and translation in multiple planes. The bimalleolar axis angles obliquely 82° (± 4°) medial to lateral in the coronal plane and defines the primary motion of the ankle. Modeling of the ankle as a simple hinge angled obliquely is helpful in understanding its function during gait. With the foot free and the leg fixed, dorsiflexion causes lateral deviation of the foot, and during plantar flexion, the foot deviates internally (Fig. 2). With the foot fixed, the obliquity of the ankle joint causes internal rotation of the tibia with plantar flexion and external rotation with dorsiflexion.

The concept of the ankle as a single-axis hinge is an oversimplification because the normal joint has significant freedom in translation and axial rotation. The anatomy of the talus is such that the articular surface is wider anteriorly than posteriorly and wider superiorly than inferiorly. A central sulcus bordered by medial and lateral talar dome eminences is present when the tibiotalar joint is viewed in the coronal plane. The diameter and axes of the medial and lateral talar dome are different. Anatomic data provided early evidence of the complex motion that occurs in the tibiotalar joint. Early models of ankle mo-

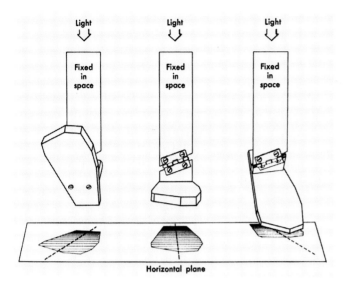

**Figure 2** The effect of the oblique orientation of the ankle joint on foot position with dorsiflexion and plantar flexion. *(Reproduced with permission from Mann RA: Biomechanics of the foot and ankle, in Mann RA, Coughlin MJ (eds): Surgery of the Foot and Ankle, ed 6. St. Louis, MO, Mosby-Year Book, 1993, p 17.)*

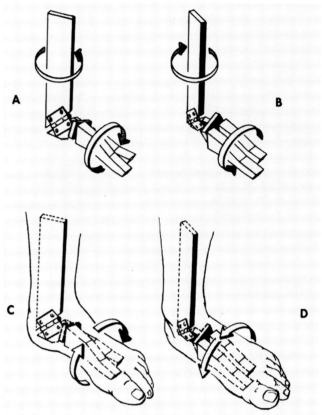

**Figure 3** The subtalar joint modeled as a mitered hinge. Rotation of the tibia causes inversion **(A)** and eversion **(B)** of the subtalar joint, and supination **(C)** and pronation **(D)** of the forefoot. *(Reproduced with permission from Mann RA: Biomechanics of the foot and ankle, in Mann RA, Coughlin MJ (eds): Surgery of the Foot and Ankle, ed 6. St. Louis, MO, Mosby-Year Book, 1993, p 21.)*

tion used a single fixed axis of rotation, and this proved useful for functional modeling during gait. However, the concept of a changing instantaneous center of rotation evolved when more accurate measurement devices became available.

Current data indicate that significant freedom of the talus within the mortise occurs throughout the entire range of motion. The contact area of the dome of the talus increases and moves anteriorly with increasing dorsiflexion. A recent study using intra-articular force sensors verified that load transmission in the medial and lateral facets increases with dorsiflexion. Conflicting data exist as to the exact path of the talar articular contact during gait, but there is increasing evidence that the talus follows a separate path in dorsiflexion than in plantar flexion.

The tibiofibular joint appears to have more function than a simple rigid support to the lateral ankle. Dorsiflexion of the ankle results in external rotation of the fibula with relation to the tibia. Other coupled motions include lateral and anterior translation with dorsiflexion. The fibula participates in static load transmission from the talus during weight bearing, but this varies depending on the position of the ankle, with increasing loads accompanying dorsiflexion. Proximal migration of the fibula occurs with dorsiflexion, and the fibula may be pulled distally during plantar flexion to deepen the mortise and add stability as tibiotalar contact decreases.

## Subtalar and Transverse Tarsal Joints
The subtalar, talonavicular, and calcaneocuboid joints functionally act in concert through a series of coupled motions to create inversion and eversion of the hindfoot

and to lock and unlock the midfoot for different phases of stance. The subtalar joint has been modeled as a single-axis hinge, which is useful in defining its function during gait. The functional axis of the joint passes from posterior to anterior medially to laterally at approximately 16° and from inferiorly to superiorly at approximately 41°. Substantial variation occurs among individuals both in the orientation of the joint and the amount of inversion and eversion. It has been suggested that the anatomy of the subtalar joint causes coupled anterior and posterior translation of the entire calcaneus through a screw-like mechanism, with anterior translation occurring during inversion. A recent study suggests that motion of the subtalar joint cannot be described about a single axis and that during loaded inversion and eversion, the joint follows different axes.

The coupled motions of the subtalar joint with the tibia have been modeled as a miter joint connected with a hinge (Fig. 3). This model effectively describes the relationship of tibial rotation to subtalar inversion and eversion as well as foot supination and pronation. Internal rotation of the tibia causes eversion of the calcaneus and pronation of the foot, and external rotation causes inversion and supination.

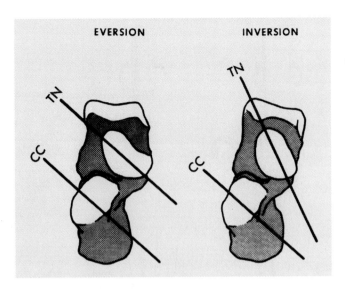

**Figure 4** Eversion and inversion of the subtalar joint locks and unlocks the transverse tarsal joint by aligning or deviating the major joint axes of the talonavicular (TN) and calcaneocuboid (CC) joints. *(Reproduced with permission from Mann RA: Biomechanics of the foot and ankle, in Mann RA, Coughlin MJ (eds): Surgery of the Foot and Ankle, ed 6. St. Louis, MO, Mosby-Year Book, 1993, p 23.)*

The talonavicular and calcaneocuboid joints function together as the transverse tarsal or Chopart's joint. The motions of these joints are affected by the position of the subtalar joint, which controls the orientation of the talonavicular and calcaneocuboid joint axes. With the subtalar joint everted, which typically accompanies the first 15% of stance phase, the major joint axes of the talonavicular and transverse tarsal joints are parallel. This allows significant motion through the transverse tarsal joint and creates flexibility through the midfoot for shock absorption and accommodation for irregular terrain. Progressive external rotation of the tibia and dorsiflexion of the ankle as the limb progresses through the gait cycle causes inversion of the subtalar joint through the mitered hinge mechanism. The change in alignment of the talus and calcaneus that accompanies inversion causes convergence of the talonavicular and calcaneocuboid joint axes, effectively locking the midfoot and creating a more efficient lever arm for push-off (Fig. 4).

Recent studies have investigated the amount of residual motion in the subtalar and transverse tarsal joints after isolated and combined arthrodeses. Isolated arthrodesis of the calcaneocuboid joint had little effect on subtalar or talonavicular joint motion. Subtalar arthrodesis diminished motion of the talonavicular and calcaneocuboid joints but still allowed dorsal and plantar flexion. Arthrodesis of the talonavicular joint dramatically decreased motion at both the subtalar and calcaneocuboid joints, demonstrating that talonavicular joint motion is highly coupled in its role during hindfoot function, particularly to the subtalar joint.

## Intertarsal and Tarsometatarsal Joints

In the normal foot, little motion occurs through the naviculocuneiform or intercuneiform articulations. Tradition-ally, the Lisfranc joint complex has also been considered to have little motion. The first tarsometatarsal (TMT) joint undergoes 3° to 4° of flexion and extension and has little motion in rotation or adduction-abduction. Hypermobility of the first TMT joint has been implicated in forefoot pathology. The fourth and fifth TMT joints have significantly greater mobility. More recently, the concept of a relatively rigid midfoot was questioned in a study that demonstrated significant variations between forefoot and hindfoot supination and pronation during progression through stance phase. This study inferred that significant motion must occur through the midfoot joint complexes to account for the variations between the forefoot and hindfoot positions at various phases of stance.

A recent anatomic study confirmed a three-level ligamentous arrangement within the TMT joint complex: dense plantar and intra-articular ligamentous constraints and a less dense dorsal ligamentous complex. Strength and stiffness testing of the TMT ligaments has demonstrated that the Lisfranc ligament is significantly stronger than the plantar ligamentous complex (which is significantly stronger than the dorsal ligamentous complex). The plantar first metatarsal-cuneiform ligament is the main restraint to dorsal angulation of the first metatarsal.

Another recent study investigated force transmission in the TMT joints with varying loads and at different foot positions. The third TMT joint was shown to bear the highest loads for all positions and loads and functioned as the keystone to force transmission through the midfoot. This is in contrast to traditional descriptions of the second TMT joint as the primary joint responsible for force transmission. Two mechanisms were described for force transmission. At low loads, contact area increased so that pressure distribution among the joints remained relatively constant. At higher loads, a mechanism involving transfer of force from the second and third TMT joints to the first and fourth-fifth TMT complexes was demonstrated. The flexibility of the first and fourth-fifth TMT complexes aids in balance and in dissipating force overloads during increased loads or radical changes in foot position.

## MTP Joints

Although significant variation exists, the second metatarsal head is typically the most distal and the fifth metatarsal head is the most proximal, creating an axis of 50° to 70°. As the foot rolls onto the metatarsal heads during the final phase of gait and toe-off, this relationship, termed the MTP break, causes coupled motions of external rotation of the tibia and inversion of the subtalar joint. Dorsiflexion of the MTP joints during push-off also acts to tighten the plantar fascia through the windlass mechanism, further inverting the hindfoot and raising the longitudinal arch. These motions during the final phase of gait act to stiffen the midfoot for a rigid platform at push-off through locking of the transverse tarsal joint.

The hallux MTP joint has been studied extensively. Normal range of motion is 30° of plantar flexion to 90° of dorsiflexion. A recent clinical study indicates that a range of motion of approximately 42° is necessary for normal gait on flat terrain. Weight bearing is actually on the sesamoids, rather than directly on the metatarsal head. The instantaneous center of rotation falls within the metatarsal head and moves dorsally with dorsiflexion. Contact area moves dorsally and diminishes substantially with dorsiflexion, which may explain why degenerative conditions of the first MTP joint tend to occur dorsally. Degenerative conditions and hallux valgus have been shown to dramatically alter the normal gliding motion of the joint and increase compression and axial load dorsally as the foot progresses into toe-off.

## Arches of the Foot

Traditionally, three arches have been described in the foot. The medial longitudinal arch consists of the first, second, and third metatarsals, the cuneiforms, navicular, talus, and calcaneus. A lesser longitudinal arch consists of the fourth and fifth metatarsals, cuboid, and calcaneus. The transverse arch spans the midfoot and across the midtarsal joints, with the second or third metatarsal base acting as a keystone to prevent collapse.

Support for the medial longitudinal arch of the foot can be described using two models, and it appears that both mechanisms are important during stance. The beam model describes the arch as a curved, segmented beam that is supported by densely connected joints. Weight applied to the arch is supported at the heel and forefoot, and applied load generates compression dorsally and tension plantarly. Clinically, this corresponds to the longitudinal arch, which is made up of the metatarsals, midfoot tarsal bones, talus, and calcaneus. As weight is applied from the leg onto the talus during standing, the forces are distributed primarily through the heel and metatarsal heads, with tension generated through the dense plantar ligaments found at the TMT, intertarsal, and talonavicular joints. Compression occurs dorsally through the bony structures (Fig. 5).

The truss model describes the arch as two beams connected superiorly by a pivot and inferiorly with a tie rod (Fig. 6). As load is applied to the beams, compression is generated in the beams, tension is generated in the tie rod, and the load is supported. Lapidus used the tie-rod model to describe the plantar fascia and the hinged-beam model to describe the tarsal bones. The plantar fascia, which is attached proximally to the calcaneus and distally to the plantar MTP capsules, is the tie rod. As load is applied from the leg through the talus, compression is generated in the tarsal bones, and the arch is supported as tension is generated in the plantar fascia.

These models account for only static support of the longitudinal arch. During gait, dynamic elevation of the

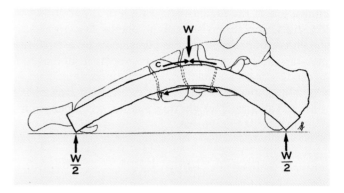

**Figure 5** Beam model of the medial longitudinal arch. Compression is generated dorsally through the tarsal bones and tension is generated in the plantar intertarsal ligaments. W = body weight, C = compression, W/2 = ½ body weight. *(Reproduced with permission from Sarrafian SK: Anatomy of the Foot and Ankle: Descriptive, Topographic, Functional, ed 2. Philadelphia, PA, Lippincott-Williams & Wilkins, 1993, p 560.)*

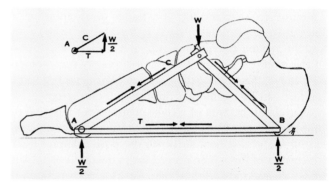

**Figure 6** Truss model of the medial longitudinal arch. Load is applied through the talus and generates compression through the tarsal bones and tension though the plantar fascia. A and B = attachment points of the plantar fascia (or the rod) in the truss model, C = compression, T = tension, W = body weight, W/2 = ½ body weight. *(Reproduced with permission from Sarrafian SK: Anatomy of the Foot and Ankle: Descriptive, Topographic, Functional, ed 2. Philadelphia, PA, Lippincott-Williams & Wilkins, 1993, p 559.)*

longitudinal arch is observed as the foot progresses toward toe-off. Passive elevation of the longitudinal arch occurs through the windlass effect, in which dorsiflexion of the toes occurs during heel rise and toe-off. Because the plantar fascia is tethered distally to the MTP joint capsules, dorsiflexion of the digits tightens the plantar fascia and raises the arch. The posterior tibialis tendon and to a lesser extent the long and short flexors of the toes also contribute to active elevation of the arch and inversion of the hindfoot during the stance phase and push-off.

Both the truss and beam models of the longitudinal arch are important in understanding the dynamics and function of the foot. Pathology of the longitudinal arch can cause significant foot dysfunction and frequently involves both mechanisms for arch support. The importance of the plantar fascia in longitudinal arch support was recently demonstrated in a cadaver study in which all or part of the fascia was transected. Division of the plantar fascia resulted in depression of the longitudinal arch and elongation of the medial base length of the foot during loading. Complete division of the plantar fascia was also shown to dramatically increase tensile loads through the metatarsals, demonstrating that as support from the truss is lost, the beam mechanism becomes more important in providing support to the arch. Compressive stress fractures and abnormal weight transmission accompany complete plantar fascia release.

## Biomechanics of Plantar Force Transmission
### Normal Pedobarograph
Analysis of foot biomechanics requires knowledge of the force distribution under the foot during normal standing and walking. Multiple devices have been developed to measure plantar pressures. The most common methods involve measurement of pressure between the foot and a force plate or between the foot and an insole sensor. These devices can produce a dynamic representation of the net force (vertical + shear forces) between the foot and the ground. Shear forces, which may cause ulceration in the neuropathic foot, are not adequately represented with the standard force plate systems. The center of force path or gait line combines information on the center of pressure and the area of weight bearing over a period of time during the stance phase. The normal center of pressure line starts at heel strike on the posterolateral heel. The center of force then progresses to the midfoot, moves under the second and third metatarsal, and terminates at the lateral border of the great toe with toe-off. Recent studies have noted a lack of medialization of force within the forefoot in the latter half of stance phase. The slowing of the gait line in the forefoot reflects the large contribution of the central metatarsal heads to weight bearing at 60% to 80% of stance phase.

### Peak Pressures
Peak pressure measurements can be a useful tool in differentiating normal from pathologic gait. During the normal gait cycle, the heel absorbs most of the load with a peak force of 80% of body weight at the beginning of the stance phase. By mid-stance these forces are distributed between the heel and the second and third metatarsals. In terminal stance phase, the hallux sustains a peak load up to 22% of body weight. Recent data suggest that the central metatarsals bear the primary propulsive forces in terminal stance phase.

It is important to realize that peak pressure measurements are dependent on several factors, some inherent to the measurement device itself. Systems vary depending on the number, size, resolution, and wear threshold of sensor cells. The type of shoe, heel height, and sole contour influence data from in-shoe devices. For example, softer, more flexible shoes decrease plantar pressures. A rocker-bottom sole can decrease peak pressures up to 30% in the forefoot, and a higher heel may increase these loads.

Peak pressures vary significantly depending on gait speed and direction. Pressures under the great toe, for instance, can be 50% greater when turning a corner compared with walking a straight line. Because of these factors, it is difficult to compare results from different pedobarographic systems. Relative peak pressures rather than absolute peak pressures appear to be more clinically relevant.

## Pathologic Entities and Changes in Force Transmission
### Diabetes and Ulceration
High peak pressures are a known risk factor for ulceration in the insensate foot. Patients with diabetes often develop neuropathy and subsequent structural deformities with associated decreased joint mobility, leading to increased plantar pressures and the likelihood of ulceration. Pressures as low as 30 $N/cm^2$ have been shown to initiate formation of ulcers in neuropathic patients. Diabetic patients with Charcot arthropathy and neuropathic ulcers have higher peak plantar pressures than patients without neuropathy or ulceration. Because of the large variability in the literature regarding threshold pressures for ulceration, it is difficult to screen patients with a "critical" value above which they are at risk for skin breakdown. Factors such as shoe wear, level of activity, deformity, repetitive stresses, and joint mobility must be taken into account. Biomechanical data have shown that peak pressures in the forefoot are decreased by Achilles tendon lengthening. Abnormalities in the integument, such as hard calluses, can increase localized pressure by as much as 30%. Repetitive stresses (cyclic loading) at relatively normal plantar pressures may also result in skin breakdown.

### Flatfoot Deformity
Many studies have investigated the biomechanics of flatfoot deformity. These studies have improved the understanding of the consequences of weakening certain anatomic structures. For example, sequential sectioning of the plantar fascia, plantar ligaments, and spring ligament may progressively destabilize the arch of the foot. Similar changes occur when the posterior tibial tendon is weakened or ruptured. The changes observed include plantar flexion and internal rotation of the talus, eversion and internal rotation of the calcaneus, and eversion of the navicular and cuboid. Eversion of the calcaneus results in pronation of the forefoot and increases load in the first metatarsal, talonavicular, and naviculocuneiform joints.

Collapse of the medial longitudinal arch produces a malalignment of the joint surfaces that alters the peak pressures and contact characteristics of the tibiotalar joint. As the hindfoot progresses into valgus, there is a 35% reduction in contact area as well as a posterior and lateral shift in the peak contact pressures. Although the mean ankle joint pressures are also increased, this does

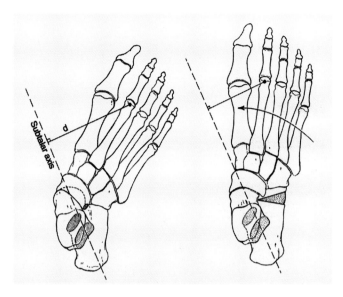

**Figure 7** Diagrams illustrating the preoperative **(A)** and postoperative **(B)** correction of the abduction deformity associated with congenital and acquired pes planovalgus using lateral column lengthening through the calcaneus. *(Reproduced with permission from Otis JC: Clinical and applied biomechanics, in Myerson MS (ed): Foot and Ankle Disorders. Philadelphia, PA, WB Saunders, 2000, p 192.)*

not occur in proportion to the decrease in contact area. A recent study demonstrated that patients with acquired flatfoot deformity have diminished ankle joint contact area and lateral subluxation of the subtalar joint complex.

### Cavovarus Deformity

Cavovarus deformity most frequently accompanies neuromuscular disease but may also be caused by trauma or by congenital conditions. The most common condition causing cavovarus deformity is Charcot-Marie-Tooth disease, in which weakness involving the tibialis anterior, peroneus brevis, and intrinsic muscles of the foot lead to alterations in foot mechanics resulting from unopposed antagonistic muscles. Weakness of the tibialis anterior tendon allows plantar flexion of the first ray by overpull of the peroneus longus tendon. Diminished peroneus brevis power allows forefoot adduction by the posterior tibial tendon, and intrinsic muscle weakness causes clawing of the lesser digits.

Structural deformities in the cavovarus foot cause alterations in force transmission during the gait cycle. Pedobarographic studies show lateralization of the gait line and increased pressures along the lateral border of the foot. Varus positioning of the calcaneus produces instability at the ankle joint during heel strike. Calcaneal inversion locks the transverse tarsal joints, leading to diminished flexibility of the foot during weight acceptance. Inversion of the subtalar joint causes forefoot supination and increased load transmission in the fourth and fifth metatarsals and calcaneocuboid joints. Clinical symptoms usually involve ankle instability, stress fractures of the lateral column, and difficulty with shoe wear.

## Biomechanical Effects of Surgical Procedures

### Calcaneal Osteotomy

Medial displacement calcaneal osteotomy is often used in conjunction with other procedures for the correction of flatfoot deformity. Sliding the calcaneal tuberosity medially shifts the Achilles force vector, creating an adduction moment at the subtalar joint complex. Similarly, the ground reaction force is shifted closer to the mechanical axis of the leg, decreasing torque forces at the subtalar joint. Biomechanical data have also shown unloading of the medial supporting structures, with decreased tension of the spring ligament and deltoid ligament during the stance phase. A recent study demonstrated that even substantial medialization causes only small changes in pressure distribution in the subtalar and tibiotalar joints, which should not cause degeneration.

Lateral column lengthening has also been used to correct forefoot abduction and improve arch height in patients with flatfoot deformity. Abduction of the forefoot creates an increased eversion moment, resulting in greater strain on the medial soft-tissue restraints (Fig. 7). The lateral column can be lengthened by creating an osteotomy between the anterior and middle facets of the calcaneus. The distal fragment is distracted, and a 1- to 1.5-cm bone block is placed into the osteotomy to maintain length. The effect is to medialize the moment arm of the forefoot-ground reaction force relative to the subtalar axis and to restore alignment of the talonavicular joint, which is usually subluxated laterally. Subsequent realignment of the joints restores the forefoot-ground as well as the heel-ground reaction forces. Biomechanical studies of lateral column lengthening of the intact foot have not shown the decreased tension in the spring ligament observed with the medial calcaneal sliding osteotomy. Concerns have been raised about using this osteotomy in adults because of its intra-articular positioning and the possibility of postoperative arthrosis of the subtalar and calcaneocuboid joints. One study demonstrated increased calcaneocuboid joint pressure after osteotomy, but a recent study demonstrated that in a flatfoot model, calcaneocuboid joint pressures were not increased above normal. In light of recent studies demonstrating minimal loss of motion at the subtalar and talonavicular joints after calcaneocuboid arthrodesis, some authors have recommended lengthening of the lateral column through distraction and arthrodesis of the calcaneocuboid joint to achieve the same biomechanical effects without the risk of subtalar or calcaneocuboid arthrosis.

### Tendon Transfer

Basic biomechanical principles of tendon transfer should be considered to ensure a satisfactory result. The most important parameters with regard to eventual joint motion are strength, excursion, moment arm, and phasic activity of the muscle to be transferred. Muscle strength

**TABLE 1 | Relative Strength and Excursion of the Extrinsic Muscles Acting On the Foot and Ankle**

| Tendon | Strength (Relative) | Excursion (cm) |
| --- | --- | --- |
| Tibialis anterior | 5.6 | 2.9 |
| Extensor digitorum longus | 1.7 | 3.1 |
| Extensor hallucis longus | 1.2 | 2.4 |
| Tibialis posterior | 6.4 | 1.6 |
| Flexor hallucis longus | 3.6 | 1.7 |
| Flexor digitorum longus | 1.8 | 1.2 |
| Achilles | 49.1 | 4.0 |
| Peroneus brevis | 2.6 | 1.4 |
| Peroneus longus | 5.5 | 1.6 |
| Peroneus tertius | 0.9 | |

*Reproduced with permission from Armegan, Ospe, Shereff M: Tendon injury and repair, in Myerson MS (ed): Foot and Ankle Disorders. Philadelphia, PA, WB Saunders, 2000, p 948.*

must be powerful enough to tolerate the expected loss of one grade that usually occurs in a transfer. The relative strength and excursion of the muscle to be transferred should be compared with those of the tendon being replaced (Table 1). Estimates of excursion are useful, but the final joint motion ultimately depends on the axis of rotation under consideration. The moment arm, or distance from the tendon pull to the center of rotation of the joint it crosses (force × distance), can be approximated by understanding the relationship of each muscle to the joint axes of the foot and ankle (Fig. 8). This allows the function of each tendon in coronal and sagittal joint motion of the foot to be determined. All muscles posterior to the ankle axis contribute to a different extent to plantar flexion based on their distance from the ankle axis, and those muscles anterior to the ankle axis (tibialis anterior, extensor hallucis longus, and extensor digitorum longus) function in dorsiflexion. Muscles medial and lateral to the subtalar axis invert (tibialis anterior and posterior, flexor digitorum longus [FDL] and flexor hallucis longus) or evert (extensor hallucis longus, extensor digitorum longus, and peroneus longus and brevis) the foot. Optimal transfer depends on having similar phasic activity between the muscle transferred and the muscle that is replaced. Nonphasic transfers generally limit joint mobility and may cause a tenodesis effect.

FDL transfer with calcaneal osteotomy for posterior tibial tendon insufficiency illustrates the application of these principles. The FDL is in phase with the posterior tibial tendon. Harvest of the FDL and transfer to the plantar and medial aspects of the navicular re-creates the moment arm of the dysfunctional posterior tibial tendon. The FDL has approximately 30% of the posterior tibial tendon strength and relatively less excursion, making isolated transfer prone to failure. Realignment of the hindfoot and/or forefoot can improve functional results by diminishing the loads required during weight bearing. A

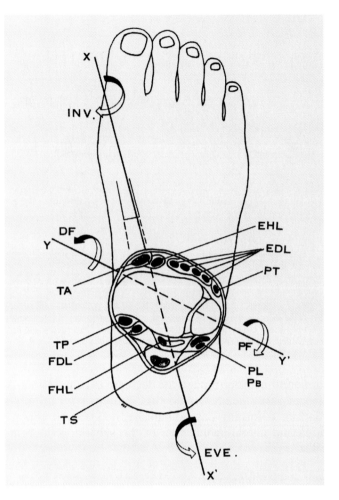

**Figure 8** Relationship of the tendons crossing the ankle joint to the axes of the subtalar (X to X¹) and tibiotalar (Y to Y¹) articulations. Tendons anterior to the ankle axis have a dorsal flexion (DF) moment, and tendons posterior to the ankle axis will create a plantar flexion (PF) moment. Tendons medial to the subtalar axis will cause inversion (INV), and tendons lateral to the subtalar axis will cause eversion (EVE). TA = tibialis anterior, TP = tibialis posterior, FHL = flexor hallucis longus, TS = Achilles tendon, EHL = extensor hallucis longus, EDL = extensor digitorum longus, PT = peroneus tertius, PL = peroneus longus, PB = peroneus brevis. *(Reproduced with permission from Sarrafian SK: Anatomy of the Foot and Ankle: Descriptive, Topographic, Functional, ed 2. Philadelphia, PA, Lippincott-Williams & Wilkins, 1993, p 551.)*

medial displacement calcaneal osteotomy reduces the antagonistic force of the Achilles tendon and decreases the strain on the medial supporting structures. Efficiency of the transferred tendon can be improved by medializing the insertion point of the transferred tendon. The navicular (and transferred tendon) can be further medialized in relation to the subtalar axis by correcting the lateral subluxation of the talonavicular joint through spring ligament reefing and/or lateral column lengthening.

## Summary

Function of the foot during gait changes from a flexible shock-absorbing structure at heel impact to a relatively rigid lever arm for efficient force transfer at push-off. An understanding of the biomechanics of the foot and ankle is necessary for evaluating foot and ankle diseases and developing principles for treatment. Study of the functional anatomy of the foot and ankle continues to improve understanding of normal and pathologic biomechanical states. Surgical reconstruction of bony deformity through osteotomy or muscular imbalance through tendon transfer attempts to normalize the weight-bearing axis of the extremity and restore function.

## Annotated Bibliography

### Gait

Christina KA, White SC, Gilchrist LA: Effect of localized muscle fatigue on vertical ground reaction forces and ankle joint motion during running. *Hum Mov Sci* 2001;20: 257-276.

This study compared vertical ground reaction forces and ankle joint motion following selective fatigue of foot dorsal flexors or invertors in running. Selective fatigue of ankle dorsal flexors resulted in increased loading rate and ankle dorsiflexion at heel contact, and selective fatigue of foot invertors resulted in decreased inversion at heel strike and diminished push-off strength.

Hunt AE, Smith RM, Torode M: Extrinsic muscle activity, foot motion and ankle joint moments during the stance phase of walking. *Foot Ankle Int* 2001;22:31-41.

The authors performed surface electromyography and kinematic analysis during the stance phase of gait in healthy adults. Patterns demonstrate that the period between heel strike and foot flat and the period between heel rise and toe-off require the most muscular activity and control. Hindfoot plantar flexors and invertors gradually change in function from foot flat (where they are contracting eccentrically) to push-off (where they are contracting concentrically). Hindfoot invertors change from eccentric to concentric action prior to plantar flexors.

Rattanaprasert U, Smith R, Sullivan M, Gilleard W: Three-dimensional kinematics of the forefoot, rearfoot, and leg without the function of tibialis posterior in comparison with normals during stance phase of walking. *Clin Biomech* 1999;14:14-23.

Three-dimensional analysis of the foot during gait was performed by comparing data from a patient with posterior tibial tendon insufficiency and normal subjects. A four-camera, three-dimensional motion analysis system with a synchronized force-plate system was used to collect data as the subjects walked on a 10-m walkway. Most major changes occurred just prior to heel-off, although no significant loss of inversion could be demonstrated.

Sammarco GJ, Hockenbury RT: Biomechanics of the foot and ankle, in Nordin M, Frankel VH (eds): *Basic Biomechanics of the Musculoskeletal System*, ed 3. Philadelphia, PA, Lippincott Williams & Wilkins, 2001, pp 222-255.

This chapter presents a detailed review of gait.

### Articular Anatomy and Kinematics

Ahn TK, Kitaoka HB, Luo ZP, An KN: Kinematics and contact characteristics of the first metatarsophalangeal joint. *Foot Ankle Int* 1997;18:170-174.

Contact area of the first MTP joint moves dorsally and diminishes with dorsiflexion of the proximal phalanx. This may explain why arthritic conditions of this joint occur predominantly at the dorsal aspect of the joint.

Arangio GA, Phillippy DC, Xiao D, Gu WK, Salathe EP: Subtalar pronation: Relationship to the medial longitudinal arch loading in the normal foot. *Foot Ankle Int* 2000; 21:216-220.

Load distribution is highly dependent on subtalar positioning. Eversion causes load in the medial column, including increased force in the talonavicular and naviculocuneiform joints. Inversion causes increased lateral load transmission.

Astion DJ, Deland JT, Otis JC, Kenneally S: Motion of the hindfoot after simulated arthrodesis. *J Bone Joint Surg Am* 1997;79:241-246.

The authors performed simulated arthrodesis of the subtalar, talonavicular, and calcaneocuboid joints in different combinations and measured the effect of these arthrodeses on the remaining joints and excursion of the posterior tibial tendon. Arthrodesis of the talonavicular joint alone or in combination with other simulated fusions had the most profound effect on remaining joint motion and in limiting posterior tibial tendon excursion. Simulated arthrodesis of the calcaneocuboid joint had little effect on subtalar motion but diminished talonavicular motion by 33%. Isolated subtalar arthrodesis diminished calcaneocuboid motion by 44%, talonavicular motion by 74%, and posterior tibial tendon excursion by 54% of the preoperative values. This study demonstrates the coupled motion of the subtalar and transverse tarsal joints and demonstrates the importance of the talonavicular joint.

de Palma L, Santucci A, Sabetta SP, Rapali S: Anatomy of the Lisfranc joint complex. *Foot Ankle Int* 1997;18:356-364.

Three functional groups of ligaments (plantar, interosseous, and dorsal) were dissected and identified. Significant variations were present, but the interosseous and plantar ligaments were consistently more substantial than the dorsal ligaments.

Hunt AE, Smith RM, Torode M, Keenan AM: Intersegment foot motion and ground reaction forces over the stance phase of walking. *Clin Biomech* 2001;16:592-600.

This study demonstrates that significant differences occur between the forefoot and hindfoot positioning at various intervals of the stance phase. Significant motion must occur through the midtarsal and tarsometatarsal joints to allow these variations in position.

Lakin RC, DeGnore LT, Pienkowski D: Contact mechanics of normal tarsometatarsal joints. *J Bone Joint Surg Am* 2001;83:520-528.

This study examined force transmission in the TMT joints in different foot positions. These authors found the third TMT joint bears the highest loads compared with the first, second, fourth, and fifth TMT joints and suggest that not the second but the third TMT joint is the keystone in force transmission of the midfoot. These authors demonstrated two mechanisms for load distribution in the TMT joints.

Leardini A, O'Connor JJ, Catani F, Giannini S: The role of the passive structures in the mobility and stability of the human ankle joint: A literature review. *Foot Ankle Int* 2000;21:602-615.

The authors performed an exhaustive review of the literature on ankle anatomy, kinematics, and biomechanics.

Leardini A, Stagni R, O'Connor JJ: Mobility of the subtalar joint in the intact ankle complex. *J Biomech* 2001; 34:805-809.

Using stereophotogrammetric techniques, a three-dimensional analysis of the coupled motion of the ankle and loaded subtalar joint was performed. Plantar flexion of the ankle was coupled with supination and inversion of the subtalar joint. Dorsiflexion of the ankle joint was coupled with pronation and eversion of the subtalar joint. Motion of the subtalar joint decreased as the ankle approached maximal dorsiflexion or plantar flexion. The loaded subtalar joint follows distinctly different axes of rotation during inversion and eversion.

Michelson JD, Checcone M, Kuhn T, Varner K: Intra-articular load distribution in the human ankle joint during motion. *Foot Ankle Int* 2001;22:226-233.

This study demonstrates increasing lateral and decreasing medial tibiotalar loading that occurs with dorsiflexion. Increased medially and laterally directed loads are directed toward the malleoli.

Nawoczenski DA, Baumhauer JF, Umberger BR: Relationship between clinical measurements and motion of the first metatarsophalangeal joint during gait. *J Bone Joint Surg Am* 1999;81:370-376.

An electromagnetic tracking device was used to measure hallucal MTP motion during clinical tests and during gait. Mean dorsiflexion during gait on level ground was 42°, which was similar to maximal active dorsiflexion while weight bearing.

Reeck J, Felten N, McCormack AP, Kiser P, Tencer AF, Sangeorzan BJ: Support of the talus: A biomechanical investigation of the contributions of the talonavicular and talocalcaneal joints, and the superomedial calcaneonavicular ligament. *Foot Ankle Int* 1998;19:674-682.

This study examined force transmission in the hindfoot in advancing positions of gait in a cadaver model. The posterior facet of the subtalar joint had the greatest contact area and force

transmission near toe-off position. The talonavicular joint, anteromedial facet of the subtalar joint, and calcaneonavicular ligament showed sequentially decreasing amounts of contact area and force transmission with advancing foot position. Loss of posterior tibial tendon tension did not significantly affect the contact forces at the talonavicular joint.

Solan MC, Moorman CT III, Miyamoto RG, Jasper LE, Belkoff SM: Ligamentous restraints of the second tarsometatarsal joint: A biomechanical evaluation. *Foot Ankle Int* 2001;22:637-641.

Mechanical testing of the ligaments of the medial Lisfranc's joint complex was performed in 20 cadaver specimens. Lisfranc's ligament was the strongest ligament, although both the plantar ligament complex and Lisfranc's ligament were significantly stronger than the thin dorsal ligaments.

Wulker N, Stukenborg C, Savory KM, Alfke D: Hindfoot motion after isolated and combined arthrodeses: Measurements in anatomic specimens. *Foot Ankle Int* 2000; 21:921-927.

This study examined residual motion in the joints of the subtalar and transverse tarsal joint complexes following isolated and combined arthrodesis in a cadaver model. Subtalar and talonavicular motion were not significantly affected by calcaneocuboid arthrodesis. Subtalar arthrodesis decreased talonavicular motion by one third. Talonavicular arthrodesis diminished subtalar motion by 75% and calcaneocuboid motion by 60%. This study demonstrates the highly interrelated motion of these joints and verifies that the talonavicular joint is critical in kinematics. This study also confirms findings by Astion and associates.

## Arches of the Foot

Chu IT, Myerson MS, Nyska M, Parks BG: Experimental flatfoot model: The contribution of dynamic loading. *Foot Ankle Int* 2001;22:220-225.

This study demonstrates that in addition to disruption of the static and dynamic supports of the longitudinal arch, dynamic loading of the foot is required to create an effective flatfoot model.

Sharkey NA, Donahue SW, Ferris L: Biomechanical consequences of plantar fascial release or rupture during gait: Part II. Alterations in forefoot loading. *Foot Ankle Int* 1999;20:86-96.

This study demonstrates that as the truss mechanism is interrupted (by sectioning of the plantar fascia), load is shifted to the metatarsals and intertarsal ligaments. Sectioning of the plantar fascia causes an 80% increase in the magnitude of strain in the dorsal aspect of the second metatarsal. This study suggests that complete release of the plantar fascia accelerates fatigue damage of the midfoot joints.

Sharkey NA, Ferris L, Donahue SW: Biomechanical consequences of plantar fascial release or rupture during gait:

Part I. Disruptions in longitudinal arch conformation. *Foot Ankle Int* 1998;19:812-820.

This study demonstrates the truss model of arch support in a cadaver model. Complete sectioning of the plantar fascia causes collapse of the longitudinal arch and elongation of the medial base length of the foot. Partial transection did not show as dramatic an effect. Loss of posterior tibial tendon function caused further depression of the arch, particularly at terminal stance.

## Biomechanics of Plantar Force Transmission

Armstrong DG, Stacpoole-Shea S, Nguyen H, Harkless LB: Lengthening of the Achilles tendon in diabetic patients who are at high risk for ulceration of the foot. *J Bone Joint Surg Am* 1999;81:535-538.

Ten patients with diabetes and chronic forefoot ulceration underwent percutaneous lengthening of the Achilles tendon. Comparison of preoperative and postoperative pedobarographic data demonstrated significant decreases in forefoot peak pressures following the procedure. Clinical ankle dorsal flexion improved significantly with the procedure.

Luger E, Nissan M, Karpf A, Steinberg E, Dekel S: Dynamic pressures on the diabetic foot. *Foot Ankle Int* 2001; 22:715-719.

This retrospective study was conducted in order to investigate the relation between increased plantar pressure and ulcers in the diabetic foot. Maximal plantar pressure is reported on various areas of the plantar aspects of the feet. An increase in maximal plantar pressure under all plantar areas except for the heels was found to be associated with an increase in the severity of the symptoms related to diabetes.

Luger EJ, Nissan M, Karpf A, Steinberg EL, Dekel S: Patterns of weight distribution under the metatarsal heads. *J Bone Joint Surg Br* 1999;81:199-202.

The authors report on peak pressure distributions under the metatarsal heads. Their findings show that there is no distal transverse metatarsal arch during the stance phase. This is important for the classification and description of disorders of the foot.

Wearing SC, Urry SR, Smeathers JE: Ground reaction forces at discrete sites of the foot derived from pressure plate measurements. *Foot Ankle Int* 2001;22:653-661.

This study provides an indirect estimate of force and accompanying temporal parameters for discrete sites of the foot in young, healthy adults walking at their preferred speed.

## Pathologic Entities and Changes in Force Transmission

Friedman MA, Draganich LF, Toolan B, Brage ME: The effects of adult acquired flatfoot deformity on tibiotalar joint contact characteristics. *Foot Ankle Int* 2001;22:241-246.

Changes in the tibiotalar contact characteristics were investigated to further develop an established model of the acquired flatfoot deformity. The flatfoot condition resulted in significant lateral shifts in global contact area and in the location of peak pressure. The lateral shift in the contact region created a local increase in mean contact pressure that may be responsible for long-term degenerative changes in patients with this deformity.

Metaxiotis D, Accles W, Pappas A, Doederlein L: Dynamic pedobarography (DPB) in operative management of cavovarus foot deformity. *Foot Ankle Int* 2000;21:935-947.

Dynamic pedobarography was performed in patients with cavovarus foot deformity, mostly originating from Charcot-Marie-Tooth disease. According to the contact pattern, the examined feet could be divided into three groups (antegrade, retrograde, and inversion contact pattern). Clinical results such as plantar callosities and "rollover avoidance gait" did not always correlate with pedobarographic data.

## Biomechanical Effects of Surgical Procedures

Arangio GA, Salathe EP: Medial displacement calcaneal osteotomy reduces the excess forces in the medial longitudinal arch of the flat foot. *Clin Biomech* 2001;16:535-539.

In a cadaveric flatfoot model, the authors demonstrate that compared with a normal foot, a cadaveric flatfoot model shifted support of a constant load from the lateral column to the medial column and medial longitudinal arch. A 10-mm medial displacement calcaneal osteotomy unloaded the medial column and shifted support back to the lateral metatarsals.

Davitt JS, Beals TC, Bachus KN: The effects of medial and lateral displacement calcaneal osteotomies on ankle and subtalar joint pressure distribution. *Foot Ankle Int* 2001;22:885-889.

This study compares the pressure distribution in the ankle and posterior facet of the subtalar joint following 1-cm medial and lateral displacement calcaneal osteotomies to the pressure distribution in the nonosteotomized foot. A 1-cm translation of the calcaneal tuberosity has only a small effect on pressure distribution in the ankle and posterior facet of the subtalar joint in a weighted cadaver model.

Momberger N, Morgan JM, Bachus KN, West JR: Calcaneocuboid joint pressure after lateral column lengthening in a cadaveric planovalgus deformity model. *Foot Ankle Int* 2000;21:730-735.

The authors show that peak pressures across the joint increased significantly from baseline in the flatfoot. However, the change in pressure from the flatfoot to the corrected foot was not significant, and in some cases, peak pressures in the corrected foot were actually lower than in the flatfoot. These findings indicate that calcaneal lengthening through an Evans osteotomy does not increase pressure across the calcaneocuboid joint beyond physiologic loads in the flatfoot.

Nyska M, Parks BG, Chu IT, Myerson MS: The contribution of the medial calcaneal osteotomy to the correction of flatfoot deformities. *Foot Ankle Int* 2001;22:278-282.

The authors found that the medial displacement osteotomy plays an important role in reducing and/or delaying the progress of flatfoot deformity. Loading of the Achilles tendon increases flatfoot deformity. Medial calcaneal osteotomy significantly decreases the arch-flattening effect of this tendon and therefore limits the potential increase of the deformity.

Otis JC, Deland JT, Kenneally S: Medial arch strain after lateral column lengthening: An in vitro study. *Foot Ankle Int* 1999;20:797-802.

Displacement gauges were used to monitor the length of the spring ligament complex following lateral column lengthening. Length of the spring ligament was unchanged after lateral column lengthening and remained functional when loaded following the procedure.

Otis JC, Deland JT, Kenneally S, Chang V: Medial arch strain after medial displacement calcaneal osteotomy: An in vitro study. *Foot Ankle Int* 1999;20:222-226.

The medial displacement calcaneal osteotomy allowed elongation of the ligament with weight bearing but at a shorter ligament length. This afforded the spring ligament protection from the levels of force experienced in the intact and lateral column-lengthened conditions.

## Classic Bibliography

Calhoun JH, Li F, Ledbetter BR, Viegas SF: A comprehensive study of pressure distribution in the ankle joint with inversion and eversion. *Foot Ankle Int* 1994;15:125-133.

Hicks JH: The mechanics of the foot: I. The joints. *J Anat* 1953;87:345-357.

Hicks JH: The mechanics of the foot: II. The plantar aponeurosis and the arch. *J Anat* 1954;88:25-30.

Hintermann B, Nigg BM, Sommer C: Foot movement and tendon excursion: An in vitro study. *Foot Ankle Int* 1994; 15:386-395.

Isman RE, Inman VT: Anthropometric studies of the human foot and ankle. *Bull Prosth Res* 1969;10:97-129.

Lapidus PW: Kinesiology and mechanical anatomy of the tarsal joints. *Clin Orthop* 1963;30:30.

Mann RA: Biomechanics of the foot and ankle, in Mann RA, Coughlin MJ (eds): *Surgery of the Foot and Ankle*, ed 6. St. Louis, MO, Mosby-Year Book, 1993, pp 3-43.

Mizel MS: The role of the plantar first metatarsal first cuneiform ligament in weightbearing on the first metatarsal. *Foot Ankle* 1993;14:82-84.

Perry J: (ed): *Gait Analysis: Normal and Pathological Function*. Thorofare, NJ, Slack Inc, 1992.

Rozema A, Ulbrecht JS, Pammer SE, Cavanagh PR: In-shoe plantar pressures during activities of daily living: Implications for therapeutic footwear design. *Foot Ankle Int* 1996;17:352-359.

Sarafian SK: Functional anatomy of the foot and ankle, in Sarrafian SK (ed): *Anatomy of the Foot and Ankle: Descriptive, Topographic, Functional*, ed 2. Philadelphia, PA, Lippincott-Williams & Wilkins, 1993, pp 474-602.

# Chapter 21

# Arthroscopy of the Ankle and Hindfoot

Bryan D. DenHartog, MD

## Introduction

Arthroscopy is a useful tool for the treatment of foot and ankle disorders. Although arthroscopy had its beginnings in the 1950s, arthroscopy of the ankle has been recognized as a surgical procedure only since the late 1970s. During the 1990s, ankle arthroscopy became an integral part of treatment for chronic ankle problems.

This chapter reviews the anatomy of the ankle and hindfoot, superficial portal anatomy, and the general techniques involved with ankle arthroscopy including instrumentation, distraction, and portal placement. The general techniques of subtalar arthroscopy, retrocalcaneal bursectomy through the scope, and endoscopic plantar fascial release are discussed and specific therapeutic indications and current developments are examined.

## Ankle Arthroscopy

### Anatomy

An understanding of the surface and intra-articular anatomy of the ankle region is essential to successful ankle arthroscopy. The normal intra-articular anatomy of the anterior and posterior joint cavities of the ankle have been well described (Fig. 1). A thorough, systematic arthroscopic examination enables the surgeon to identify and document intra-articular pathologic changes.

The superficial anatomy must be used as a guide to correctly place the arthroscopic portals. Neurovascular and tendinous structures are most at risk for injury; therefore, important anatomic landmarks including the peroneus tertius tendon, the anterior tibial tendon, the dorsalis pedis artery, the greater saphenous vein, and the ankle joint line should be outlined with a skin marker.

The topographic anatomy of the superficial peroneal nerve and its branches is important because of their proximity to the anterolateral (AL) portal (Fig. 2). Approximately 6.5 cm proximal to the tip of the fibula, the superficial peroneal nerve divides into the intermediate and medial dorsal cutaneous branches. Frequently, these branches (particularly the intermediate branch) can be seen beneath the skin when the fourth toe is plantar flexed while the forefoot is pulled into plantar flexion and

adduction. The intermediate dorsal cutaneous nerve passes superficial to the inferior extensor retinaculum, crosses anterior to the common extensor tendons of the fourth and fifth toes, and then runs in the direction of the space between the second and third and the third and fourth metatarsals before it divides into dorsal digital branches. The medial terminal branch of the superficial peroneal nerve is the medial dorsal cutaneous nerve that crosses the anterior aspect of the ankle superficial to the common extensor tendons. The nerve courses adjacent to the lateral border of the extensor hallucis longus tendon and divides over or just distal to the inferior extensor retinaculum into the dorsal digital branches that are located on the medial side of the hallux and the second web space. The AL portal is usually located between the intermediate and medial branches of the superficial peroneal nerve.

### Arthroscopic Portals

The safest and most commonly used portals for arthroscopic entry are the anteromedial (AM), AL, and posterolateral (PL) portals (Fig. 3). The AM portal is established first; it is the safest and easiest to locate because it is relatively devoid of any major neurovascular structures. The AM portal is made just medial to the tendon of the anterior tibialis at, or just proximal to, the joint line. The greater saphenous vein and nerve are at risk for injury when establishing this portal. An injection of saline with a 22-gauge needle helps to establish the exact location of the AM portal. Once the ankle joint has been distended with saline, the incision for the portal should be made vertically and through the skin only. Deeper anatomic layers are bluntly dissected with a small hemostat followed by a blunt obturator that penetrates the joint capsule. This will protect the saphenous nerve and vein.

The AL portal is established after the arthroscope has been placed in the AM portal. The location of this portal often can be determined by transilluminating the skin with the arthroscope from the AM portal, allowing visualization of the neurovascular and tendinous structures. A 22-gauge, 1.5-inch needle is placed just lateral to the tendon of the peroneus tertius at, or just proximal to, the

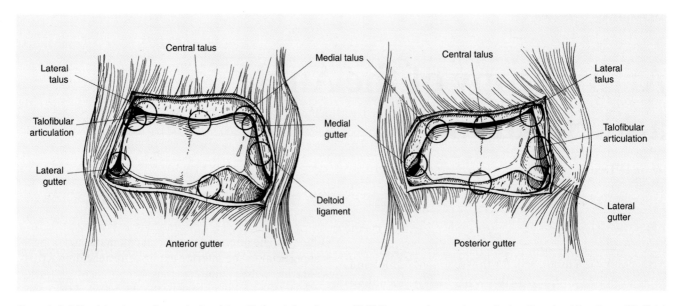

Figure 1 **Left**, The eight-point anterior examination of the ankle through the arthroscope. **Right**, The seven-point posterior examination. *(Reproduced from Stetson WB, Ferkel RD: Ankle arthroscopy: I. Techniques and complications. J Am Acad Orthop Surg 1996;4:17-23.)*

level of the joint line. The branches of the superficial peroneal nerve are most at risk for injury.

Entry at the PL portal is made just lateral to the Achilles tendon, 1.0 to 1.5 cm proximal to the tip of the fibula, and can be made under direct visualization from the AM portal by looking in a posterior direction through the notch of Hardy. A 22-gauge needle is placed just lateral to the Achilles tendon at a 45° angle toward the medial malleolus. Neurovascular structures at risk for injury at this portal are the lesser saphenous vein and the sural nerve.

Other ankle arthroscopic portals have been described but are not recommended. The anterocentral portal is made between the tendons of the extensor digitorum longus and extensor hallucis longus; however, use of this portal is not recommended because of its proximity to the dorsalis pedis artery and deep peroneal nerve. The posterocentral portal is made just below the joint line of the ankle to the middle of the Achilles tendon. Because of the limited scope and range of motion offered by this portal and the possibility for irritation of the Achilles tendon, the use of this approach is not advised. Use of the posteromedial (PM) portal for arthroscopic entry can be risky because of its proximity to the medial neurovascular structures. A recent study reported that the PM approach can be safely used if it is kept lateral to the flexor hallucis longus (FHL). A transmalleolar portal can be used to drill an osteochondritis dissecans lesion either medially or laterally. A small joint guide is helpful in directing the tip of the Kirschner wire to the lesion (Fig. 4). Also, a transtalar portal can be used through the sinus tarsi or the medial talus for drilling a talar dome cyst.

## Instrumentation

A standard 4.0-mm, 30° angle scope can be used for ankle arthroscopy, but a 2.7-mm, 30° short scope is preferred because the short lever arm allows better control of the scope. Also recommended are 2.0- and 2.7-mm motorized burrs and shavers, mini probes, and a 2.7-mm grasper and pituitary rongeur for retrieving loose bodies. An Acufex (Smith & Nephew, Andover, MA) 4.5-mm curet is helpful for débriding talar dome defects. A 0.25-inch (6-mm) curved osteotome is helpful for removing anterior tibial spurs.

An arthroscopic pump allows improved distention of the joint. However, when using the 2.7-mm scope, it is advisable to avoid pressures of more than 90 mm Hg because higher pressures can cause large amounts of fluid to extravasate into the retinacular soft tissues.

## Patient Positioning

The position of the patient depends on the surgeon's preference. Placing the patient supine with the hip flexed and a bump under the ipsilateral hip to keep the foot in neutral rotation, which allows easy access to either anterior portal, is the most commonly used position. A support under the calf lifts the foot and ankle off the operating table, thus improving access to all portals during the arthroscopic procedure. An alternate method of positioning is flexion of the knee over the end of the operating table, allowing for some distraction of the joint by gravity; however, it is somewhat more difficult to access the posterior portals with this technique. A thigh tourniquet can be used to minimize intra-articular bleeding for improved visibility.

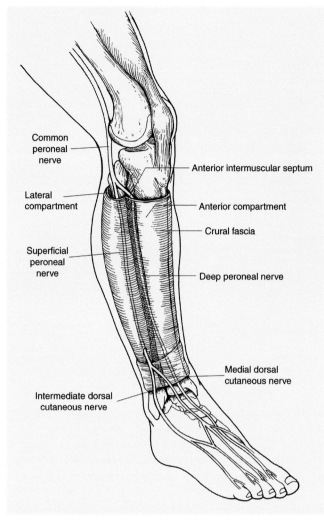

**Figure 2** The superficial branch of the peroneal nerve divides into the medial dorsal cutaneous nerve and the intermediate dorsal cutaneous nerve as it penetrates the fascia of the lateral compartment. *(Reproduced from Stetson WB, Ferkel RD: Ankle arthroscopy: I. Techniques and complications.* J Am Acad Orthop Surg *1996;4:17-23.)*

## Ankle Distraction

The use of distraction during arthroscopic ankle surgery depends on the type of procedure to be done, the degree of laxity of the ankle joint, and the location of the pathologic tissue to be removed. Invasive distraction involves use of threaded Steinmann pins placed in the tibia and the calcaneus or the talus on the medial or the lateral side of the ankle (Fig. 5, *A*). The distraction device can be attached medially or laterally. Invasive distraction is recommended only if the ankle is quite stiff and when prolonged and marked distraction is required. It is not recommended for competitive athletes because the pinholes can act as a stress riser for several months postoperatively, making the tibia particularly vulnerable to fracture.

Noninvasive distraction can be applied manually by an assistant or with the use of a noninvasive distraction device, such as a clove-hitch-type device wrapped over the anterior aspect of the midfoot and posterior aspect of

the heel (Fig. 5, *B*). Approximately 90% to 95% of ankle arthroscopic procedures can be done without invasive distraction.

### Pathology and Specific Portals for Specific Lesions

Soft-tissue lesions account for approximately 30% to 50% of ankle joint lesions. Precise clinical diagnosis is often not readily apparent. However, patients may have persistent ankle pain after an injury, despite prolonged nonsurgical treatment. Findings from radiographs, CT, and technetium Tc 99m bone scans usually are normal. MRI can assist in identifying soft-tissue lesions particularly in the coronal (frontal) plane.

### Synovitis

The ankle joint synovium may become inflamed and hypertrophied secondary to inflammatory arthritides, infection, crystalline arthropathies, and degenerative or neuropathic changes. Trauma and overuse also can cause generalized inflammation of the joint lining.

Initial treatment should consist of limited weight bearing, anti-inflammatory medications, and/or intra-articular injections of corticosteroids. Nonsurgical treatment that has proved unsuccessful after at least 3 months is an indication for arthroscopic partial synovectomy and lysis of adhesions. In most patients this procedure can provide dramatic relief of pain.

### Anterior Soft-Tissue Impingement

Anterior soft-tissue impingement, or AL impingement of the ankle, is believed to be caused by one or more inversion injuries to the ankle joint. It most commonly occurs in the superior portion of the anterior talofibular ligament, but can also be localized to the distal portion of the anteroinferior tibiofibular ligament (meniscoid lesion). The pain persists despite adequate rest, healing, and rehabilitation. Ankle tenderness usually originates from the lateral gutter of the ankle joint.

AL synovial tissue and redundant ligamentous tissue may cause joint irritation and pain, or may be secondary to an isolated tear of the anterior talofibular ligament and/or syndesmosis. Adjacent talar or fibular chondromalacia and inflammatory synovitis may occur in association with these lesions. A basket forceps or power shaver aids arthroscopic débridement of inflamed synovium and inflamed capsular ligamentous tissue. The rehabilitation program is delayed 2 to 3 weeks to avoid reinflammation of the joint. Patients may resume athletic activities when pain has subsided and normal range of motion and strength have returned. Good to excellent results are obtained in 75% to 90% of patients who undergo arthroscopic removal of the impinging tissue.

### Syndesmotic Impingement

Impingement in the syndesmotic interval secondary to injury of the syndesmosis can lead to pain and disability.

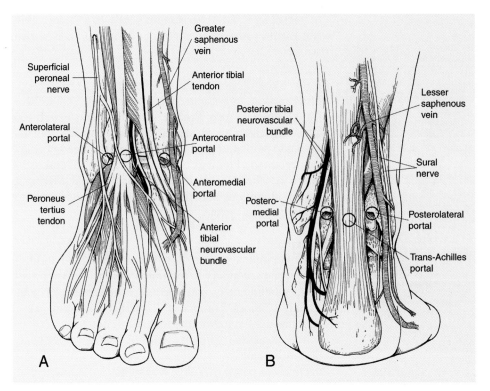

Figure 3 **A,** location of the anteromedial, anterolateral, and anterocentral portals. The central portal should be avoided. **B,** The posterolateral portal is established just lateral to the Achilles tendon, approximately 1.0 to 1.5 cm proximal to the distal tip of the fibula. The posteromedial and trans-Achilles portals are also shown but not recommended. *(Reproduced from Stetson WB, Ferkel RD: Ankle arthroscopy: I. Techniques and complications.* J Am Acad Orthop Surg *1996;4:17-23.)*

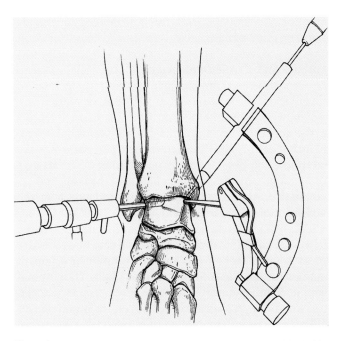

Figure 4 Transmalleolar drilling can be useful in treating chronic osteochondral lesions that are not loose. For medial lesions, a small-joint drill guide is inserted through the anteromedial portal, and the arthroscope is inserted through the anterolateral portal. *(Reproduced from Stetson WB, Ferkel RD: Ankle arthroscopy: II. Indications and results.* J Am Acad Orthop Surg *1996;4:24-34.)*

The injury usually involves the anteroinferior tibiofibular ligament followed by synovitis and scarring in this area, including the distal tibiofibular joint. A tear of the anteroinferior tibiofibular ligament can produce increased laxity, allowing the talar dome to extrude anteriorly in

dorsiflexion and cause soft-tissue impingement. The patient typically has tenderness along the syndesmosis and more proximally on the interosseous membrane and may have tenderness on squeeze testing and ankle external rotation. If nonsurgical treatment fails, arthroscopic débridement of the anteroinferior tibiofibular ligament and the tibiofibular joint is indicated. If a separate, anteroinferior tibiofibular ligament fascicle is seen, it should be removed (Bassett's ligament). Approximately 20% of the syndesmotic ligament is intra-articular, and excision of this portion of the ligament has no significant negative effects on long-term outcome provided a competent anterior talofibular ligament remains.

### Osteochondral Lesions of the Talus
Lesions of the talar dome can range from a small defect in the articular surface to subchondral cysts or osteochondral fragments. These chondral lesions may be the result of an acute trauma, such as an ankle sprain, or degenerative changes caused by repetitive microtrauma; 10% of lesions are bilateral with no associated history of trauma. These nontraumatic bilateral lesions are more common medially, and medial lesions are more common than lateral lesions. Symptoms include swelling, pain, and occasional catching or locking. Radiographs often appear normal or show only very subtle findings; therefore, most authors advocate staging these lesions on the basis of the CT or MRI appearance. Arthroscopic treatment is recommended for those lesions that remain symptomatic despite nonsurgical treatment. These lesions are débrided and osteochondral fragments are removed through an en-

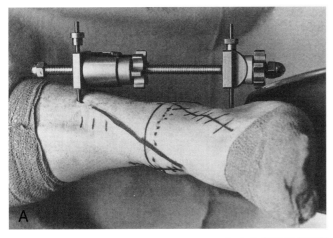

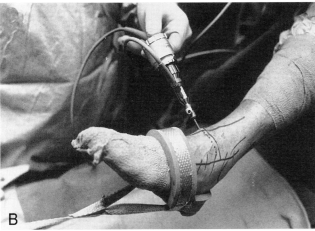

Figure 5 **A,** Invasive distraction device placed laterally with pins in the tibia and calcaneus. **B,** Clove-hitch-type device wrapped over the anterior aspect of the midfoot and the posterior aspect of the heel for noninvasive distraction. *(Reproduced from Stetson WB, Ferkel RD: Ankle arthroscopy: I. Techniques and complications. J Am Acad Orthop Surg 1996;4:17-23.)*

larged arthroscopic portal when necessary. Improved distraction techniques have allowed greater access to the joint and adequate débridement and curettage of the bed of the osteochondral defect. If the fragments are large (> 1 cm) and the overlying articular cartilage is healthy, drilling of the lesion is recommended. For medial lesions that are difficult to access, a small-joint drill guide is inserted through the AM portal and a 0.062-inch Kirschner wire is drilled through the medial malleolus into the lesion. If there is sufficient underlying bone, the base of the lesion is débrided and the piece is reattached with absorbable pins or screws through a medial malleolar osteotomy. However, most chronic lesions are loose, nonviable, and occasionally displaced and must be excised. After excision, curettage and abrasion or drilling is done. If the crater is large, bone grafting should be considered.

The beneficial role of ankle arthroscopy in the treatment of all grade 1 and lateral grade 2 osteochondral defects of the talus is established. However, less favorable outcomes have been found for stage 2 medial lesions and all stage 3 lesions. Good to excellent results overall are achieved in approximately 84% of patients; however, results were worse in patients with preexisting arthritis. Results of arthroscopic treatment are as good as or better than those with open techniques.

### Loose Bodies
Loose bodies may be chondral or osteochondral in origin and usually are a result of trauma. They can occur with synovial chondromatosis or synovial osteochondromatosis and can be freely floating within the joint or fixed to synovium or scar tissue. Symptoms include catching or locking, swelling, pain, and decreased range of motion. It is important to localize the lesion preoperatively to facilitate the surgical approach and lesion removal. Radiographs and CT are helpful if there is bone in the lesion. After the loose body has been removed, the joint surfaces should be carefully inspected to locate its source. If a chondral or osteochondral defect is found, it should be débrided.

### Anterior Osteophytes (Spurs)
Osteophytes are usually secondary to trauma or degenerative changes. The anterior lip of the distal tibia is the most common location for these osteophytes; however, they may occur anywhere in the ankle joint. Often a reciprocal lesion forms on the anterior neck of the talus. This combination spur often is caused by repetitive and forceful dorsiflexion of the ankle and is termed anterior impingement syndrome. There is a high incidence of spurs in football players (nearly 45%) and in dancers (approximately 50%). Usually the patient has persistent pain in the anterior aspect of the ankle, and the lateral radiograph depicts an anterior tibiotalar spur. A lateral, weight-bearing view taken with the ankle in dorsiflexion may show the abutment between the anterior tibial spur and the talus. Most of these lesions are located anterolaterally and are readily seen on the lateral radiograph of the foot and ankle. However, if an AM osteophyte is suspected, a lateral radiograph with the ankle externally rotated 20° to 30° may show it.

A single injection of corticosteroid accompanied by a heel lift will sometimes eliminate or reduce the pain. A classification system for anterior ankle osteophytes based on the size of the spur and the presence of associated arthritis was developed (Fig. 6). It was found that patients who were treated arthroscopically recovered in approximately half the time of those treated with arthrotomy. Results are generally good or excellent with spur excision and scar removal in patients with minimal joint arthritis. When removing the osteophytes anteriorly, adequate visibility is essential. Extreme care should be taken to prevent injury to the neurovascular structures. The shaver or burr should never be directed dorsally into the soft tissue. A 0.25-inch (6-mm), curved osteotome can be used through the AM and AL portals to detach the osteophytes, and a grasper can be used to remove the fragments.

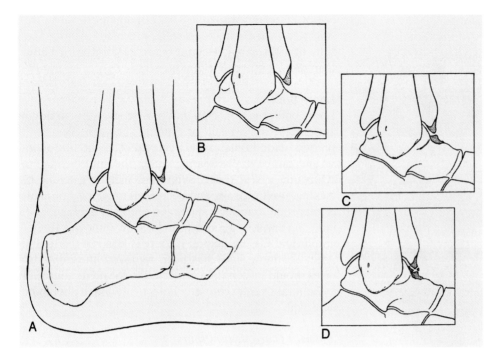

Figure 6 A classification system that grades the degree of spur formation and helps predict the time to recovery and whether a patient would benefit from athroscopic removal of the spur. **A,** Grade I: Synovial impingement up to 3-mm tibial span. **B,** Grade II: Tibial span > 3 mm. **C,** Grade III: Significant tibial exostosis with or without fragmentation; secondary spur formation on dorsum of talus. **D,** Grade IV: Pantalocrural arthritic destruction (not suitable candidates for arthroscopic débridement). *(Reproduced with permission from Scranton PE, McDermott JE: Anterior tibiotalar spurs: A comparison of open versus arthroscopic débridement. Foot Ankle 1992; 13:124-129.)*

### Traumatic and Degenerative Arthritis

Long-term studies of arthroscopy for treatment of degenerative joint disease of the ankle have shown little benefit from this procedure.

### Aftercare

A soft compressive dressing with or without a plaster splint is applied to allow the soft tissues to rest until portal closure occurs. Range-of-motion exercises begin approximately 7 to 10 days postoperatively. Weight bearing is delayed 7 to 8 days, depending on the size of the lesion.

### Arthrodesis

The results of arthroscopic ankle arthrodesis, when done for an appropriate indication by an experienced surgeon, appear to be as good as or better than those obtained by open methods. The arthroscopic technique is not suitable for correction of varus or valgus deformities of more than 13°, malrotation of the ankle, anterior posterior translation of the tibiotalar joint, or in the presence of significant bone loss, active infection, reflex sympathetic dystrophy, or neuropathic destruction of the tibiotalar joint. However, for osteoarthritic joints with minimal deformity, arthroscopic ankle arthrodesis has fusion rates that are comparable to those of open procedures, with faster healing time, better cosmetic results, less postoperative pain, and shorter hospital stays.

It is important to débride all hyaline cartilage and underlying avascular subchondral bone from the talus and tibial plafond, as well as from the medial and lateral gutters. Internal fixation is required to maintain anatomic position. It is important during débridement to maintain the normal contour of the talar dome and tibial plafond

and to remove as little bone as possible to adequately prepare the joint surfaces for arthrodesis. Avoiding squaring of tibiotalar surfaces helps prevent varus or valgus deformity.

The use of invasive distraction and an arthroscopic pump provides maximal exposure of the joint. Fixation of the fusion is usually accomplished with percutaneous transarticular 6.5- or 7.0-mm cannulated screws through the medial and lateral malleoli. Three screws can be used if more fixation is required, especially in osteoporotic bone.

Arthroscopic arthrodesis of the ankle is a technically difficult procedure with a significant learning curve for the surgeon. The expense of the arthroscopic equipment and the inability to correct significant ankle deformities are other disadvantages. Arthroscopic arthrodesis also makes it more difficult to obtain a congruent fusion surface as well as to posteriorly displace the talus, which improves gait.

Advantages of arthroscopic ankle arthrodesis (in a carefully selected group of patients) over the open methods are earlier fusion, a shorter hospital stay, less pain, and diminished morbidity.

### Acute Ankle Fractures

The role of ankle arthroscopy in evaluation and treatment of acute ankle fractures is still unclear. Arthroscopy can be used to assess adequacy of reduction in minimally displaced talar neck and triplane fractures of the distal tibia. Ankle arthroscopy is contraindicated in open fractures and in those with neurovascular compromise or massive soft-tissue swelling.

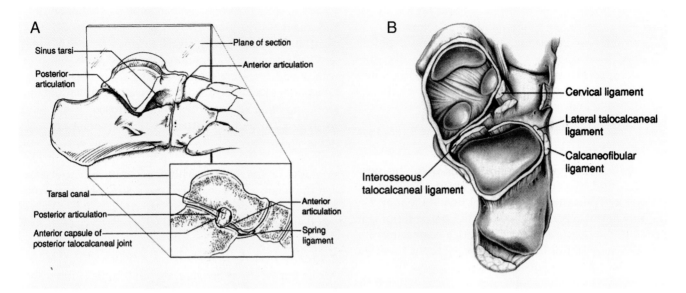

Figure 7   **A,** The sinus tarsi and tarsal canal separate the anterior and posterior articulations of the subtalar joint. The plane of section helps to show the anatomy more clearly. (Insert) After sectioning, the tarsal canal and the subtalar articulations are more clearly seen. *(Reproduced with permission from Ferkel RD: Subtalar arthroscopy, in Ferkel RD (ed): Arthroscopic Surgery: The Foot and Ankle. Philadelphia, PA, Lippincott-Raven, 1996, pp 231-254. Illustration by Susan Brust.)* **B,** Axial view of the subtalar joint showing the deep and peripheral ligaments. Note the location of the interosseous talocalcaneal, lateral talocalcaneal, and calcaneofibular ligaments. *(© Richard D. Ferkel.)*

## Complications

A wide range of complications are associated with arthroscopy of the foot and ankle. In a recent, comprehensive study, the incidence of complications reported from ankle arthroscopy was 9.8%. The most frequent and persistent complication was neurologic injury (49%); at 10-year follow-up, numbness at the incision site was also noted. All other complications associated with ankle arthroscopy were temporary and resolved within 6 months.

Other complications include injury to the neurovascular, tendinous, and ligamentous tissues; skin slough; sinus formation; infection; compartment syndrome (from extravasated fluids); reflex sympathetic dystrophy; thrombophlebitis; and articular cartilage damage. Proper patient selection and careful preoperative evaluation including skin, nerve, and vascular status are important to avoid complications. Other protective measures include a thorough knowledge of foot and ankle anatomy, invasive distraction, and proper pin position; careful portal placement; the use of interchangeable cannulae for arthroscope and instrumentation; the use of small joint instrumentation; the administration of perioperative antibiotics; limited surgical time and tourniquet use; the use of skin sutures in portal wounds; and brief postoperative immobilization to allow incision healing.

## Hindfoot Arthroscopy

Hindfoot arthroscopy involving the subtalar joint has been advocated when assessment of the articular surfaces of the subtalar joint is needed and for chronic pain, adhesions, osteochondral lesions, loose bodies, and degenerative or inflammatory synovitic conditions of this joint.

## Anatomy

The subtalar joint has two articulations, anterior and posterior, which are divided by the sinus tarsi and tarsal canal (Fig. 7). The saddle-shaped posterior joint includes the posterior talar and calcaneal facets. It has a convex upward orientation and its motion is that of a mitered hinge. The anterior subtalar joint includes the inferior navicular bone and the anterior aspect of the calcaneus, along with the plantar calcaneonavicular (spring) ligament. These two articulations are separated by the tarsal canal, which is formed by the inferior talar sulcus and the superior calcaneal sulcus. The lateral opening of the tarsal canal is called the sinus tarsi. The ligament of the tarsal canal (interosseous talocalcaneal ligament) is the most important ligament uniting the talus and the calcaneus because it prevents eversion, heel valgus, and depression of the longitudinal arch. The ligament of the tarsal canal is a broad band that originates from the sulcus calcanei on the floor of the tarsal canal, runs obliquely upward and medially at a 45° angle, and inserts into the inferior surface of the talus. This structure is readily seen during diagnostic subtalar arthroscopy.

There is a thin capsular envelope over the subtalar joint that does not appear to communicate with other joints. The anterior and middle subtalar joints are anatomically small and usually are not associated with the pathology of the posterior subtalar joint.

Indications for subtalar arthroscopy include persistent pain, swelling, stiffness, and locking or catching that are resistant to nonsurgical treatment. Arthroscopic procedures include débridement of chondromalacia or osteoarthritis, excision of loose bodies and/or osteophytes, synovectomy, débridement of osteochondral lesions of the talus, and excision of a symptomatic os trigonum.

Absolute contraindications to subtalar arthroscopy include localized infection and severe degenerative joint disease, especially with deformity. Relative contraindications include a poorly vascularized extremity, a very stiff arthrofibrotic joint, and severe edema that makes localization of bony landmarks difficult.

### Portals, Instrumentation, and Technique

With the patient supine or in the lateral decubitus position, standard working portals for the subtalar joint are anterior and posterior on the lateral side of the foot. The anterior portal placement is located 2 cm anterior and 1 cm distal to the tip of the fibula, with a posterior portal placed 2 cm posterior and 1 cm proximal to the tip of the fibula. The subtalar joint is first injected with 10 mL of saline solution through a spinal needle. The entering technique is similar to that described for the ankle. A 2.7- or 1.9-mm arthroscope is used with a 30° lens; a 70° lens is recommended for examination of the posterior facet. The anterior portal is typically used for inflow and introduction of the arthroscope, and the posterior portal initially is used for outflow. Great care must be taken when placing the posterior portal to avoid entry in the ankle joint. In particularly tight joints, a 1.9-mm, 30° arthroscope is used. For most patients, a 2.9-mm shaver and burr are adequate, but smaller 1.9- and 2.0-mm blades are available for very tight joints. Noninvasive distraction usually is applied. However, invasive distraction with pins inserted laterally in the tibia and the calcaneus can be used to increase joint exposure in patients with arthrofibrosis or when arthroscopic fusion is done.

Several authors recently have described the efficacy and safety of coaxial posterior subtalar portals (PL and PM). Care, however, must be taken to keep the PM portal lateral to the FHL.

Once bony anatomy has been outlined, the joint is distended through the PL portal, which is located at approximately 0.5 cm proximal to the tip of the fibula just lateral to the Achilles tendon. Entering is done in the same manner as with ankle arthroscopy in that only the skin is incised and subcutaneous tissue is separated bluntly using a small hemostat. The AL portal is used as the initial viewing portal. The scope then is switched to the PL portal to complete the diagnostic examination, and the AL portal is used for inflow. The performance of diagnostic subtalar arthroscopy requires a reproducible and systematic method of anatomic review to consistently examine the entire subtalar joint.

### Pathology

The types of pathology encountered in the subtalar joint include arthrofibrosis and osteochondral and chondral injuries. In one study of 50 patients who underwent diagnostic subtalar and ankle arthroscopy for chronic pain af-

ter ankle sprain, 29 patients had subtalar pathology, five had degenerative joint disease and underwent débridement and chondroplasty, five had sinus tarsi syndrome and underwent débridement of the sinus tarsi, and four with chondromalacia underwent intra-articular shaving. One patient had a loose body removed from the subtalar joint, and two patients underwent arthroscopic resection for arthrofibrosis. Four patients with symptomatic os trigonum underwent arthroscopic excision, and one patient underwent excision and drilling for an osteochondral lesion of the talus. Patients with degenerative joint disease had the poorest prognosis; however, 86% of the patients who had arthroscopic subtalar joint surgery had good or excellent results.

### Aftercare

At the end of the procedure, the limb is placed in a soft bulky compressive dressing with a posterior or sugar-tong splint. Five days postoperatively, the sutures are removed and the limb is placed in a compressive stocking and a stirrup ankle support. Weight bearing is then increased as tolerated depending on the type of procedure performed and the patient's comfort. Physical therapy is instituted emphasizing range of motion, strengthening, and proprioceptive training. The patient may return to athletic activities when full range of motion and strength, normal proprioception, and freedom from pain have been achieved.

## Other Arthroscopic Procedures

### Os Trigonum and Stieda's Process

Excision of the os trigonum and Stieda's process is an advanced arthroscopic technique and has been reported to be a good alternative to open treatment for patients who require surgical intervention. Compared with open incisions, properly placed arthroscopic portals offer a low risk of skin necrosis, incisional neuromas, and cutaneous scarring.

Typically, subtalar arthroscopy using the standard portals is done first. The borders of the os trigonum are identified using a small blunt probe. The os trigonum is then removed using a banana knife, a full-radius power shaver, and a reverse-angled curet and extracted using a grasper through an enlarged posterior portal. The PM portal can be used with the patient prone if care is taken to avoid injury to the FHL and posterior tibial neurovascular bundle by remaining lateral to this tendon.

In a 3- to 5-month follow-up study of 11 patients who underwent arthroscopic excision of the os trigonum in the supine position with a distraction device applied, it was reported that all patients had recovered fully at 3 months, there were no major complications, and all showed significant improvement. The aftercare protocol is similar to that after subtalar and ankle arthroscopy.

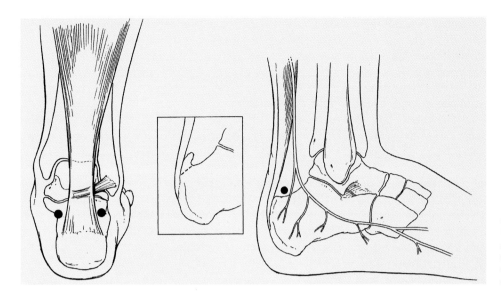

**Figure 8** Portals used for arthroscopic débridement of the retrocalcaneal bursa and Haglund's deformity. *(Reproduced with permission from Frey C: Foot and ankle arthroscopy and endoscopy, in Myerson M (ed):* Foot and Ankle Disorders. *Philadelphia, PA, WB Saunders, 2000, vol 2, pp 1477-1511.)*

## Retrocalcaneal Bursectomy

The retrocalcaneal bursa is a horseshoe-shaped structure located between the posterosuperior tuberosity of the calcaneus and the Achilles tendon. Occasionally, an inflamed retrocalcaneal bursa with Haglund's deformity is refractory to conservative care, and excision of the Haglund's deformity and bursectomy are necessary. This procedure has been described as an open procedure but also can be done endoscopically. Open procedures to remove the retrocalcaneal bursa and accompanying calcaneal exostosis have been described using single and double incisions and also a posterior splitting incision of the Achilles tendon. The medial and lateral borders of the Achilles tendon are easy to palpate in all patients. The posterosuperior aspect of the calcaneus is also easy to locate. The Achilles tendon inserts on the posterior margin of the calcaneus approximately 2 cm distal to its posterosuperior margin. The sural nerve usually runs 7 mm anterior to the lateral margin of the Achilles tendon. The calcaneal branch of the lateral plantar nerve is at risk for injury with a medial portal.

### Technique

Endoscopy of the bursa is approached using portals just medial and lateral to the Achilles tendon at the level of the retrocalcaneal bursa (Fig. 8). A 3-mm vertical incision is made in the skin and the subcutaneous tissue is spread with a small hemostat. The bursa is then entered with a blunt trocar, and small joint shavers and burrs are used to remove the bursa and the Haglund's bony deformity, starting at the posterosuperior aspect of the calcaneus and moving inferiorly 2 to 4 cm toward the attachment of the Achilles tendon. Experience with this technique is limited. There is no definitive study to show that this technique is more effective than the open technique at relieving symptoms of retrocalcaneal bursitis. After the procedure is completed, a compressive dressing is applied. Five days postoperatively, the sutures are removed and weight bearing is increased as tolerated.

## Endoscopic Plantar Fascia Release

Heel pain remains one of the most common orthopaedic foot problems, and it has multiple causes, including plantar fasciitis; proper diagnosis is crucial for effective treatment. The differential diagnosis includes tendinitis of the FHL or flexor digitorum tendon, fat pad atrophy and inflammation, tarsal tunnel syndrome, entrapment of the first branch of the lateral plantar nerve, neuroma of the medial calcaneal nerve, stress fracture of the calcaneus, and midfoot plantar fasciitis. When appropriate nonsurgical measures have failed to relieve pain, plantar fascia release may be indicated if the plantar fascia is the main source of pain.

Open release of part of the plantar fascial origin remains the usual surgical technique. However, endoscopic release of the plantar fascia is an alternative. Several structures, including the medial plantar nerve, the lateral plantar nerve and artery, the nerve to the adductor digiti minimi, the medial calcaneal nerve, and one or more of the intrinsic muscles of the foot, particularly the medial head of the quadratus plantae, are potentially at risk when the endoscopic technique is used for plantar fascia release, especially because most of these structures are not visible during the procedure.

### Instrumentation

A standard 4-mm, 30° wide-angle video arthroscope is used for the plantar fascial release. A Chow 2-mm, two-portal endoscopic device (Smith & Nephew, Andover, MA), the Agee one-portal endoscopic device (3M, St. Paul, MN), or the Instratek (Instratek, Houston, TX) two-portal endoscopic device can be used for this procedure.

### Technique

The procedure is done with the patient supine on the operating table. A general, regional, or local anesthetic can be used, and a tourniquet is recommended. A small incision is placed just anterior and inferior to the inferior aspect of the medial calcaneal tubercle. Through a vertical skin incision, blunt dissection is done with a small, straight hemostat to the level of the medial edge of the plantar fascia. Care is taken to avoid the medial calcaneal branches of the posterior tibial nerve and lateral plantar nerve. A small Freer elevator is used to create a small channel inferior to the plantar fascia. A trocar-cannula system is then placed through the channel and passed to the lateral aspect of the foot. The tip of the trocar is palpated under the lateral skin of the heel and a small incision is made to allow the trocar to pass through the lateral heel. The trocar is removed from the cannula, and a probe followed by a retrograde knife are introduced through the lateral portal. The retrograde knife is brought medially to the medial aspect of the plantar fascia after identifying its edge with a probe. The retrograde knife is then pulled laterally, incising the medial one third to one half of the plantar fascia under direct vision. The endoscopic cannula has a marker to facilitate measuring the amount of fascia to be severed. Several passes may be necessary with the retrograde knife to assure that the full depth of the plantar fascia has been released.

### Aftercare

After the procedure is completed, a compression dressing is applied. The patient is instructed to bear weight as tolerated on the first postoperative day. The patient can wear a well-cushioned heel and begin a stretching program 2 weeks after the procedure.

Complications include midtarsal pain, particularly in the lateral cuneocuboid and calcaneocuboid joints and lateral sinus tarsi, as well as nerve damage and partial loss of height of the medial longitudinal arch. Even with a good result, it often takes 6 to 12 months to fully recover from the surgery, which is comparable to results achieved with the open technique. Endoscopic release of the plantar fascia should still be considered an alternative to the open technique and should be done only by a surgeon experienced in advanced arthroscopic techniques. This technique has been used successfully in many patients.

### Summary

Although not as well established as arthroscopy of the knee and shoulder, arthroscopy of the foot and ankle can be useful for specific conditions in selected patients. Ankle arthroscopy can be used for synovectomy, correction of soft-tissue and bone impingement, treatment of osteochondral lesions, and removal of loose bodies and osteophytes. Hindfoot arthroscopy has been used to successfully treat arthrofibrosis, osteochondral and chondral injuries, retrocalcaneal bursitis, and plantar fasciitis. Knowledge of the complex anatomy of the foot and an-

kle is essential, as is experience with arthroscopic equipment and techniques.

## Annotated Bibliography

### Ankle Arthroscopy

Acevedo JI, Busch MT, Ganey TM, Hutton WC, Ogden JA: Coaxial portals for posterior ankle arthroscopy: An anatomic study with clinical correlation on 29 patients. *Arthroscopy* 2000;16:836-842.

Results from a cadaveric study of 10 ankles and retrospective study of 29 arthroscopic synovectomies to determine trajectory, minimal safe distances, and complications using PM and PL portals suggested that the technique of using coaxial portals is safe, effective, and reproducible.

Ferkel RD, Small HN, Gittins JE: Complications in foot and ankle arthroscopy. *Clin Orthop* 2001;391:89-104.

This article presents an excellent review of the authors' 10-year experience with 612 ankle arthroscopy procedures. The overall complication rate was 9.8%. The most common complication was neurologic, which accounted for 49% of the complications.

Lahm A, Erggelet C, Steinwachs M, Reichelt A: Arthroscopic management of osteochondral lesions of the talus: Results of drilling and usefulness of magnetic resonance imaging before and after treatment. *Arthroscopy* 2000;16: 299-304.

This article presents the results of a review of 42 patients who underwent arthroscopic treatment for osteochondritis dissecans of the talus. Results showed that drilling with a Kirschner wire was as successful as cancellous grafting of a lesion. Long-term results in preventing arthrosis is unknown.

Loren GJ, Ferkel RD: Arthroscopic assessment of occult intra-articular injury in acute ankle fractures. *Arthroscopy* 2002;18:412-421.

Forty-eight consecutive patients with acute unstable ankle fractures underwent ankle arthroscopy followed by open reduction and internal fixation. It was concluded that arthroscopy is a valuable tool in identifying and treating intra-articular damage and may provide prognostic information regarding functional outcomes for these injuries.

Schimmer RC, Dick W, Hintermann B: The role of ankle arthroscopy in the treatment strategies of osteochondritis dissecans lesions of the talus. *Foot Ankle Int* 2001;22: 895-900.

A retrospective study of 36 cases of osteochondritis dissecans of the talus is presented. Results showed that apart from enabling the various minimally invasive surgical treatment options, ankle arthroscopy helped define the treatment strategy and avoid unnecessary treatment of stable lesions.

Sitler DF, Amendola A, Baily CS, Thain LMF, Spouge A: Posterior ankle arthroscopy: An anatomic study. *J Bone Joint Surg Am* 2002;84:763-769.

This cadaveric study suggested that, with the patient prone, arthroscopic equipment may be introduced into the posterior ankle without gross injury to the posterior neurovascular structures. The authors recommend remaining lateral to the FHL tendon.

Takao M, Ochi M, Naito K, et al: Arthroscopic diagnosis of tibiofibular syndesmosis disruption. *Arthroscopy* 2001; 17:836-843.

The results of this study in which 38 patients with distal fibular fractures underwent ankle arthroscopy to determine whether tibiofibular syndesmosis disruption was present showed that ankle arthroscopy is necessary for the correct diagnosis of tibiofibular syndesmosis disruption.

Thordarson DB, Bains R, Shepherd LE: The role of ankle arthroscopy on the surgical management of ankle fractures. *Foot Ankle Int* 2001;22:123-125.

In this prospective, randomized study, 19 patients were surgically treated for ankle fracture; in some patients the treatment was supplemented with ankle arthroscopy. With an average follow-up of 21 months, no difference in Medical Outcomes Study 36-Item Short Form scores was seen between those that received arthroscopy and those that did not.

### Hindfoot Arthroscopy

Frey C: Foot and ankle arthroscopy and endoscopy, in Myerson M (ed): *Foot and Ankle Disorders.* Philadelphia, PA, WB Saunders, 2000, vol 2, pp 1477-1511.

This chapter presents a comprehensive overview of the indications, technique, and results of arthroscopy and endoscopy of the foot and ankle.

Marumoto JM, Ferkel RD: Arthroscopic excision of the os trigonum: A new technique with preliminary clinical results. *Foot Ankle Int* 1997;18:777-784.

After arthroscopic excision of the os trigonum, all 11 patients had improved American Orthopaedic Foot and Ankle Society scores, with no complications.

Williams MM, Ferkel RD: Subtalar arthroscopy: Indications, technique, and results. *Arthroscopy* 1998;14:373-381.

In this excellent retrospective study of 50 patients who underwent subtalar arthroscopy, results showed that 86% of patients had good to excellent relief of preoperative pain.

### Other Arthroscopic Procedures

Jerosch J: Endoscopic release of plantar fasciitis: A benign procedure? *Foot Ankle Int* 2000;21:511-513.

A case report of a patient with recurrent pain after endoscopic plantar fascial release, secondary to a stress reaction of the calcaneus, is presented.

Lundeen RO, Aziz S, Burks JB, Rose JM: Endoscopic plantar fasciotomy: A retrospective analysis of results in 53 patients. *J Foot Ankle Surg* 2000;39:208-217.

In this retrospective study of patients who underwent an isolated endoscopic plantar fasciotomy, findings showed that 81.1% were satisfied and 18.9% were unsatisfied with the surgical outcome.

Ogilvie-Harris DJ, Lobo J: Endoscopic plantar fascia release. *Arthroscopy* 2000;16:290-298.

The results of a clinical study of 53 patients (65 feet) at 2-year follow-up are presented. Endoscopic plantar fascial release effectively relieved heel pain in 89% of patients.

O'Malley MJ, Page A, Cook R: Endoscopic plantar fasciotomy for chronic heel pain. *Foot Ankle Int* 2000;21:505-510.

In this retrospective review of 20 feet treated with endoscopic plantar fasciotomy for chronic heel pain, there was complete relief of pain in 9 feet, and symptoms improved in another 9 feet. There were no nerve injuries.

## Classic Bibliography

Amendola A, Petrik J, Webster-Bogaert S: Ankle arthroscopy: Outcome in 79 consecutive patients. *Arthroscopy* 1996;12:565-573.

Branca A, Di Palma L, Bucca C, Visconti CS, Di Mille M: Arthroscopic treatment of anterior ankle impingement. *Foot Ankle Int* 1997;18:418-423.

Cooper PS, Murray TF Jr: Arthroscopy of the foot and ankle in the athlete. *Clin Sports Med* 1996;15:805-824.

Drez D Jr, Guhl JF, Gollehon DL: Ankle arthroscopy: Technique and indications. *Foot Ankle* 1981;2:138-143.

Feiwell LA, Frey C: Anatomic study of arthroscopic portal sites of the ankle. *Foot Ankle* 1993;14:142-147.

Ferkel RD, Heath DD, Guhl JF: Neurological complications of ankle arthroscopy. *Arthroscopy* 1996;12:200-208.

Ogilvie-Harris DJ, Gilbart MK, Chorney K: Chronic pain following ankle sprains in athletes: The role of arthroscopic surgery. *Arthroscopy* 1997;13:564-574.

Scranton PE Jr, McDermott JE: Anterior tibiotalar spurs: A comparison of open versus arthroscopic debridement. *Foot Ankle* 1992;13:125-129.

Stetson WB, Ferkel RD: Ankle arthroscopy: I. Technique and complications. *J Am Acad Orthop Surg* 1996;4:17-23.

Stetson WB, Ferkel RD: Ankle arthroscopy: II. Indications and results. *J Am Acad Orthop Surg* 1996;4:24-34.

Van Dijk CN, Scholte D: Arthroscopy of the ankle joint. *Arthroscopy* 1997;13:90-96.

# Index

*f* indicates figure
*t* indicates table